Advancements in Lung Cancer Surgical Treatment and Prognosis

Advancements in Lung Cancer Surgical Treatment and Prognosis

Guest Editors

Sai Yendamuri
Kenneth Patrick Seastedt

MDPI Basel • Beijing • Wuhan • Barcelona • Belgrade • Novi Sad • Cluj • Manchester

Guest Editors
Sai Yendamuri
Department of Thoracic Surgery
Roswell Park Comprehensive
Cancer Center
Buffalo, NY
USA

Kenneth Patrick Seastedt
Department of Thoracic Surgery
Roswell Park Comprehensive
Cancer Center
Buffalo, NY
USA

Editorial Office
MDPI AG
Grosspeteranlage 5
4052 Basel, Switzerland

This is a reprint of the Special Issue, published open access by the journal *Cancers* (ISSN 2072-6694), freely accessible at: https://www.mdpi.com/journal/cancers/special_issues/R7242D8BB2.

For citation purposes, cite each article independently as indicated on the article page online and as indicated below:

Lastname, A.A.; Lastname, B.B. Article Title. *Journal Name* **Year**, *Volume Number*, Page Range.

ISBN 978-3-7258-7298-5 (Hbk)
ISBN 978-3-7258-7299-2 (PDF)
https://doi.org/10.3390/books978-3-7258-7299-2

Contents

cancers

Article

Minimally Invasive Total Versus Partial Thymectomy for Early-Stage Thymoma

Alexander Pohlman [1,2,3], Bilal Odeh [1,2], Irene Helenowski [1], Julia M. Coughlin [1,2], Wissam Raad [1,2], James Lubawski [1,2] and Zaid M. Abdelsattar [1,2,4,*]

1 Stritch School of Medicine, Loyola University Chicago, Maywood, IL 60153, USA; ihelenowski@luc.edu (I.H.); julia.coughlin@lumc.edu (J.M.C.)
2 Department of Thoracic and Cardiovascular Surgery, Loyola University Medical Center, Maywood, IL 60153, USA
3 Department of Surgery, University of Illinois Chicago, Chicago, IL 60612, USA
4 Department of Veterans Affairs, Edward Hines Jr. VA Hospital, Hines, IL 60141, USA
* Correspondence: zaid.abdelsattar@lumc.edu; Tel.: +1-(708)-327-2449

Simple Summary: Total thymectomy is the current standard for the treatment of early-stage thymoma. However, recent studies have raised partial thymectomy as an option and brought attention to the thymus's potential role in protection against autoimmune disease, development of extra-thymic malignancy and overall mortality. Therefore, it's unclear if an organ-sparing approach is an equivalent alternative. In this context, we compare partial versus total thymectomy for early-stage thymoma using a national database. We demonstrate that partial- and total-thymectomy have similar short- and long-term outcomes. These results may help better inform patients of their surgical options within shared decision making discussions with their surgeon.

Abstract

Background/Objectives: Total thymectomy is currently the gold standard operation for treating thymoma. However, recent studies have suggested the potential health consequences of thymus removal in adults, including possible increased autoimmune disease and all-cause mortality. In this context, we assess oncologic outcomes following total vs. partial thymectomy for early-stage thymoma. **Methods**: We identified patients diagnosed with WHO types A–B3 thymoma between 2010–2021 from a national hospital-based dataset. We excluded patients with stage II or higher disease, open resections and perioperative chemo-/radiation therapy. We stratified patients into total and partial thymectomy cohorts. We used propensity score matching to minimize confounding, Kaplan–Meier analysis to estimate survival, and Cox proportional hazards to identify associations. **Results**: Of 1598 patients with early-stage thymoma, 495 (31.0%) underwent partial and 1103 (69.0%) total thymectomy. Patients undergoing partial thymectomy were similar in sex (female 53.7% vs. 53.4%; $p = 0.914$), race (white 74.5% vs. 74.0%; $p = 0.921$), comorbidities (0 in 77.0% vs. 75.5%; $p = 0.742$), and tumor size (48.7 mm vs. 50.4 mm; $p = 0.455$) compared to total thymectomy. There were no differences in 30-day (0.8% vs. 0.6%, $p = 0.747$) or 90-day mortality (0.8% vs. 0.8%, $p > 0.999$), which persisted after matching. Moreover, 10-year survival was similar in both unmatched ($p = 0.471$) and matched cohorts ($p = 0.828$). Partial thymectomy was not independently associated with survival (aHR = 1.00, $p = 0.976$). **Conclusions**: In patients with early-stage thymoma, partial and total thymectomy were associated with similar short- and long-term outcomes. In light of recent attention to the role of the thymus gland, the results add important insights to shared decision-making discussions.

Keywords: thymoma; total thymectomy; partial thymectomy; minimally invasive surgery

1. Introduction

The role of the thymus gland in adults is not clear, particularly since the thymus naturally involutes with age. However, a recent study in the *New England Journal of Medicine* (*NEJM*) examined the health consequences of thymectomy, demonstrating worse all-cause mortality and higher rates of autoimmune disease [1]. However, ability to definitively draw these conclusions is limited by the design of the study. In patients with thymoma, the Society of Thoracic Surgeons currently recommends total thymectomy for all thymomas, except in high-risk patients in whom a partial thymectomy may be considered [2]. The rationale behind total thymectomy stems from previous studies that demonstrated that all fatty tissue may harbor microscopic foci of thymic cells, which could give rise to recurrent thymoma [3].

With the newfound interest in preserving the thymus, understanding the comparative effectiveness of a partial thymectomy (also referred to as a thymomectomy) compared to a total thymectomy (also called a thymothymectomy) is needed on two fronts. The first of these concerns the question of whether total thymectomy is truly a better oncologic operation for early-stage thymoma compared to partial thymectomy. Previous studies on this topic have shown mixed results. For example, a multicenter, international study revealed similar post-op complication rates and slightly improved five-year survival and freedom from recurrence with total thymectomy [4]. However, in that study, only 6% of patients underwent partial thymectomy. Studies with larger sample sizes showed similar five-year disease-free survival [5–8]. However, these studies included heterogeneous populations, various foreign institutions, and a blend of surgical techniques (minimally invasive and open), and they spanned multiple decades due to the rarity of the disease. Therefore, these results are not easily generalizable, which, in conjunction with the mixed nature of the results, led to poor evidence for current practice. On the other hand, the recent findings of increased all-cause mortality associated with total thymectomy may be over-emphasized, as discussed in a recent review of the literature [9]. This leaves surgeons without clear evidence-based recommendations for current practice; they are left to decide between two opposing theoretical benefits: remove the entire thymus to prevent recurrence or preserve part of the thymus to prevent the reported occurrences of extra-thymic malignancy and/or auto-immune disease.

In this context, we conduct a comparative effectiveness study using the largest hospital-based national dataset on this topic. Specifically, we examine short- and long-term outcomes in patients with early-stage thymoma undergoing a minimally invasive partial or total thymectomy. We hypothesize that partial thymectomy will have similar long-term outcomes to total thymectomy. The results are important for shared decision making for patients afflicted with thymoma.

2. Materials and Methods

2.1. Data Source

This study was reviewed and deemed exempt by the Loyola University Chicago institutional review board (IRB 219066, 10 January 2025). For this retrospective cohort study, we used data from the National Cancer Database (NCDB), which is a prospective national cancer registry that collects data from ~1500 Commission on Cancer accredited centers across the US, capturing ~70% of all cancer cases. The thymus malignancy participant user file was utilized and included patient demographics, tumor characteristics (such as histology and size), tumor node metastasis (TNM) staging, administered treatment, and short- and long-term outcomes associated with each case [10].

2.2. Patient Population

We identified adult patients with World Health Organization (WHO) types A–B3 thymoma using site code C379 and histology codes 8580–8585 undergoing partial or total thymectomy (site-specific surgery codes 30 and 40, respectively). All patients underwent minimally invasive surgery. Any patients with invasive disease requiring en bloc resections were not included. Patients with TNM stage II or higher were excluded. The NCDB does not contain Masaoka staging data. In patients without complete American Joint Committee on Cancer (AJCC) staging data and to ensure the inclusion of only stage I disease, any patients with nodal or metastatic disease and perioperative chemo- or radiation-therapy were excluded. Open resections were also excluded, as these are more likely to be associated with total thymectomy and thus may confound results. Figure 1 shows a consort-type algorithm.

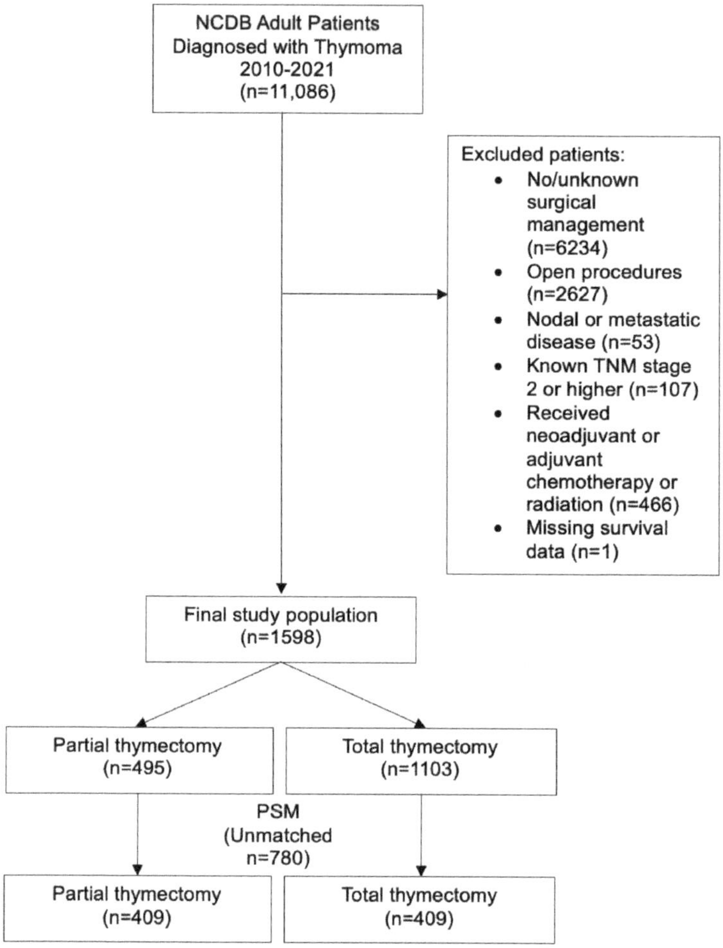

Figure 1. Consort diagram for the creation of the study population. NCDB—National Cancer Database, TNM–tumor node metastasis.

2.3. Main Exposure and Independent Variables

The main exposure variable was the extent of resection. Patients were stratified into two cohorts: partial thymectomy and total thymectomy. Other independent variables included age, sex, race, ethnicity, comorbidity index, tumor size, histology, primary insurance payer, median income quartiles, and facility type (academic vs. nonacademic).

2.4. Outcome Variables

The primary long-term outcome of this study was 10-year overall survival, measured in months from initial diagnosis. Short-term outcomes were 30-day mortality, 90-day mortality, resection margins, length of stay, and unplanned readmission within 30 days. Resection margins were categorized as either negative (R0) or positive (R1/R2). Resection margins were drawn from final pathology reports for each case.

2.5. Statistical Analysis

Baseline clinical and demographic characteristics were compared between partial and total thymectomy groups using Fisher's exact tests for categorical variables and the Wilcoxon rank–sum test for continuous variables.

Short-term outcomes, including 30-day mortality, 90-day mortality, resection margins, length of stay and unplanned readmission, were compared between the two groups. The Wilcoxon rank–sum test was used to assess differences in length of stay and Fisher's exact tests, or Chi-squared tests in computationally intensive cases, were used for differences in mortality, resection margins, and readmission.

Individual factors affecting long-term survival were compared using Cox proportional hazards analysis on unmatched data. Factors affecting survival in the Cox analysis, in addition to basic tumor and patient characteristics, were included in the propensity score match; this included age, sex, race, ethnicity, comorbidities, insurance status, median income, histology, tumor size, and facility type. These were used in a multivariable probit regression to calculate propensity scores for each patient. Patients in both groups were matched 1:1 using the nearest neighbor method without replacement. A caliper of 0.5 was used, as this was just below 20% of the propensity score standard deviation, which is consistent with prior studies and recommendations [11,12]. All standardized bias was reduced to $|<10\%|$, indicating balance. Unmatched patients were dropped from the analysis.

After matching, short-term outcomes were again compared with the same statistical tests used on the unmatched groups. Long-term outcomes were compared using Kaplan–Meier survival analysis in both unmatched and matched groups to estimate 5- and 10-year survival with a log-rank test for significance.

Statistical analyses were performed using Stata version 17.0SE (StataCorp LLC, College Station, TX, USA) and R 4.3.1 (R Foundation for Statistical Computing, Vienna, Austria). All tests were two-sided using a p value < 0.05. Confidence intervals were reported to a 95% confidence level.

3. Results

After fitting the inclusion criteria, there were 1598 patients with early-stage thymoma who underwent minimally invasive surgery. Of those, 495 (31.0%) underwent partial thymectomy and 1103 (69.0%) underwent total thymectomy. The robotic approach was more common (69.8% of cases) than thoracoscopy. Patients undergoing partial thymectomy in the unmatched cohorts were similar in terms of sex (female 53.7% vs. 53.4%; $p = 0.914$), race (white 74.5% vs. 74.0%; $p = 0.921$), comorbidities (0 in 77.0% vs. 75.5%; $p = 0.742$), and tumor size (48.7 mm vs. 50.4 mm; $p = 0.455$) compared to total thymectomy. Age was slightly higher in the partial thymectomy group (63.7 vs. 61.1 years old, $p < 0.001$). Academic centers tended to have a higher proportion of partial thymectomies than nonacademic centers (33.2% vs. 28.8%), but this was not statistically significant ($p = 0.058$). A full summary of the demographic and clinical characteristics of the two groups can be seen in Table 1.

Table 1. Baseline patient and tumor characteristics in patients undergoing partial versus total thymectomy in unmatched and matched analyses.

	Unmatched				Matched			
	Partial Thymectomy (N = 495)	**Total Thymectomy (N = 1103)**	***p*-Value**	**Standardized Bias | % |**	**Partial Thymectomy (N = 409)**	**Total Thymectomy (N = 409)**	***p*-Value**	**Standardized Bias | % |**
Sex, female	266(53.7%)	589(53.4%)	0.914	2.9%	226(55.3%)	224(54.8%)	0.944	0.1%
Age, mean (SD)	63.7(12.2)	61.1(13.3)	<0.001	17.6%	63.4(12.2)	63.4(12.1)	0.970	0.2%
Race			0.921	4.6%			0.990	2.6%
White	369(74.5%)	816(74.0%)			306(74.8%)	308(75.3%)		
Black	62(12.5%)	151(13.7%)			52(12.7%)	53(13.0%)		
Asian	48(9.7%)	103(9.3%)			39(9.5%)	36(8.8%)		
Other	16(3.2%)	33(3%)			12(2.9%)	12(2.9%)		
Ethnicity, Hispanic	36(7.3%)	83(7.5%)	0.918	4.2%	28(6.9%)	26(6.4%)	0.888	2.0%
Charlson-Deyo Index			0.742	6.0%			0.953	2.4%
0	381(77.0%)	833(75.5%)			313(76.5%)	317(77.5%)		
1	77(15.6%)	189(17.1%)			63(15.4%)	60(14.7%)		
2+	37(7.5%)	81(7.3%)			33(8.1%)	32(7.8%)		
Tumor Size, mm (SD)	48.7(26.4)	50.4(28.0)	0.455	7.0%	48.4(26.7)	49.6(26.6)	0.512	4.3%
Histology			0.587	9.4%			>0.999	2.5%
Type A	71(14.3%)	151(13.7%)			62(15.2%)	59(14.4%)		
Type AB	182(36.8%)	380(34.5%)			148(36.2%)	148(36.2%)		
Type B1	71(14.3%)	185(16.8%)			57(13.9%)	57(13.9%)		
Type B2	80(16.2%)	193(17.5%)			69(16.9%)	71(17.4%)		
Type B3	32(6.5%)	55(5%)			23(5.6%)	24(5.9%)		
Thymoma, NOS	59(11.9%)	139(12.6%)			50(12.2%)	50(12.2%)		
Primary Payor			0.063	18.4%			0.986	5.8%
Private Insurance	221(44.6%)	530(48.1%)			190(46.5%)	187(45.7%)		
Medicare	239(48.3%)	458(41.5%)			191(46.7%)	189(46.2%)		
Medicaid/Government	26(5.2%)	89(8.1%)			17(4.2%)	20(4.9%)		
Not Insured	5(1%)	20(1.8%)			3(0.7%)	3(0.7%)		
Unknown	4(0.8%)	6(0.5%)			4(1.0%)	4(1%)		
Median Income Quartiles			0.330	11.1%			0.707	3.1%
<$30,000	26(6.1%)	81(8.9%)			25(6.1%)	26(6.4%)		
$30,000–$34,999	59(13.9%)	112(12.3%)			57(13.9%)	54(13.2%)		
$35,000–$45,999	103(24.3%)	219(24.1%)			101(24.7%)	98(24.0%)		
≥$46,000	235(55.6%)	496(54.6%)			226(55.3%)	231(56.5%)		
Center Type			0.058	13.1%			0.622	3.9%
Academic	264(53.3%)	531(48.1%)			224(54.8%)	232(56.7%)		
Non-academic	231(46.7%)	572(51.9%)			185(45.2%)	177(43.3%)		
Approach			0.135				0.937	
Robotic	333(67.3%)	783(71.0%)			277(67.7%)	280(68.5%)		
VATS	162(32.7%)	320(29.0%)			132(32.3%)	129(31.5%)		

SD—standard deviation, mm—millimeters, NOS—not otherwise specified, VATS—video-assisted thoracoscopic surgery.

3.1. Unmatched Analysis

All short-term outcomes were similar between partial and total thymectomy groups. There were no differences in 30-day mortality (0.8% vs. 0.6%, $p = 0.747$), 90-day mortality (0.8% vs. 0.8%, $p > 0.999$), length of stay (2 days vs. 2 days, $p = 0.943$), unplanned readmissions (1.6% vs. 2.2%, $p = 0.564$), or positive margin rates (9.9% vs. 8.5%, $p = 0.386$). All short-term outcomes can be seen in Table 2.

Next, Cox proportional hazards analysis was used to see how individual variables affected overall survival, as shown by the adjusted hazard ratios (aHR) listed in Table 3. Partial thymectomy had no impact on survival compared to total thymectomy (aHR 1.00, $p = 0.976$). Factors associated with worse survival included increasing age (aHR = 1.06, $p < 0.001$), a Charlson–Deyo comorbidity index of 2 + (aHR 2.91, $p < 0.001$) and Hispanic ethnicity (aHR 2.20, $p = 0.022$). On the other hand, undergoing thymectomy at an academic center was associated with improved survival (aHR 0.66, $p = 0.030$). Kaplan–Meier survival analysis in the unmatched cohorts revealed no difference in 10-year survival between the two groups ($p = 0.471$).

Table 2. Short-term outcomes in patients undergoing partial versus total thymectomy in unmatched and matched analyses.

	Unmatched Cohort			Matched Cohort		
	Partial Thymectomy	Total Thymectomy	*p* Value	Partial Thymectomy	Total Thymectomy	*p* Value
30-Day Mortality	4 (0.8%)	7 (0.6%)	0.747	4 (1.0%)	4 (1.0%)	>0.999
90-Day Mortality	4 (0.8%)	9 (0.8%)	>0.999	4 (1.0%)	4 (1.0%)	>0.999
Resection Margins			0.386			0.905
Positive	47 (9.9%)	90 (8.5%)		38 (9.7%)	40 (10.1%)	
Negative	428 (90.1%)	963 (91.5%)		356 (90.3%)	356 (89.9%)	
Length of Stay, median days (IQR)	2 (1–3)	2 (1–3)	0.943	2 (1–3)	2 (1–3)	0.315
Readmission within 30 days	8 (1.6%)	24 (2.2%)	0.564	7 (1.7%)	7 (1.7%)	>0.999

IQR—interquartile range.

Table 3. Cox proportional hazards model predicting overall survival.

Variable		aHR	*p*-Value	95% CI
Partial Thymectomy		1.00	0.976	(0.68–1.48)
Negative Margins(R0)		0.91	0.761	(0.54–1.58)
Tumor Size(mm)		1.01	0.004	(1.00–1.01)
Age		1.06	<0.001	(1.04–1.08)
Sex (Female)		0.76	0.146	(0.53–1.10)
Histology				
	A		Reference	
	AB	0.93	0.773	(0.55–1.57)
	B1	0.74	0.392	(0.38–1.46)
	B2	0.96	0.899	(0.51–1.82)
	B3	1.53	0.243	(0.75–3.12)
	NOS	0.91	0.790	(0.46–1.81)
Race				
	White		Reference	
	Black	1.07	0.810	(0.59–1.96)
	Asian	0.91	0.775	(0.47–1.77)
	Other	0.98	0.981	(0.24–4.06)
Hispanic		2.20	0.022	(1.12–4.31)
Academic Center		0.66	0.030	(0.46–0.96)
Charlson-Deyo Index				
	0		Reference	
	1	0.93	0.788	(0.58–1.51)
	2+	2.91	<0.001	(1.73–4.88)

aHR—adjusted hazard ratio, CI—confidence interval, R0—negative resection margin, NOS—not otherwise specified.

When specifically comparing robotic to thoracoscopic thymectomies, there were only minor differences in demographics and tumor characteristics. The two groups were similar in terms of age (62.0 vs. 61.9, p = 0.962), sex (female 54.0% vs. 52.3%, p = 0.548), race (white 74.5% vs. 73.4%, p = 0.862), comorbidities (Charlson–Deyo Index = 0 in 74.6% vs. 79.0%, p = 0.131), and tumor size (48.9 vs. 53.0 mm, p = 0.209). The only statistically significant difference was in the primary insurance provider (private: 48.4% robotic vs. 43.8% thoracoscopic, p = 0.032). There were higher readmission rates in the thoracoscopic group (3.1% vs. 1.5%, p = 0.035), but all other short-term outcomes were similar, including 30-day mortality (0.8% vs. 0.4%, p = 0.521), R0 resections (91.8% vs. 89.3%, p = 0.125), and median length of stay (2 vs. 2 days, p = 0.978). All demographics and short-term outcomes of the robotic and thoracoscopic groups can be seen in Supplemental Table S1.

3.2. *Propensity Score Matched Analysis*

After propensity score matching, the two groups were similar in all measured areas, and all measured standardized bias was < | 10% | . The Love plot comparing standardized bias before and after matching is shown in Supplemental Figure S1, and bihistograms of propensity scores before and after matching are shown in Supplemental Figure S2. All demographics and the standardized bias of the matched cohorts can be seen in Table 1 for comparisons to unmatched groups.

The similarities in short- and long-term outcomes persisted after matching. Perioperative outcomes, including 30- and 90-day mortality were similar (1.0% vs. 1.0%, $p > 0.999$) as were length of stay (2 days vs. 2 days, $p = 0.315$) and unplanned readmission rates (1.7% vs. 1.7%, $p > 0.999$). Full results can be seen in Table 2 for comparison to unmatched data.

Oncologic outcomes were similar in the matched cohorts. R0 resection rates were similar (90.3% vs. 89.9%, $p = 0.905$), as were 5- and 10-year survival rates, as shown in Figure 2. Survival at 5 years was 93.6% partial vs. 90.8% total thymectomy ($p = 0.237$) and at 10 years it was 75.8% partial vs. 85.8% total ($p = 0.828$).

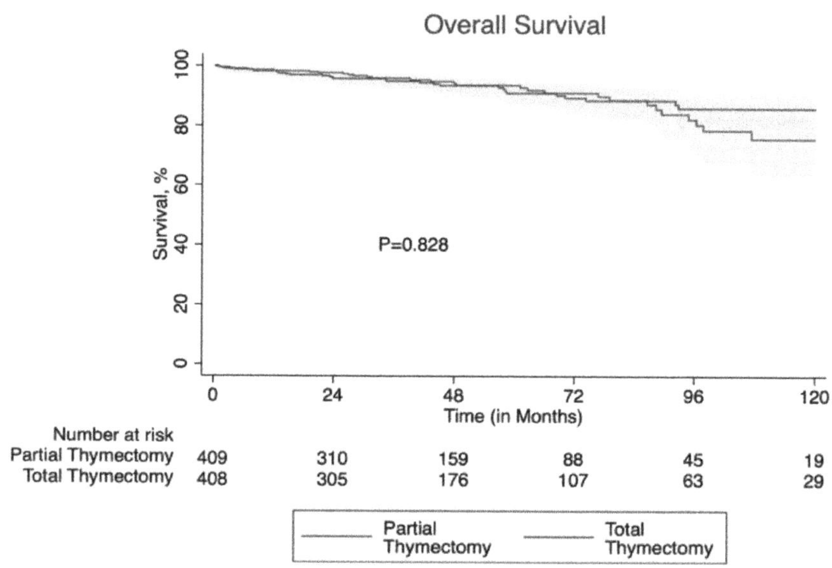

Figure 2. Kaplan–Meier survival curve comparing 10-year survival of partial versus total thymectomy after propensity score matching.

4. Discussion

In this national hospital-based study of patients with early-stage thymoma undergoing minimally invasive surgery, we found that partial thymectomy had similar peri-operative outcomes, similar rates of R0 resection, and similar 5- and 10-year survival when compared to total thymectomy. Thus, partial thymectomy can be viewed as a safe and effective operation for early-stage thymoma. Likewise, patients undergoing total thymectomy did not have worse overall survival as a consequence of the surgical removal of the thymus, as suggested by recent studies [1]. These findings are important for shared decision making, particularly at a time where the role of the thymus is being revisited.

In this study, short-term outcomes were nearly identical between partial and total thymectomy. In undertaking this study, we did not think there would be a difference in perioperative outcomes, as all included patients underwent a minimally invasive operation for early-stage disease by design. The low peri-operative mortality rate of ~1% and short length of stay are similar to those reported in other studies that have established the role of minimally invasive thymectomy [13]. In addition, rates of positive margins did not differ between groups and are similar to those found in previous studies [14]. Complete resection and negative margins have previously been associated with improved long-term survival and decreased recurrence [15,16]. It is important to note that previous studies have shown no difference in rates of negative margins between open and minimally invasive techniques, so we would not expect the inclusion of open cases to change these results [14,17].

The primary outcome in this study was long-term survival. In the present study, 5- and 10-year overall survival were similar in patients undergoing partial versus total thymectomy, and there was no difference in the multivariable Cox proportional hazards analysis (partial thymectomy aHR = 1.00). It is important to note that 10-year survival was slightly lower in the partial thymectomy group (75.8% vs. 85.8%), but the difference was not statistically significant, and the reverse was true at 5 years (93.6% partial vs. 90.8% total thymectomy). As this is overall survival and not cancer-specific or disease-free survival, it is difficult to comment further on the cause of this finding. However, given that the two survival curves cross at several time points, significance is not likely. Prior studies are in line with our findings of similar survival, although they were limited to non-homogenous populations, a mix of open and minimally invasive techniques, and a smaller proportion of partial thymectomies [8,18,19]. Thus, our study adds more evidence to existing literature, particularly regarding minimally invasive thymectomy.

The Society of Thoracic Surgeons' consensus statement states that patients who are high-risk for surgery may undergo a partial thymectomy rather than a total thymectomy [2]. This recommendation may stem from other studies that have shown fewer post-operative complications, such as decreased pleural drainage and decreased hospital stay with partial thymectomy [18]. While we are not able to capture these specific complications in our study, we found that hospital length of stay and perioperative mortality were identical. Again, this is not surprising, as both groups underwent a minimally invasive operation. In addition, both groups had similar comorbidity burdens prior to surgery.

There may be other benefits outside of the surgical and oncologic treatment course for preserving part of the thymus. A recent study in the NEJM found that removal of the thymus gland was associated with increased rates of autoimmune disease, extra-thymic malignancy and all-cause mortality [1]. However, there is concern that the results of this NEJM study may be over-interpreted.

A review by Kaminski et al. highlights important methodological issues within the NEJM study, including selection bias and potential confounding factors [1,9]. The NEJM article was a case–control study that compared patients undergoing cardiac procedures to those undergoing thymectomy, as is typically for thymic malignancy. Therefore, this is a non-comparable control group that does not help us to identify how the thymus or associated thymic pathology directly affects mortality, extra-thymic malignancy or autoimmune disease. Additionally, most deaths occurred within one year of surgery, indicating that a mortality difference was likely a product of the innate risks of surgery rather than a protective effect of the thymus. Finally, a high percentage of patients developed autoimmunity, likely indicating pre-existing bias in the study population [9]. Given these concerns, the role of the thymus in adults is still unclear. However, regardless of the ongoing debate surrounding the role of the thymus, if an organ-sparing approach does not compromise oncologic outcomes, then it would make sense to consider organ preservation as an option during discussion with patients.

There may be other considerations outside the scope of this study that may also impact a surgeon's decision to resect the entire thymus versus a portion of it. One is in cases of myasthenia gravis, where removal of the entire thymus has been shown to be beneficial for patients' symptoms and recurrence of disease regardless of the presence of thymoma [20,21]. Therefore, we do not believe that the results of this study should change the treatment course for myasthenic patients. However, patients with thymoma, but without myasthenia gravis or other neoplastic syndromes, may be eligible for a partial thymectomy. Some studies have suggested that partial thymectomy may confer lower operative complications or make it more likely that a surgeon will pursue a minimally invasive approach [8,18,22]. Another instance where partial thymectomy may be considered is a small well-circumscribed 2 cm thymoma on the inferior- and peripheral-most portion of the thymus without any involvement of the pericardium or diaphragm. It is not clear that such tumors really require the resection of the thymic horns superiorly, including all thymic tissue to the contralateral pleural space. There are valid theoretical benefits for either approach, removing the entire thymus to prevent thymoma recurrence or preserve part of the thymus to prevent the reported increase in incidence of extra-thymic malignancy and/or autoimmune disease.

This study has a few limitations. First and foremost, this is an observational study using data from a national database, which collects data from Commission-on-Cancer-accredited centers. Due to the exclusion of non-accredited centers, this introduces potential selection bias and may limit generalizability. The retrospective nature of the study does not allow us to determine direct causation, or to account for all potential confounding factors or errors in hospital reporting. In particular, the NCDB does not collect data on cases of myasthenia gravis, specific location within the thymus or macroscopic morphology, so these individual variables could not be factored into the analysis directly. However, we did factor in the overall comorbidity burden, microscopic tumor morphology, and stage. We believe that the partial and total thymectomy groups being similar in almost all demographic and clinical characteristics, in addition to our propensity score matching and inclusion of only minimally invasive operations, make the results as robust as possible. That said, thymoma is an uncommon disease and a randomized trial is unlikely to happen, making this national database an appropriate data source to answer this question. Second, the NCDB does not provide data on recurrence or disease-free survival. Thymomas are slow-growing tumors with the potential for multifocal, synchronous disease and recurrence. Therefore, further studies may be needed to assess recurrence with both resection extents. However, the absence of an overall survival difference is reassuring. Prior smaller studies have shown no difference in recurrence rates between partial and total thymectomy [23,24]. Additionally, median time to recurrence in prior studies was ~52 months, which falls well within our study period [23]. Therefore, if these recurrences played a clinically significant role in survival, it is likely that we would have seen that effect within our 10-year study period. Third, we do not have information on certain operative factors, such as operative time, estimated blood loss or chest tube duration, so we cannot fully compare the surgical burden between groups. Similarly, the database does not contain granular data on complications and reasons for readmission. Institutional studies where individual patient charts and notes are accessible may be better suited for studying more specific details. Notwithstanding these limitations, we believe our results are important to practicing thoracic surgeons and can help improve shared decision making when discussing operative options with patients.

5. Conclusions

In this largest US-hospital-based national study on partial versus total thymectomy, patients with early-stage thymoma undergoing partial thymectomy had comparable perioperative outcomes and long-term survival to those undergoing total thymectomy. In light of recent attention to the potential importance of the thymus gland, patients without myasthenia gravis who are eligible for minimally invasive resection of early-stage thymomas should be counseled on their options for optimal shared-decision making.

Supplementary Materials: The following supporting information can be downloaded at: https://www.mdpi.com/article/10.3390/cancers17152518/s1, Table S1: Demographics and short-term outcomes of robotic and thoracoscopic surgery for early-stage thymoma; Figure S1: Love plot comparing standardized bias before and after propensity score matching for all covariates; Figure S2: (**A**) Bihistogram before propensity score matching; (**B**) Bihistogram after propensity score matching.

Author Contributions: Conceptualization, Z.M.A.; methodology, Z.M.A., A.P., B.O., I.H., J.M.C., W.R. and J.L.; validation, B.O., J.M.C., W.R. and J.L.; formal analysis, A.P. and I.H.; data curation, A.P.; writing—original draft preparation, A.P., B.O., I.H., J.M.C., W.R., J.L. and Z.M.A.; writing—review and editing, A.P. and Z.M.A.; visualization, A.P.; supervision Z.M.A. All authors have read and agreed to the published version of the manuscript.

Funding: This research received no external funding.

Institutional Review Board Statement: This study was reviewed and deemed exempt by the Loyola University Chicago institutional review board (IRB 219066, 10 January 2025).

Informed Consent Statement: Not applicable.

Data Availability Statement: Data are available directly from the National Cancer Database to those at CoC-accredited institutions. Data may also be made available from the corresponding author upon reasonable request.

Conflicts of Interest: The authors declare no conflicts of interest.

Abbreviations

The following abbreviations are used in this manuscript:

WHO	World Health Organization
NEJM	*New England Journal of Medicine*
NCDB	National Cancer Database
TNM	Tumor node metastasis
AJCC	American Joint Committee on Cancer
aHR	Adjusted hazard ratio

References

1. Kooshesh, K.A.; Foy, B.H.; Sykes, D.B.; Gustafsson, K.; Scadden, D.T. Health Consequences of Thymus Removal in Adults. *N. Engl. J. Med.* **2023**, *389*, 406–417. [CrossRef]
2. Liou, D.Z.; Berry, M.F.; Brown, L.M.; Demmy, T.L.; Huang, J.; Khullar, O.V.; Padda, S.K.; Shah, R.D.; Taylor, M.D.; Toker, S.A.; et al. The Society of Thoracic Surgeons Expert Consensus Document on the Surgical Management of Thymomas. *Ann. Thorac. Surg.* **2024**, *118*, 975–1004. [CrossRef]
3. Zielinski, M.; Kuzdzal, J.; Szlubowski, A.; Soja, J. Comparison of late results of basic transsternal and extended transsternal thymectomies in the treatment of myasthenia gravis. *Ann. Thorac. Surg.* **2004**, *78*, 253–258. [CrossRef] [PubMed]
4. Guerrera, F.; Falcoz, P.E.; Moser, B.; van Raemdonck, D.; Bille, A.; Toker, A.; Spaggiari, L.; Ampollini, L.; Filippini, C.; Thomas, P.A.; et al. Thymomectomy plus total thymectomy versus simple thymomectomy for early-stage thymoma without myasthenia gravis: A European Society of Thoracic Surgeons Thymic Working Group Study. *Eur. J. Cardio-Thorac. Surg.* **2021**, *60*, 881–887. [CrossRef]

5. Gu, Z.; Fu, J.; Shen, Y.; Wei, Y.; Tan, L.; Zhang, P.; Han, Y.; Chen, C.; Zhang, R.; Li, Y.; et al. Thymectomy versus tumor resection for early-stage thymic malignancies: A Chinese Alliance for Research in Thymomas retrospective database analysis. *J. Thorac. Dis.* **2016**, *8*, 680–686. [CrossRef]
6. Narm, K.S.; Lee, C.Y.; Do, Y.W.; Jung, H.S.; Byun, G.E.; Lee, J.G.; Kim, D.J.; Hwang, Y.; Park, I.K.; Kang, C.H.; et al. Limited thymectomy as a potential alternative treatment option for early-stage thymoma: A multi-institutional propensity-matched study. *Lung Cancer* **2016**, *101*, 22–27. [CrossRef]
7. Voulaz, E.; Perroni, G.; Russo, A.; Patirelis, A.; Mangiameli, G.; Alloisio, M.; Ambrogi, V. Thymomectomy versus complete thymectomy in early-stage non-myasthenic thymomas: A multicentric propensity score-matched study. *Interact. Cardiovasc. Thorac. Surg.* **2022**, *35*, ivac167. [CrossRef]
8. Nakagawa, K.; Yokoi, K.; Nakajima, J.; Tanaka, F.; Maniwa, Y.; Suzuki, M.; Nagayasu, T.; Asamura, H. Is Thymomectomy Alone Appropriate for Stage I (T1N0M0) Thymoma? Results of a Propensity-Score Analysis. *Ann. Thorac. Surg.* **2016**, *101*, 520–526. [CrossRef]
9. Kaminski, H.J.; Kusner, L.L.; Cutter, G.R.; Le Panse, R.; Wright, C.D.; Perry, Y.; Wolfe, G.I. Does Surgical Removal of the Thymus Have Deleterious Consequences? *Neurology* **2024**, *102*, e209482. [CrossRef]
10. The American College of Surgeons. National Cancer Database. 2021. Available online: https://www.facs.org/quality-programs/cancer-programs/national-cancer-database/ (accessed on 3 December 2024).
11. Austin, P.C. Optimal caliper widths for propensity-score matching when estimating differences in means and differences in proportions in observational studies. *Pharm. Stat.* **2011**, *10*, 150–161. [CrossRef]
12. Lunt, M. Selecting an appropriate caliper can be essential for achieving good balance with propensity score matching. *Am. J. Epidemiol.* **2014**, *179*, 226–235. [CrossRef] [PubMed]
13. Jurado, J.; Javidfar, J.; Newmark, A.; Lavelle, M.; Bacchetta, M.; Gorenstein, L.; D'Ovidio, F.; Ginsburg, M.E.; Sonett, J.R. Minimally invasive thymectomy and open thymectomy: Outcome analysis of 263 patients. *Ann. Thorac. Surg.* **2012**, *94*, 974–981. [CrossRef] [PubMed]
14. Burt, B.M.; Nguyen, D.; Groth, S.S.; Palivela, N.; Ripley, R.T.; Makris, K.I.; Farjah, F.; Cornwell, L.; Massarweh, N.N. Utilization of Minimally Invasive Thymectomy and Margin-Negative Resection for Early-Stage Thymoma. *Ann. Thorac. Surg.* **2019**, *108*, 405–411. [CrossRef]
15. Strobel, P.; Bauer, A.; Puppe, B.; Kraushaar, T.; Krein, A.; Toyka, K.; Gold, R.; Semik, M.; Kiefer, R.; Nix, W.; et al. Tumor recurrence and survival in patients treated for thymomas and thymic squamous cell carcinomas: A retrospective analysis. *J. Clin. Oncol.* **2004**, *22*, 1501–1509. [CrossRef]
16. Safieddine, N.; Liu, G.; Cuningham, K.; Ming, T.; Hwang, D.; Brade, A.; Bezjak, A.; Fischer, S.; Xu, W.; Azad, S.; et al. Prognostic factors for cure, recurrence and long-term survival after surgical resection of thymoma. *J. Thorac. Oncol.* **2014**, *9*, 1018–1022. [CrossRef]
17. Burt, B.M.; Yao, X.; Shrager, J.; Antonicelli, A.; Padda, S.; Reiss, J.; Wakelee, H.; Su, S.; Huang, J.; Scott, W. Determinants of Complete Resection of Thymoma by Minimally Invasive and Open Thymectomy: Analysis of an International Registry. *J. Thorac. Oncol.* **2017**, *12*, 129–136. [CrossRef]
18. Papadimas, E.; Tan, Y.K.; Luo, H.; Choong, A.; Tam, J.K.C.; Kofidis, T.; Mithiran, H. Partial Versus Complete Thymectomy in Non-Myasthenic Patients With Thymoma: A Systematic Review and Meta-Analysis of Clinical Outcomes. *Heart Lung Circ.* **2022**, *31*, 59–68. [CrossRef]
19. Pulle, M.V.; Asaf, B.B.; Puri, H.V.; Bishnoi, S.; Kumar, A. Meta-Analysis of Limited Thymectomy versus Total Thymectomy for Masaoka Stage I and II Thymoma. *J. Chest Surg.* **2021**, *54*, 127–136. [CrossRef]
20. Wolfe, G.I.; Kaminski, H.J.; Aban, I.B.; Minisman, G.; Kuo, H.C.; Marx, A.; Strobel, P.; Mazia, C.; Oger, J.; Cea, J.G.; et al. Randomized trial of thymectomy in myasthenia gravis. *N. Engl. J. Med.* **2016**, *375*, 511–522. [CrossRef]
21. Lucchi, M.; Ricciardi, R.; Melfi, F.; Duranti, L.; Basolo, F.; Palmiero, G.; Murri, L.; Mussi, A. Association of thymoma and myasthenia gravis: Oncological and neurological results of the surgical treatment. *Eur. J. Cardiothorac. Surg.* **2009**, *35*, 812–816. [CrossRef]
22. Hess, N.R.; Sarkaria, I.S.; Pennathur, A.; Levy, R.M.; Christie, N.A.; Luketich, J.D. Minimally invasive versus open thymectomy: A systematic review of surgical techniques, patient demographics, and perioperative outcomes. *Ann. Cardiothorac. Surg.* **2016**, *5*, 1–9. [CrossRef] [PubMed]
23. Bae, M.K.; Lee, S.K.; Kim, H.Y.; Park, S.Y.; Park, I.K.; Kim, D.J.; Chung, K.Y. Recurrence after thymoma resection according to the extent of the resection. *J. Cardiothorac. Surg.* **2014**, *9*, 51. [CrossRef] [PubMed]
24. Xu, C.; Zhang, Q.; Li, J.; Qiu, H.; Zhu, K.; Chen, D.; Jin, Z.; Zhang, J.; Zhang, B.; Witharana, P.; et al. Prognosis and surgical outcomes of the total thymectomy versus thymomectomy in non-myasthenic patients with early-stage thymoma: A systematic review and meta-analysis. *Asian J. Surg.* **2023**, *46*, 3455–3463. [CrossRef] [PubMed]

cancers

MDPI

Article

Sex-Based Differences in Lung Cancer Incidence: A Retrospective Analysis of Two Large US-Based Cancer Databases

Kalyan Ratnakaram [1], Sai Yendamuri [1,*], Adrienne Groman [2] and Sukumar Kalvapudi [1]

1 Department of Thoracic Surgery, Roswell Park Comprehensive Cancer Center, Elm and Carlton Streets, Buffalo, NY 14263, USA; kalyan.ratnakaram@roswellpark.org (K.R.); skalvapudi@utmck.edu (S.K.)

2 Department of Biostatistics and Bioinformatics, Roswell Park Comprehensive Cancer Center, Elm and Carlton Streets, Buffalo, NY 14263, USA; adrienne.groman@roswellpark.org

* Correspondence: sai.yendamuri@roswellpark.org; Tel.: +1-716-845-8675

Simple Summary: In recent years, researchers have begun to investigate the relation between sex and cancer. We wanted to look at the relation between sex and non-small cell lung cancer among high-risk patients to see if this relationship needs further exploration. In order to do this, we chose to look at large publicly available databases that contained information on lung cancer incidence. Our research found indications that females have an elevated risk of lung cancer incidence in comparison with males within high-risk populations. These results suggest that the difference in sex-specific cancer biomechanisms should be further investigated and explored.

Abstract: Background/Objectives: Non-small cell lung cancer (NSCLC) has seen a relative rise in incidence among females versus males in recent years, although males still have a higher overall incidence. However, it is unclear whether this trend is consistent across all populations. Therefore, we retrospectively examined this relationship in two large high-risk clinical cohorts. **Methods:** First, we analyzed lung cancer incidence among individuals with a smoking history of over 40 pack-years in the National Lung Screening Trial (NLST). Then, we investigated the incidence of second primary NSCLC in patients who underwent lobectomy for previous stage I lung cancer using the Surveillance, Epidemiology, and End Results (SEER) database. We performed both univariate and multivariable time-to-event analyses to investigate the relationship between sex and lung cancer incidence. **Results:** In the NLST cohort (n = 37,627), females had a higher risk of developing primary NSCLC than males (HR = 1.11 [1.007–1.222], p = 0.035) after adjusting for age and pack-year history. In the SEER cohort (n = 19,327), females again exhibited an increased risk of developing a second primary lung cancer (HR = 1.138 [1.02–1.269], p = 0.021), after adjusting for age, race, grade, and histology. **Conclusions**: Our analysis reveals that females have a modestly higher lung cancer incidence than males in high-risk populations. These findings underscore the importance of further researching the underlying cellular processes that may cause sex-specific differences in lung cancer incidence.

Keywords: NSCLC; lung cancer incidence; sex disparities; NLST; SEER

1. Introduction

Lung cancer, the second most prevalent malignancy worldwide, is the leading cause of cancer-related deaths in both sexes. In the United States alone, an estimated 234,000 new cases and 125,000 deaths are projected for 2024, underscoring the significant public health challenge posed by lung cancer [1]. Cigarette smoking is recognized as the primary cause of lung cancer, with all histological subtypes linked to this habit [2]. Nonetheless, other factors also seem to influence lung cancer risk.

Epidemiological studies have consistently documented sex differences in the incidence and outcomes of lung cancer. Historically, males have exhibited a higher age-standardized incidence rate of lung cancer than females [3,4]. From 2015 to 2019, the incidence of lung cancer was 27% higher in males than in females [5]. Males were also diagnosed at a more advanced stage than females, leading to a poorer prognosis [6]. Much of this disparity is attributed to the higher smoking prevalence among males [7].

However, over the last two decades, a decline in smoking prevalence in the United States has led to a decrease in the incidence of lung cancer [8]. Since 2006, the annual incidence rates of lung cancer have decreased by 2.6% in males and 1.1% in females [5]. This has resulted in a relative increase in female lung cancer rates when compared to male rates. Recent studies have also indicated a rise in lung cancer diagnoses among young females compared to their male counterparts [9]. Nevertheless, despite these trends, lung cancer incidence remains higher in males in the overall population compared to females [10].

For our study, we chose to look at individuals at high risk of developing lung cancer. Risk factors for lung cancer are numerous and include age, history of smoking, prior diagnosis of malignant tumors, and occupational exposure to asbestos. Of these, smoking is the biggest risk factor for lung cancer [11]. Another important factor is age, as older individuals are more likely to develop lung cancer [11]. Selection criteria for all randomized controlled trials for lung cancer screening include smoking history and age to target higher risk individuals [12]. For example, the NLST required a 30 pack-year smoking history and participants aged over 55 as inclusion criteria [12]. Additionally, prior malignancy, although less studied, is associated with an increased risk of new lung cancer, as highlighted by the National Comprehensive Cancer Network (NCCN) and the American Association for Thoracic Surgery (AATS), which advocate for lower screening thresholds in patients with a history of malignancy [13].

Most previous epidemiological studies have focused on lung cancer incidence and sex-related differences in the general population, not specifically in high-risk populations. To explore the relationship between sex and lung cancer incidence in high-risk populations, we retrospectively performed time-to-event analyses of two publicly available clinical cohorts: the National Lung Screening Trial (NLST) and the Surveillance, Epidemiology, and End Results (SEER) databases. This information is necessary in determining whether additional research into the sex-specific physiological mechanisms that relate to lung cancer is worthwhile.

2. Materials and Methods

We conducted a retrospective analysis to explore the association between sex and lung cancer incidence, utilizing data from two sizable clinical cohorts: the National Lung Screening Trial database and the Surveillance, Epidemiology, and End Results database.

2.1. NLST Analysis

The NLST was a randomized controlled trial sponsored by the U.S. National Cancer Institute (NCI) aimed at assessing the efficacy of low-dose helical computed tomography (CT) screening in reducing lung cancer mortality among individuals at high risk [11] We used this publicly available database to examine sex-based disparities in primary lung cancer incidence.

Patient recruitment for the NLST occurred between August 2002 and April 2004. Demographic information was gathered, and participants were monitored for lung cancer occurrence throughout the trial. The NLST inclusion criteria comprised a smoking history of $\geq$30 pack-years, cessation of smoking within $\leq$15 years for former smokers, absence of prior lung cancer or other life-threatening cancers within the preceding five years, and no symptoms indicative of lung cancer such as hemoptysis or unexplained weight loss [14]. This initial screening resulted in the enrollment of 53,354 eligible participants aged 55 to 74.

For our investigation, we focused solely on patients with a smoking history exceeding 40 pack-years and those diagnosed with non-small cell lung carcinoma (NSCLC), leading to a final cohort of 37,627 individuals. We limited our patient population to those with a 40-pack-year smoking history to emulate high-risk patients and to ensure a higher incidence rate of lung cancer for the time-to-event analysis. Case selection strategy for the NLST cohort is given in Figure 1A. Details including patient age, sex, race, smoking behavior, pack-year history, and lung cancer incidence were collected from the NLST database. To conduct time-to-event analysis, the start date was defined as the date of enrollment in the trial, extending until either the last follow-up date or the date of primary lung cancer development.

The database was accessed on 11 August 2023 at the url: https://cdas.cancer.gov/nlst/.

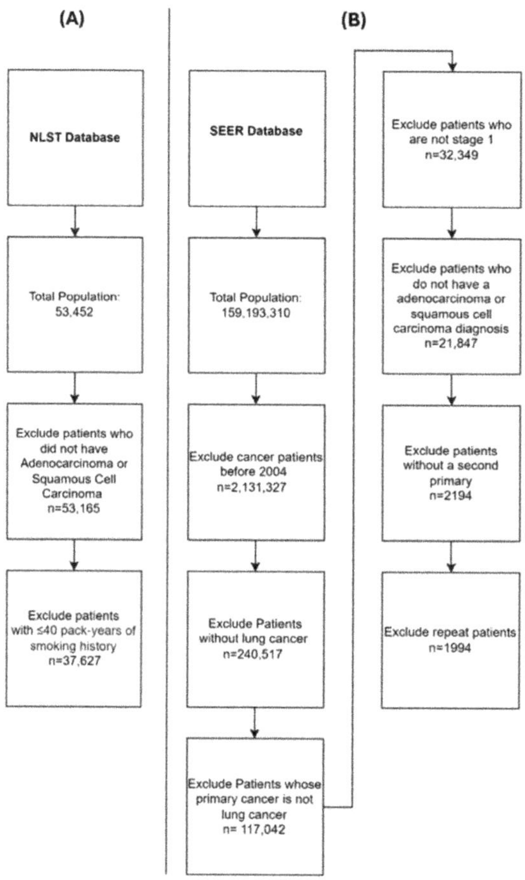

Figure 1. Study Selection Criteria. (**A**)—selection criteria for the NLST database. (**B**)—selection criteria for the SEER database.

2.2. SEER Analysis

The SEER Program database, overseen by the National Cancer Institute (NCI), encompasses 18 cancer registries, covering approximately 48% of the U.S. population [15]. This comprehensive database contains information regarding patient demographics, primary tumor characteristics, and follow-up data, including survival outcomes.

To identify individuals at high risk for developing lung cancer, we chose people with treated primary lung cancer and followed them to see if they developed a second lung cancer. We therefore looked at patients diagnosed with primary lung cancer between 2004 and 2020 within the SEER database. Patients with a history of any other malignancy were excluded as well as histologies other than adenocarcinoma or squamous cell carcinoma. We wanted to select patients who developed a second primary lung cancer and not recurrence of lung cancer. Subsequently, we refined our cohort to include only those with stage I disease who underwent lobectomy. We specifically selected patients with prior stage I NSCLC who underwent lobectomies, as stage I NSCLC generally has a lower recurrence rate than more advanced stages. Lobectomies are also regarded as the most effective treatment for early-stage non-small cell lung cancer [16]. Furthermore, we concentrated exclusively on these two histological subtypes, which represent the most prevalent forms of NSCLC, accounting for approximately 70% of all lung cancer cases [17]. This approach also ensured consistency between the two databases. The selection process yielded a final cohort comprising 19,327 patients (Figure 1B). Data regarding patient age, sex, race, grade of first primary lung cancer, and histology of first primary lung cancer were extracted from the SEER database. Follow-up was conducted until death, the last follow-up date, or the occurrence of a second primary lung cancer. For time-to-event analysis, the date of primary lung cancer diagnosis was defined as the starting point, extending until either the occurrence of a second primary lung cancer or the date of the last follow-up.

The database was accessed on 15 May 2023 at https://seer.cancer.gov/.

2.3. Statistical Analysis

Continuous data were presented as means with standard deviation and categorical data as numerical values and percentages. Independent *t*-tests were used to compare group differences for continuous variables and chi-squared tests for categorical variables.

Time-to-event univariate Cox proportional hazards modeling was used to identify significant associations between various clinical characteristics and either incidence of primary lung cancer (NLST) or incidence of second primary lung cancer (SEER). Time to last follow-up and either time to incidence of lung cancer (NLST) or time to incidence of second primary (SEER) was used as the time variable. To control confounding factors, multivariate Cox proportional hazards modeling was conducted using a stepwise backward elimination method to develop the final model, with a tolerance of $p < 0.1$ at each step.

Statistical analyses were performed using the IBM SPSS statistical software version 28.0.1.0. Plotting was performed using GraphPad Prism version 10.1.2. For all analyses, $p < 0.05$ was considered statistically significant.

3. Results

3.1. NLST

A total of 37,627 patients were examined in the NLST database, with a mean age of 62 (standard deviation (SD) = 5.1). Most of the cohort was Caucasian (92%), with former and current smokers comprising an even split (50.7% former smokers, 49.3% current smokers). The overall incidence of primary lung cancer was 4.7% (1781 out of 37,627).

For the purposes of this analysis, we compared males (n = 23,662, 62.9%) to females (n = 13,965, 37.1%) in the cohort. Males tended to be slightly older (male vs. female, *p*-value; 62.2 vs. 61.8, $p < 0.01$) and were less likely to be current smokers (47.8% vs. 52%, $p < 0.01$) than females, yet they had a higher pack-year history (66.9% vs. 60.6%, $p < 0.01$) (Table 1). The mean follow-up time for males was 2273 (95% CI: 2266–2280) days and for females was 2300 (95% CI: 2292–2308) days. The incidence rate of primary lung cancer per 1000 person-years was 7.57 (95% CI: 7.23–7.93) in the overall population, 7.48 (95% CI: 7.05–7.93) in males, and 7.72 (95% CI: 7.16–8.32) in females.

Subsequently, univariate time-to-event Cox proportional hazards modeling was employed to explore the associations between age, sex, and pack-years with lung cancer incidence. Increasing patient age (Hazard Ratio (HR) = 1.076 [95% Confidence Interval (CI) = 1.066–1.085], $p < 0.01$) and pack-year history (HR = 1.007 [1.006–1.009], $p < 0.01$) were predictive of decreased time to lung cancer development. Patient sex was not significantly associated with time to lung cancer (female vs. male, HR = 1.033 [0.939–1.137], $p = 0.502$). Multivariable time-to-event Cox proportional hazards modeling, incorporating age, sex, and pack-years as covariates, along with the interaction between sex and pack-years, revealed that females had a significantly higher rate of lung cancer development than males

(HR = 1.11 [1.007–1.222], $p = 0.035$) after adjusting for age and pack-year history (Table 2). Age and pack-year history were also retained in the final model, but the interaction between sex and pack-years was eliminated.

Table 1. Overall Patient Characteristics of the NLST Cohort as well as Differences Between Males and Females.

Variable	Overall n = 37,627	Male n = 23,662 (62.9%)	Female n = 13,965 (37.1%)	*p*-Value
Age	62 (5.1)	62.2 (5.1)	61.8 (5)	**<0.001**
Race				**<0.001**
Caucasian	34,552 (92.4%)	21,658 (92.1%)	12,894 (93%)	
African American	1389 (3.7%)	833 (3.5%)	556 (4%)	
Other	1434 (3.8%)	1014 (4.3%)	420 (3%)	
Smoking Status				**<0.001**
Former	19,060 (50.7%)	12,360 (52.2%)	6700 (48%)	
Current	18,567 (49.3%)	11,302 (47.8%)	7265 (52%)	
Pack-years	64.6 (23.6)	66.9 (25.1)	60.6 (20.4)	**<0.001**

Age, race, smoking status, and pack-years in the NLST cohort. Age and pack-years are given as mean (standard deviation). Numerical values as well as percentages are used for the categorical variables. Age and pack-year history were compared using independent *t*-tests and the other variables were compared using chi-squared tests. Significant *p*-values are bolded. n = number.

Table 2. Univariate and Multivariate Time-to-Event Cox Proportional Hazards Analyses for the NLST Cohort.

Variable	Univariate HR 95% (95% CI)	*p*-Value	Multivariate HR (95% CI)	*p*-Value
Age	1.076 (1.066–1.085)	**<0.001**	1.073 (1.063–1.082)	**<0.001**
Sex				
Female vs. Male	1.033 (0.939–1.137)	0.502	1.11 (1.007–1.222)	**0.035**
Pack-years	1.007 (1.006–1.009)	**<0.001**	1.006 (1.005–1.008)	**<0.001**

Univariate time-to-event analyses were performed to investigate the association between age, sex, and pack-year history with risk of developing lung cancer in the NLST cohort. All variables used in the univariate analysis were inputted into the multivariate analysis to account for confounding. Additionally, the interaction between sex and pack-years was inputted as an additional covariate. Age, sex, and pack-years were significant in the final analysis. The interaction between sex and pack-years was eliminated. Significant *p*-values are bolded. HR = Hazard Ratio. CI = Confidence Interval.

3.2. SEER

A total of 19,327 patients with stage I NSCLC who underwent lobectomy were included from the SEER database. The mean age of the cohort was 70.5 (SD 9.8), with the majority being Caucasian (81.3%). In the overall population, 47.5% had well/moderately well-differentiated tumors, and 22.4% had poorly differentiated tumors prior to surgery. Most patients were diagnosed with adenocarcinoma (64.8%). During the follow-up period, 9.6% of the cohort (1862 out of 19,327) developed a second primary lung cancer.

Between the two groups, an equal number of males (n = 9175, 47.5%) and females (n = 10,152, 52.5%) were observed. Males were more likely to have poorly differentiated primaries (25.4% vs. 19.6%, p <0.01) and squamous cell carcinoma (42.7% vs. 28.3%, $p < 0.01$) prior to lobectomy compared to females (Table 3).

Univariate time-to-event Cox hazard analysis revealed that only squamous histology (HR = 1.181 [1.073–1.3], p <.01) and female sex (HR = 1.12 [1.022–1.228], $p = 0.016$) significantly predicted earlier onset of second primary lung cancer diagnosis. A multivariable analysis incorporating age, sex, race, grade, and histology as covariates retained only sex and histology in the final model (Table 4). The mean follow-up time for males was 51 (95% CI: 50–52) months and for females was 58 (95% CI: 57–59) months. The incidence rate of second primary cancer per 1000 person-years was 22 (95% CI: 21.1–23) in the overall population, 16 (14.9–17.1) in males, and 30.1 (28.4–31.8) in females.

Table 3. Overall Patient Characteristics of the SEER Cohort as well as Differences Between Males and Females.

Variable	Overall n = 19,327	Male n = 9175 (47.5%)	Female n = 10,152 (52.5%)	*p*-Value
Age	70.5 (9.8)	70.4 (9.4)	70.9 (10.1)	0.086
Race				**0.005**
Caucasian	15,721 (81.3%)	7400 (80.7%)	8321 (82%)	
Non-Caucasian	1568 (8.1%)	738 (8%)	830 (8.2%)	
Unknown	2038 (10.5%)	1037 (11.3%)	1001 (9.9%)	
Grade				**<0.001**
Well/Moderately Well Differentiated	9175 (47.5%)	4131 (45%)	5044 (49.7%)	
Poorly Differentiated	4325 (22.4%)	2332 (25.4%)	1993 (19.6%)	
Unknown	5827 (30.1%)	2712 (29.6%)	3115 (30.7%)	
Histology				**<0.001**
Adenocarcinoma	12,528 (64.8%)	5254 (57.3%)	7274 (71.7%)	
Squamous Cell Carcinoma	6799 (35.2%)	3921 (42.7%)	2878 (28.3%)	

Age, race, tumor grade of first primary, and tumor histology of first primary in the SEER cohort. Age is given as mean (standard deviation). Numerical values as well as percentages are used for the categorical variables. Age was compared using independent *t*-test, and the other variables were compared using chi-squared tests. Significant *p*-values are bolded. n = number.

Table 4. Univariate and Multivariate Time-to-Event Cox Proportional Hazards Analyses for the SEER Cohort.

Variable	Univariate HR (95% CI)	*p*-Value	Multivariate HR (95% CI)	*p*-Value
Age	0.998 (0.993–1.002)	0.369	-	-
Sex				
Female vs. Male	**1.12 (1.022–1.228)**	**0.016**	**1.138 (1.02–1.269)**	**0.021**
Race				
Non-Caucasian vs. Caucasian	0.907 (0.764–1.078)	0.267	-	-
Grade				
Poorly Differentiated vs. Well/Moderately Well Differentiated	1.071 (0.959–1.196)	0.226	-	-
Histology				
Squamous Cell Carcinoma vs. Adenocarcinoma	**1.181 (1.073–1.3)**	**<0.001**	**1.171 (1.046–1.311)**	**0.006**

Univariate time-to-event analyses were performed to investigate the association between age, sex, race, grade of first primary lung cancer, and histology of first primary with risk of developing second primary lung cancer in the SEER cohort. All variables used in the univariate analysis were inputted into the multivariate analysis to account for confounding. Only sex and histology were retained in the multivariate analysis. Significant *p*-values are bolded. HR = Hazard Ratio. CI = Confidence Interval.

4. Discussion

Lung cancer incidence has displayed a concerning trend in recent decades, with a consistent rise among females compared to males. Data spanning 2001–2019 show a steady decrease in male lung cancer rates, while female lung cancer rates reached a peak around 2006 before also declining, albeit at a slower pace than males [8]. Despite this, males still exhibit a higher overall incidence than females. This prompted an investigation into whether this pattern held true even within high-risk populations. The main aim of this study was to systematically compare lung cancer incidence in high-risk populations and explore sex-based differences. Our findings, based on two large publicly available databases—the NLST and SEER databases—indicate that females are at a higher risk of developing lung cancer than males, even after accounting for confounding factors such as age, smoking history, and histology (Figure 2). While previous studies have investigated sex-based disparities in lung cancer incidence, this study is potentially the first to assess sex differences in high-risk populations specifically.

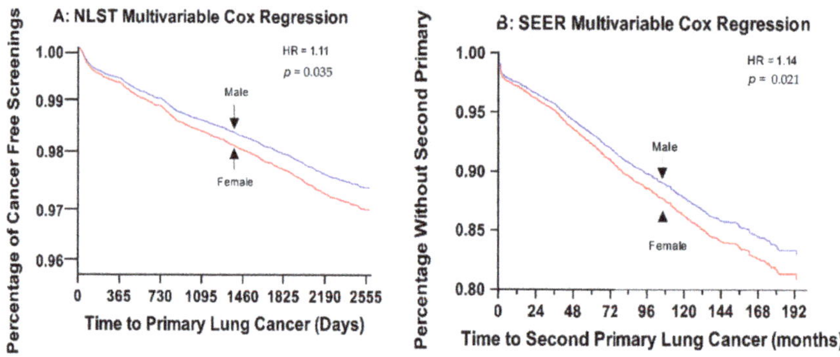

Figure 2. Multivariate Cox Regression Graphs for both the NLST and SEER Databases. (**A**) Multivariable cox proportional hazards model for time to primary lung cancer in the NLST database. Final model includes sex, age, and number of pack-years. (**B**) Multivariable cox proportional hazards model for second primary lung cancer in the SEER database. Final model includes sex and histopathology.

The disparity in lung cancer incidence between sex can be partially attributed to differences in smoking behavior. Historically, females began smoking in larger numbers later than males and were slower to quit [7,18]. This aligns with data indicating a slower decline in lung cancer rates in females, as well as an increase in lung cancer diagnoses in young females [18,19]. To further investigate the association between gender and lung cancer incidence, as well as its relation to smoking, we examined the NLST database. Initial univariate Cox proportional time-to-event analysis did not reveal significant sex differences in lung cancer risk. However, multivariable analysis, after adjusting for the number of pack-years and age, identified female sex as an independent risk factor for lung cancer incidence. Thus, for the same number of pack-years smoked, females had an 11% higher risk of developing lung cancer than males. This finding is consistent with previous studies [20–23]. For instance, Zang et al. found that at every level of tobacco exposure, the risk of lung cancer in females was 1.2- to 1.5-fold higher than in males, suggesting that females have a higher relative risk of lung cancer than males with the same level of smoke exposure [23]. Additionally, Harris et al. found that females, compared to males, face a higher risk of lung cancer at the same level of smoking for both major forms of lung cancer, with a 70% higher risk for squamous cell carcinoma and a 50% higher risk for adenocarcinoma [21].

Well-documented differences in smoking patterns exist between males and females. Although females began smoking in larger numbers later than males and have been slower to quit, males still consume a greater overall quantity of tobacco products [24]. Consistent with this, in our selected NLST cohort, we discovered that females were more likely to be current smokers than males but had a lower pack-year history. Females tend to start smoking at a later age, smoke less frequently, inhale less deeply, and are less likely to smoke harmful non-menthol cigarettes than males. Despite reduced intensity of smoking, females exhibit a higher risk of lung cancer for a given pack-year history than males [20,23,25,26]. This suggests that a more effective metric should be implemented—perhaps pack-years is not the most accurate measure of cigarette smoke exposure when considering females. A potentially better metric, such as total duration smoked, might be a more suitable measure for screening guidelines. For instance, a 2018 study of the Norwegian population by Hansen et al. found that when smoking amount was measured as a continuous variable, female smokers had a greater risk of lung cancer than male smokers [20].

To corroborate the elevated incidence of lung cancer in high-risk females relative to high-risk males, we employed the SEER database. We examined patients with a history of prior stage I lung cancer who had undergone successful lobectomy and conducted a time-to-event analysis to ascertain the onset of a second primary. A multivariable analysis revealed that females had a 14% higher chance of developing a second primary compared to males, even after adjusting for confounders such as age, race, grade, and histology. One of the most significant risk factors for developing a second primary is continued smoking. Regrettably, data regarding smoking history were not available from the SEER database, and the absence of these data is a limitation of our study. While there is extensive data reporting on overall lung cancer incidence and sex differences, there is a scarcity of data concerning the incidence of second primary specifically. In a 2017 study of the SEER database by Thakur et al., females were found to have a higher standardized incidence ratio of second primary lung cancer than males [27]. This novel and intriguing finding that females are at a higher risk of developing a second primary warrants further investigation into the underlying risk factors.

Several potential mechanisms underpin the increased risk of lung cancer in females. One potential mechanism is estrogen-induced carcinogenesis, mediated by the altered metabolism of tobacco carcinogens [28]. Nicotine-derived nitrosamine ketones (NNKs), a group of extensively studied tobacco carcinogens, significantly contribute to the carcinogenic potential of cigarette smoke. Female sex hormones have been demonstrated to inhibit safe NNK metabolism, thereby promoting carcinogenesis [29]. Furthermore, estrogen can be metabolized into catechol estrogens through the increased activity of cytochrome P450 1B1 (CYP1B1) [30]. CYP1B1 expression is amplified by cigarette smoking, and it has been shown in animal models that female mice exposed to cigarette smoke exhibit increased CYP1B1 activation compared to male mice [31]. These catechol estrogens are subsequently activated into semiquinone and quinone intermediates, leading to the formation of harmful DNA adducts that promote mutagenesis and inhibit DNA repair [28,30,32]. However, these observed differences cannot be entirely attributed to variations in smoking patterns, as females appear to develop lung cancer at higher rates even after controlling for smoking. For instance, females who have never smoked seem to develop lung cancer at rates that exceed those of their male counterparts [33]. One explanation is that the changing patterns of lung cancer histology as well as endogenous genetic variations between the two sexes may contribute to these disparities [29].

Over the last few decades, there has been an increasing trend of adenocarcinoma compared to squamous cell carcinoma. This rising incidence of adenocarcinoma may be partially associated with increased smoking of low-tar filter cigarettes allowing for smaller particles to travel more distally within lungs. Adenocarcinoma surpassed squamous cell carcinoma as the most frequently diagnosed lung cancer in males [10]. Adenocarcinoma also exhibits a less rapid decline compared to squamous cell carcinoma in response to cigarette smoking cessation [10]. Females have been reported to carry a higher frequency of mutations in critical driver genes such as epidermal growth factor receptor (EGFR), anaplastic lymphoma kinase (ALK), Kirsten rat sarcoma (KRAS) genes, and tumor protein 53 (TP53), thereby increasing susceptibility to adenocarcinoma [8,34]. This heightened susceptibility to adenocarcinoma could account for the relative incidence of lung cancer in females compared to males. Endogenous genetic variations in females also may be responsible for increased lung cancer in females. Polymorphisms in the cytochrome P450 1A1 gene, defects in DNA repair, overexpression of the X-linked gastrin-releasing peptide receptor, and mutations in p53 have been linked to increased lung cancer pathogenesis in females [34].

Finally, exposure-related factors, including increased exposure to secondhand smoke and environmental carcinogens, may also contribute to the elevated risk in females [10]. Unfortunately, population-based quantification of secondhand smoke exposure is challenging, and there is a lack of robust data. An observational study of patients diagnosed with lung cancer in France found that 78% of nonsmoker females had environmental exposure to tobacco smoke compared to only 21% of nonsmoker males [35]. Another analysis of 37 studies found that females whose spouses smoked had a 24% increased risk of developing lung cancer [36]. Risk factors like asbestos and radon, which are known to contribute to lung carcinogenesis, have been inadequately studied in women, despite their increased exposure at home [10]. Indoor cooking fumes are another possible gender-role-dependent risk factor. One meta-analysis from Asia demonstrated that females who cook with wood or coal at home have increased odds of developing lung cancer compared to those who do not [37]. Cooking oil fumes also contain polycyclic aromatic hydrocarbons (PAHs), which are known to be carcinogenic. The effect of PAHs on lung carcinogenesis is especially seen in women from developing countries, due to improper ventilation [38]. Further investigation into these non-cigarette smoking-induced pathways of lung carcinogenesis is needed to address the disproportionate risk to females.

The limitations of our study must be acknowledged. As a retrospective analysis, our study was constrained by the data available from two databases. We could only adjust for covariates present in the datasets, and we lacked information on patients' overall health and socioeconomic status, both of which are known to influence cancer rates. This absence may have confounded our results. In the NLST database, we used pack-years as a numerical variable, which assumes a linear relationship between pack-years and lung cancer incidence. While some studies suggest a linear dose–response between cigarette smoking and lung cancer risk [39–41], others indicate that this relationship may vary depending on daily consumption [42]. For those with lower daily consumption, the relationship is suggested to be logarithmic, while at higher levels of smoking, the relationship appears more linear [43]. Unfortunately, there is limited research specifically examining pack-years as opposed to cigarettes smoked per day. This presents a limitation in our study, as assuming linearity may not fully capture the complexities of smoking behavior and its impact on lung cancer risk. In the SEER database, we used patients with prior lung cancer as surrogates for high-risk individuals to observe the development of second lung cancers. This approach has limitations, as distinguishing between recurrence and new primary cancers is challenging. Additionally, the SEER database lacks data on smoking, a significant confounder in lung cancer studies. Although race was included as a covariate, the databases primarily comprised patients of Caucasian descent, which limits the study's applicability to more diverse populations [44,45]. Furthermore, we lacked data on occupation-related lung cancer and passive smoking, both of which differentially affect males and females. This underscores the need for further research in these areas. Finally, this study's generalizability may be limited, as both SEER and NLST are US-based.

5. Conclusions

Numerous epidemiological studies indicate that the incidence of lung cancer is higher in males than in females, although there has been a relative increase in lung cancer risk in females over the past few decades. However, most of these studies have concentrated on the general population. When examining high-risk patients specifically, we find that females are at a higher risk for developing lung cancer than males, even after adjusting for confounding factors such as age and smoking history. Notably, we discovered that females are at an elevated risk of developing a second primary compared to males. The increased incidence of lung cancer in females compared to males in high-risk populations necessitates a deeper understanding of the potential underlying mechanisms. Conducting further epidemiological and biological research into sex-specific differences in lung cancer incidence will lead to a better understanding of how sex plays a role in lung cancer.

Author Contributions: K.R. performed formal analysis, investigation, and wrote the original draft. S.Y. conceptualized the study, came up with the methodology, and provided administrative resources. A.G. collected patient data, performed formal analysis, and provided validation. S.K. assisted with data curation and analysis, generated figures, and assisted writing the original draft. All authors have read and agreed to the published version of the manuscript.

Funding: This work was funded by the National Cancer Institute (grant number: P30CA016056; used for access to Roswell Park Biostatistics Shared Resource). The funders had no role in the design of this study or the decision to publish the work. The content is solely the responsibility of the authors and does not necessarily represent the official views of Roswell Park Comprehensive Cancer Center.

Institutional Review Board Statement: This study was conducted according to the principles of the Declaration of Helsinki and approved by the Institutional Review Board of Roswell Park Comprehensive Cancer Center.

Informed Consent Statement: This study utilizes publicly available de-identified data, obviating the need for IRB approval and patient consent.

Data Availability Statement: Data for this study were extracted from two publicly available clinical databases: the National Lung Screening Trial (NLST) and Surveillance, Epidemiology, and End Results (SEER).

Acknowledgments: We thank the Roswell Park Biostatistics Shared Resource for assistance with database curation and analysis.

Conflicts of Interest: The authors report no proprietary or commercial interest in any product mentioned or concept discussed in this article. The funding sponsors had no role in the choice of research project; design of the study; in the collection, analyses, or interpretation of data; in the writing of the manuscript; or in the decision to publish the results.

References

1. Siegel, R.L.; Giaquinto, A.N.; Jemal, A. Cancer statistics, 2024. *CA A Cancer J. Clin.* **2024**, *74*, 12–49. [CrossRef] [PubMed]
2. Bade, B.C.; Dela Cruz, C.S. Lung Cancer 2020: Epidemiology, Etiology, and Prevention. *Clin. Chest Med.* **2020**, *41*, 1–24. [CrossRef] [PubMed]
3. Patel, M.I.; McKinley, M.; Cheng, I.; Haile, R.; Wakelee, H.; Gomez, S.L. Lung cancer incidence trends in California by race/ethnicity, histology, sex, and neighborhood socioeconomic status: An analysis spanning 28 years. *Lung Cancer* **2017**, *108*, 140–149. [CrossRef]
4. Lewis, D.R.; Check, D.P.; Caporaso, N.E.; Travis, W.D.; Devesa, S.S. US lung cancer trends by histologic type. *Cancer* **2014**, *120*, 2883–2892. [CrossRef]
5. Siegel, R.L.; Miller, K.D.; Wagle, N.S.; Jemal, A. Cancer statistics, 2023. *CA A Cancer J. Clin.* **2023**, *73*, 17–48. [CrossRef] [PubMed]
6. May, L.; Shows, K.; Nana-Sinkam, P.; Li, H.; Landry, J.W. Sex Differences in Lung Cancer. *Cancers* **2023**, *15*, 3111. [CrossRef]
7. Ragavan, M.V.; Patel, M.I. Understanding Sex Disparities in Lung Cancer Incidence: Are Women more at Risk? *Lung Cancer Manag.* **2020**, *9*, LMT34. [CrossRef]
8. Fu, Y.; Liu, J.; Chen, Y.; Liu, Z.; Xia, H.; Xu, H. Gender disparities in lung cancer incidence in the United States during 2001–2019. *Sci. Rep.* **2023**, *13*, 12581. [CrossRef]
9. Jemal, A.; Miller, K.D.; Ma, J.; Siegel, R.L.; Fedewa, S.A.; Islami, F.; Devesa, S.S.; Thun, M.J. Higher Lung Cancer Incidence in Young Women Than Young Men in the United States. *N. Engl. J. Med.* **2018**, *378*, 1999–2009. [CrossRef]
10. Gee, K.; Yendamuri, S. Lung cancer in females-sex-based differences from males in epidemiology, biology, and outcomes: A narrative review. *Transl. Lung Cancer Res.* **2024**, *13*, 163–178. [CrossRef]
11. Marcus, M.W.; Raji, O.Y.; Field, J.K. Lung cancer screening: Identifying the high risk cohort. *J. Thorac. Dis.* **2015**, *7*, S156–S162. [CrossRef] [PubMed]
12. Bach, P.B.; Mirkin, J.N.; Oliver, T.K.; Azzoli, C.G.; Berry, D.A.; Brawley, O.W.; Byers, T.; Colditz, G.A.; Gould, M.K.; Jett, J.R.; et al. Benefits and harms of CT screening for lung cancer: A systematic review. *JAMA* **2012**, *307*, 2418–2429. [CrossRef] [PubMed]
13. Wu, G.X.; Nelson, R.A.; Kim, J.Y.; Raz, D.J. Non–Small Cell Lung Cancer as a Second Primary Among Patients with Previous Malignancy: Who Is at Risk? *Clin. Lung Cancer* **2017**, *18*, 543–550.e543. [CrossRef] [PubMed]
14. Tammemägi, M.C.; Katki, H.A.; Hocking, W.G.; Church, T.R.; Caporaso, N.; Kvale, P.A.; Chaturvedi, A.K.; Silvestri, G.A.; Riley, T.L.; Commins, J.; et al. Selection Criteria for Lung-Cancer Screening. *N. Engl. J. Med.* **2013**, *368*, 728–736. [CrossRef]
15. Murphy, P.K.; Sellers, M.E.; Bonds, S.H.; Scott, S. The SEER Program's longstanding commitment to making cancer resources available. *J. Natl. Cancer Inst. Monogr.* **2024**, *2024*, 118–122. [CrossRef]
16. Mahvi, D.A.; Liu, R.; Grinstaff, M.W.; Colson, Y.L.; Raut, C.P. Local Cancer Recurrence: The Realities, Challenges, and Opportunities for New Therapies. *CA A Cancer J. Clin.* **2018**, *68*, 488–505. [CrossRef] [PubMed]

17. Tian, S. Classification and survival prediction for early-stage lung adenocarcinoma and squamous cell carcinoma patients. *Oncol. Lett.* **2017**, *14*, 5464–5470. [CrossRef] [PubMed]
18. Jemal, A.; Ma, J.; Rosenberg, P.S.; Siegel, R.; Anderson, W.F. Increasing lung cancer death rates among young women in southern and midwestern States. *J. Clin. Oncol.* **2012**, *30*, 2739–2744. [CrossRef]
19. Jeon, J.; Holford, T.R.; Levy, D.T.; Feuer, E.J.; Cao, P.; Tam, J.; Clarke, L.; Clarke, J.; Kong, C.Y.; Meza, R. Smoking and Lung Cancer Mortality in the United States From 2015 to 2065: A Comparative Modeling Approach. *Ann. Intern. Med.* **2018**, *169*, 684–693. [CrossRef]
20. Hansen, M.S.; Licaj, I.; Braaten, T.; Langhammer, A.; Le Marchand, L.; Gram, I.T. Sex Differences in Risk of Smoking-Associated Lung Cancer: Results from a Cohort of 600,000 Norwegians. *Am. J. Epidemiol.* **2017**, *187*, 971–981. [CrossRef]
21. Harris, R.E.; Zang, E.A.; Anderson, J.I.; Wynder, E.L. Race and Sex Differences in Lung Cancer Risk Associated with Cigarette Smoking. *Int. J. Epidemiol.* **1993**, *22*, 592–599. [CrossRef] [PubMed]
22. Risch, H.A.; Howe, G.R.; Jain, M.; Burch, J.D.; Holowaty, E.J.; Miller, A.B. Are female smokers at higher risk for lung cancer than male smokers? A case-control analysis by histologic type. *Am. J. Epidemiol.* **1993**, *138*, 281–293. [CrossRef]
23. Zang, E.A.; Wynder, E.L. Differences in lung cancer risk between men and women: Examination of the evidence. *J. Natl. Cancer Inst.* **1996**, *88*, 183–192. [CrossRef]
24. Cornelius, M.E.; Loretan, C.G.; Wang, T.W.; Jamal, A.; Homa, D.M. Tobacco Product Use Among Adults—United States, 2020. *MMWR Morb. Mortal. Wkly. Rep.* **2022**, *71*, 397–405. [CrossRef]
25. Xu, F.H.; Xiong, D.; Xu, Y.F.; Cao, S.M.; Xue, W.Q.; Qin, H.D.; Liu, W.S.; Cao, J.Y.; Zhang, Y.; Feng, Q.S.; et al. An epidemiological and molecular study of the relationship between smoking, risk of nasopharyngeal carcinoma, and Epstein-Barr virus activation. *J. Natl. Cancer Inst.* **2012**, *104*, 1396–1410. [CrossRef]
26. Giovino, G.A.; Villanti, A.C.; Mowery, P.D.; Sevilimedu, V.; Niaura, R.S.; Vallone, D.M.; Abrams, D.B. Differential trends in cigarette smoking in the USA: Is menthol slowing progress? *Tob. Control* **2015**, *24*, 28. [CrossRef] [PubMed]
27. Thakur, M.K.; Ruterbusch, J.J.; Schwartz, A.G.; Gadgeel, S.M.; Beebe-Dimmer, J.L.; Wozniak, A.J. Risk of Second Lung Cancer in Patients with Previously Treated Lung Cancer: Analysis of Surveillance, Epidemiology, and End Results (SEER) Data. *J. Thorac. Oncol.* **2018**, *13*, 46–53. [CrossRef] [PubMed]
28. Gasperino, J. Gender is a risk factor for lung cancer. *Med. Hypotheses* **2011**, *76*, 328–331. [CrossRef]
29. Stapelfeld, C.; Dammann, C.; Maser, E. Sex-specificity in lung cancer risk. *Int. J. Cancer* **2020**, *146*, 2376–2382. [CrossRef]
30. Sarabia, S.F.; Zhu, B.T.; Kurosawa, T.; Tohma, M.; Liehr, J.G. Mechanism of cytochrome P450-catalyzed aromatic hydroxylation of estrogens. *Chem. Res. Toxicol.* **1997**, *10*, 767–771. [CrossRef]
31. Ben-Zaken Cohen, S.; Paré, P.D.; Man, S.F.; Sin, D.D. The growing burden of chronic obstructive pulmonary disease and lung cancer in women: Examining sex differences in cigarette smoke metabolism. *Am. J. Respir. Crit. Care Med.* **2007**, *176*, 113–120. [CrossRef]
32. Newbold, R.R.; Liehr, J.G. Induction of uterine adenocarcinoma in CD-1 mice by catechol estrogens. *Cancer Res.* **2000**, *60*, 235–237.
33. Pinheiro, P.S.; Callahan, K.E.; Medina, H.N.; Koru-Sengul, T.; Kobetz, E.N.; Gomez, S.L.; de Lima Lopes, G. Lung cancer in never smokers: Distinct population-based patterns by age, sex, and race/ethnicity. *Lung Cancer* **2022**, *174*, 50–56. [CrossRef]
34. Ragavan, M.; Patel, M.I. The evolving landscape of sex-based differences in lung cancer: A distinct disease in women. *Eur. Respir. Rev.* **2022**, *31*, 210100. [CrossRef]
35. Clément-Duchêne, C.; Vignaud, J.M.; Stoufflet, A.; Bertrand, O.; Gislard, A.; Thiberville, L.; Grosdidier, G.; Martinet, Y.; Benichou, J.; Hainaut, P.; et al. Characteristics of never smoker lung cancer including environmental and occupational risk factors. *Lung Cancer* **2010**, *67*, 144–150. [CrossRef]
36. Hackshaw, A.K.; Law, M.R.; Wald, N.J. The accumulated evidence on lung cancer and environmental tobacco smoke. *BMJ* **1997**, *315*, 980–988. [CrossRef]
37. Hosgood, H.D., III; Boffetta, P.; Greenland, S.; Lee, Y.-C.A.; McLaughlin, J.; Seow, A.; Duell, E.J.; Andrew, A.S.; Zaridze, D.; Szeszenia-Dabrowska, N. In-home coal and wood use and lung cancer risk: A pooled analysis of the International Lung Cancer Consortium. *Environ. Health Perspect.* **2010**, *118*, 1743–1747. [CrossRef]
38. North, C.M.; Christiani, D.C. Women and Lung Cancer: What is New? *Semin. Thorac. Cardiovasc. Surg.* **2013**, *25*, 87–94. [CrossRef]
39. Ai, F.; Zhao, J.; Yang, W.; Wan, X. Dose–response relationship between active smoking and lung cancer mortality/prevalence in the Chinese population: A meta-analysis. *BMC Public Health* **2023**, *23*, 747. [CrossRef]
40. Chen, J. A Comparative Analysis of Lung Cancer Incidence and Tobacco Consumption in Canada, Norway and Sweden: A Population-Based Study. *Int. J. Environ. Res. Public Health* **2023**, *20*, 6930. [CrossRef]
41. Ruano-Ravina, A.; Figueiras, A.; Montes-Martínez, A.; Barros-Dios, J.M. Dose–response relationship between tobacco and lung cancer: New findings. *Eur. J. Cancer Prev.* **2003**, *12*, 257–263. [CrossRef]
42. Law, M.; Morris, J.; Watt, H.; Wald, N. The dose-response relationship between cigarette consumption, biochemical markers and risk of lung cancer. *Br. J. Cancer* **1997**, *75*, 1690–1693. [CrossRef]
43. Lubin, J.H.; Caporaso, N.E. Cigarette Smoking and Lung Cancer: Modeling Total Exposure and Intensity. *Cancer Epidemiol. Biomark. Prev.* **2006**, *15*, 517–523. [CrossRef]

44. Cranford, H.M.; Koru-Sengul, T.; Lopes, G.; Pinheiro, P.S. Lung Cancer Incidence by Detailed Race-Ethnicity. *Cancers* **2023**, *15*, 2164. [CrossRef]
45. Schabath, M.B.; Cress, D.; Munoz-Antonia, T. Racial and Ethnic Differences in the Epidemiology and Genomics of Lung Cancer. *Cancer Control* **2016**, *23*, 338–346. [CrossRef] [PubMed]

cancers

MDPI

Article

Musculoskeletal Disorders Related to Upper Limb Disability after One-Year Lung Cancer Resection

Javier Martín Núñez [1], Julia Raya Benítez [2], Florencio Quero Valenzuela [3], Andrés Calvache Mateo [1], Alba Navas Otero [1], Alejandro Heredia Ciuró [1,*] and Marie Carmen Valenza [1]

[1] Department of Physiotherapy, Faculty of Health Sciences, University of Granada, 18071 Granada, Spain; javimn@ugr.es (J.M.N.); andrescalvache@ugr.es (A.C.M.); albanavas@ugr.es (A.N.O.); cvalenza@ugr.es (M.C.V.)
[2] Department of Nursing, Faculty of Health Sciences, University of Granada, 18071 Granada, Spain; juliarb@ugr.es
[3] Thoracic Surgery Department, Hospital Virgen de las Nieves de Granda, 18014 Granada, Spain
* Correspondence: ahc@ugr.es; Tel.: +349-58-248-035

Simple Summary: Lung resection is the main curative treatment for lung cancer, but it can cause several tissue and organ disorders. While cardiovascular, pulmonary, and muscular disturbances post-surgery have been studied, long-term upper limb impairment has not been extensively explored despite its impact on patient independence. This study aimed to characterize upper limb impairment in survivors of lung cancer one year after surgery. In an observational trial, 76 patients with lung cancer who had undergone surgery were compared to 74 healthy controls. Our results revealed significant differences in active shoulder mobility, pain hypersensitivity, neural tissue mechanosensitivity, and upper limb exercise capacity. These results indicate that survivors of lung cancer experience significant upper limb musculoskeletal disorders and functional impairment one year post-resection, which can limit their functionality and quality of life.

Abstract: Lung resection represents the main curative treatment in lung cancer; however, this surgical process leads to several disorders in tissues and organs. Previous studies have reported cardiovascular, pulmonary, and muscular disturbances that affect the functional capacity of these patients in the short, mid, and long term. However, upper limb impairment has been scarcely explored in the long term, despite the relevance in the independence of the patients. The aim of this study was to characterize the upper limb impairment in survivors of lung cancer one year after pulmonary resection. In this observational trial, patients who underwent lung cancer surgery were compared to control, healthy subjects matched by age and gender. Upper limb musculoskeletal disorders (shoulder range of motion, pain pressure threshold, nerve-related symptoms) and functional capacity (upper limb exercise capacity) were evaluated one-year post-surgery. A total of 76 survivors of lung cancer and 74 healthy subjects were included in the study. Significant differences between groups were found for active shoulder mobility ($p < 0.05$), widespread hypersensitivity to mechanical pain ($p < 0.001$), mechanosensitivity of the neural tissue ($p < 0.001$), and upper limb exercise capacity ($p < 0.001$). Patients who undergo lung cancer surgery show upper limb musculoskeletal disorders and upper limb functional impairment after a one-year lung resection. This clinical condition could limit the functionality and quality of life of patients with lung cancer.

Keywords: lung cancer; pulmonary surgical procedures; musculoskeletal disorders; upper limb; disability

1. Introduction

Pulmonary resection represents the main treatment for patients with lung cancer [1]. This approach consists of removing the tumor of lung tissue, preventing it from growing into adjacent tissues [2]. Although in recent years pulmonary resection procedures have undergone a major evolution with less invasive and quick techniques [3], they are still associated with a high incidence of postoperative complications [4].

Patients with lung cancer accept complications as a possible risk of the surgery process; however, they are not expected to have disability issues [5]. The disability rate in these patients has become a major health problem due to the current high prevalence accompanying increased survival in recent years. In this sense, survivors of lung cancer reported that the causes of disability often do not resolve after lung resection, and disability issues remain between 3 and 6 months and up to 5 years after lung surgery [6]. For these reasons, achieving a functional lifestyle and a high quality of life has become one of the main long-term therapeutic goals [7].

Pain and shoulder dysfunction are the most common disability issues after lung resection, affecting the quality of life of patients with lung cancer [8]. Shoulder impairment has been widely explored [9] and has been associated with several upper limb musculoskeletal disorders [10]. The most reported have been shoulder pain [11], limited range of motion, and functional disturbances from the upper limbs, including limitations in the ability to perform activities of daily living, lifting above shoulder level, or performing sports activities [12].

Previous studies have observed that upper limb musculoskeletal disorders are still present one month after lung resection [10], being reported in more than 20% of patients with lung cancer [13]. However, there are uncertain results when these sequelae are studied after six months of surgery [14–16]. Considering the close relationship reported between upper limb impairment and disability in survivors of lung cancer, this lack of knowledge is worrisome due to the remarkable rates of disability in long-term survivors of lung cancer [17].

In this line, no previous studies have explored upper limb musculoskeletal disorders in patients who underwent lung cancer surgery in the long term. Therefore, the aim of this study was to explore and characterize the upper limb musculoskeletal disorders suffered by survivors of lung cancer one year after lung resection.

2. Materials and Methods

We conducted a single-blind observational study in which patients undergoing lung resection were compared to healthy subjects matched by age and gender. Sample size calculation was performed with G*Power 3.1.9.2 software based on the data of a previous study published by the research group [10], adopting statistical power of 95%, $\alpha = 0.05$, and allocation ratio between groups = 1, resulting in a calculated sample size of 146 (73 per group). However, 87 participants per group were recruited to allow for a dropout rate of 20%.

Patients with lung cancer were recruited from the Thoracic Surgery Service of the "Hospital Universitario Virgen de las Nieves de Granada" (HVN) between October 2019 and February 2020. Healthy subjects were recruited from the general community through announcements at the University of Granada (Spain). Assessors were blinded before evaluations were scheduled and other team members booked the patients' visits. Informed consent was obtained from all included participants. This study protocol was developed according to STROBE guidelines and was reviewed and approved by the Granada Provincial Research Ethics Committee (Spain), with the code: FISIOLUNG: 12 March 2018 [18].

The inclusion criteria included the following: survivors of lung cancer aged 18–80 years who had undergone resection surgery one year ago, were informed about the study purpose, and signed the informed consent. Exclusion criteria included the following: cognitive impairment, mental instability, orthopedic pathologies that limited the test performance or neurologic pathologies that could limit the patient's comprehension or expression or could make it difficult to perform the physical assessment.

Data collection was carried out one-year after surgery, consistently conducted by pre-trained investigators. Inclusion criteria were confirmed, and a structured interview and initial assessment were conducted. Pertinent medical history data including anthropometric measurements, comorbidities (evaluated using the Charlson comorbidities index) [19], length of stay, surgical duration, and spirometry values (forced expiratory volume in the first second (FEV-1)) [20] were retrieved.

The main outcomes included upper limb musculoskeletal disorders (shoulder range of motion, pain pressure threshold, nerve-related symptoms) and functional capacity, which was studied with upper limb exercise capacity.

Active shoulder mobility was evaluated using a laser-guided digital goniometer (Halo, Halo Medical Devices, Subiaco, Western Australia) and expressed in degrees [21]. The assessment included the following movements: flexion, extension, adduction, abduction, and internal and external rotations of both arms. Patients stood while the researcher instructed and supervised the execution of these movements, ensuring correct posture and correcting any compensations. The reliability of this tool has demonstrated a high accuracy (intra-class correlation coefficient > 0.90) [22].

Widespread hypersensitivity to mechanical pain was measured by assessing pain tolerance thresholds to pressure (PPT) [23], which were measured with a digital algometer (Model Mark-10 M3-20 Series, Copiague, NY, USA). This algometer consisted of a circular platform with an area of 1 cm^2 rubber tip and a range from 0 to 12 kg. The subjects were instructed to press a switch immediately when the sensation of pain was the highest tolerable. The mean of the three trials was calculated for the main analysis. Algometry measuring PPT exhibited high intra- and inter-rater reliability {intraclass correlation coefficient = 0.80–0.97)} [24,25]. The PPTs were assessed bilaterally in random order at a local point of the anterior deltoid muscle and a distal pain-free point on the flexor carpi longus muscle, to determine the widespread pressure hypersensitivity [26,27].

Neurodynamics testing was used to assess neural tolerance to movement. Passive neurodynamics tests were performed according to the process described by Butler [28], in nerves which have been used in previous thoracic cancer studies [29]: median, ulnar, and radial nerves. Neurodynamics tests were conducted bilaterally, following a standardized sequence until reaching the end of the range or symptom reproduction. Shoulder and elbow range of motion (ROM) at the conclusion of the tests were measured using a standard goniometer based on a previously reported procedure [30].

The unsupported upper limb exercise (UULEX) test, devised by Takahashi et al. [31], is an incremental test to measure peak unsupported arm exercise capacity. Participants lift a barbell from their lap to the highest point they can reach in levels, continuing until exhaustion. The total score is determined by the total duration of the test in seconds. Self-reported dyspnea and upper limb fatigue were evaluated using a modified version of the Borg scale [32], with a minimum clinically important difference (MCID) set at 1 score.

Statistical Analysis

The statistical package SPSS version 27.0 (International Business Machines, Armonk, NY, USA) was used to analyze the data obtained. Descriptive statistics (mean ± SD) or percentages (%) were used to describe sample baseline characteristics. The Kolmogorov–Smirnov test was performed to assess continuous data normality, prior to statistical analysis. T-Student's test for unpaired samples was employed to perform the data analysis, comparing test results between case and control subjects. A p value of less than 0.05 was considered statistically significant. A 95% confidence interval was used for statistical analysis.

3. Results

A total of 90 potential patients with lung cancer were initially invited to participate in the study, 80 were considered eligible based on meeting inclusion criteria and consented to participate. A total of four patients with lung cancer and two healthy subjects were excluded during the assessment because drop out or physical limitations. Finally, 76 participants completed the evaluation process. Additionally, 85 healthy control subjects, matched for age and gender, were recruited, with 76 consenting and meeting inclusion criteria, and 74 completing the evaluation. Participant distribution is illustrated in Figure 1.

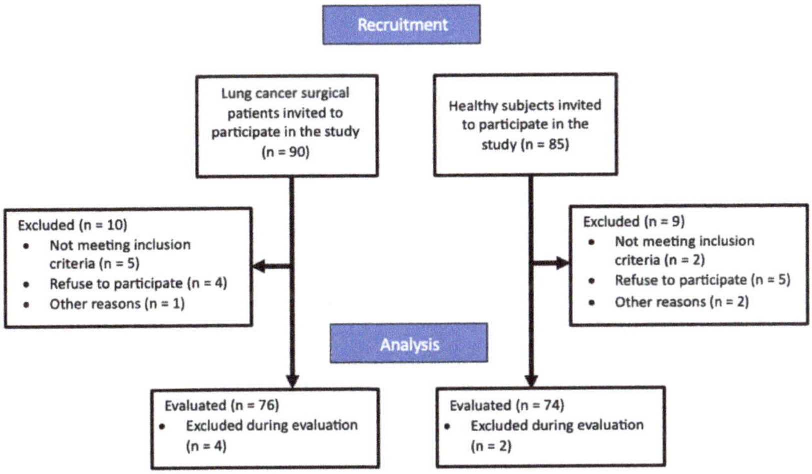

Figure 1. Flow diagram for distribution of participants.

The baseline characteristics of the sample are presented in Table 1. The mean age of the groups was 58.98 ± 13.34 in the lung resection group and 58.75 ± 11.01 in the control group ($p = 0.856$). Both groups presented a similar sex distribution (84.3%; 85%; $p = 0.785$), and similar BMI ($p = 0.614$). There were no significant differences in the associated comorbidities according to the Charlson index ($p = 0.705$) and FEV-1 values ($p = 0.764$). The duration of the lung resection was around 156.78 min, and the hospital stay 6.82 ± 2.03 days.

Table 1. Baseline characteristics of the sample.

Variables	Resection Group (n = 76)	Control Group (n = 74)	*p*
Sex distribution (% male)	64 (84.3%)	63 (85%)	0.785
Age (years)	58.98 ± 13.34	58.75 ± 11.01	0.856
BMI (kg/m^2)	27.58 ± 12.5	29.35 ± 15.47	0.614
Charlson Index	4.55 ± 2.51	4.47 ± 1.99	0.705
FEV1%	80.44 ± 23.63	81.02 ± 24.55	0.764
Surgery duration (minutes)	156.78 ± 24.3	-	-
Length of stay	6.82 ± 2.03	-	-

Variables were expressed as mean ± Standard Deviation or Percentage (%). BMI: body mass index; FEV1%: Forced expiratory volume in the first second.

Table 2 shows the results of the between-groups comparison of the upper limb musculoskeletal disorders. Active shoulder range of motion showed significant differences in favor of the control group for flexion of the intervened side ($p = 0.033$), and the abduction of the no intervened side ($p < 0.001$) and external rotation ($p < 0.001$). Adduction and internal rotation of both sides also showed significant differences ($p < 0.05$).

The abduction of the intervened side and external rotation were minor in the lung resection group; however, no significant differences were found. The flexion of the no intervened side, and extension of both upper limbs were similar between groups.

The assessment of the pain pressure threshold showed significant differences in the intervened side ($p = 0.004$) and no intervened side ($p < 0.001$) anterior deltoid muscle, and both flexor carpi longus muscles ($p < 0.001$), with higher values for the control groups.

Significant differences were also found during neurodynamics testing. The median nerve showed significant differences for the intervened ($p = 0.001$) and no intervened ($p < 0.001$) upper limb, in a similar way to the radial nerve ($p < 0.001$) ($p = 0.007$). The ulnar nerve presented significant differences in the no intervened side to surgery ($p = 0.007$), but no significant differences appeared on the intervened side, although the control group showed a wider range of motion.

Table 2. Musculoskeletal disorders in patients with lung resected cancer and healthy control subjects.

	Resection Group (n = 76)	Control Group (n = 74)	*p*
AROM			
Flexion (°)			
Intervened Side	152.42 ± 3.60	159.36 ± 16.58	0.033 *
No Intervened Side	166.00 ± 12.01	162.52 ± 12.20	0.252
Extension (°)			
Intervened Side	50.00 ± 6.88	52.16 ± 9.64	0.300
No Intervened Side	51.50 ± 8.45	50.60 ± 8.86	0.679
Abduction (°)			
Intervened Side	159.14 ± 34.80	165.84 ± 17.44	0.261
No Intervened Side	166.28 ± 15.00	180.00 ± 0.00	<0.001 **
Adduction (°)			
Intervened Side	18.85 ± 3.41	36.52 ± 24.45	<0.001 **
No Intervened Side	18.00 ± 3.12	31.08 ± 20.52	0.003 *
Internal Rotation (°)			
Intervened Side	37.42 ± 7.90	51.92 ± 20.91	0.001 *
No Intervened Side	34.00 ± 7.64	52.32 ± 18.23	<0.001 **
External Rotation (°)			
Intervened Side	77.14 ± 6.87	81.56 ± 12.79	0.095
No Intervened Side	72.33 ± 9.09	83.20 ± 9.31	<0.001 **
Pain Pressure Threshold			
Deltoid (kg)			
Intervened Side	4.19 ± 3.24	5.78 ± 2.13	0.004 *
No Intervened Side	3.63 ± 2.76	5.94 ± 2.12	<0.001 **
Carpal Long flexor muscle (kg)			
Intervened Side	4.44 ± 3.46	6.68 ± 2.86	<0.001 **
No Intervened Side	4.26 ± 3.43	6.79 ± 2.83	<0.001 **
Neurodynamic test			
Median (°)			
Intervened Side	122.41 ± 36.07	141.04 ± 30.41	0.001 *
No Intervened Side	123.45 ± 28.51	141.30 ± 27.36	<0.001 **
Ulnar (°)			
Intervened Side	114.52 ± 17.51	119.05 ± 42.98	0.421
No Intervened Side	123.63 ± 22.66	137.71 ± 35.83	0.007 *
Radial (°)			
Intervened Side	75.47 ± 24.24	95.48 ± 38.63	<0.001 **
No Intervened Side	70.98 ± 30.72	84.45 ± 27.48	0.007 *

Variables were expressed as mean ± standard deviation. Significant results are expressed as * $p < 0.05$ and ** $p < 0.001$. AROM: active range of motion; °: grades; kg: kilograms.

Table 3 shows the results of the UULEX test. The groups showed significant differences in the achieved level ($p < 0.001$) and the spent time ($p < 0.001$), in favor of the control group. However, the fatigue and dyspnea reported at the end of the test did not show significant differences ($p = 0.194$ and $p = 0.694$, respectively).

Table 3. Functional capacity of patients with lung resected cancer and healthy control subjects.

	Resection Group (n = 76)	Control Group (n = 74)	*p*
UULEX level	3.94 ± 2.88	6.81 ± 1.61	<0.001 **
UULEX weight (grames)	505.88 ± 631.01	454.77 ± 667.37	0.649
UULEX time (seconds)	362.11 ± 272.82	529.43 ± 157.79	<0.001 **
UULEX Fatigue Post	4.88 ± 2.34	4.24 ± 3.27	0.194
UULEX Dyspnea Post	2.34 ± 1.18	2.24 ± 1.17	0.694

Variables were expressed as mean ± standard deviation. Significant results are expressed as ** $p < 0.001$. UULEX: unsupported upper limb exercise test.

4. Discussion

This study aimed to characterize upper musculoskeletal impairment in survivors of lung cancer one year after lung resection. Our results showed the presence of musculoskeletal disorders in the upper limbs and limited functional capacity one year after undergoing pulmonary resection. These results were in line with previous studies that reported post-thoracotomy painful syndrome even one year after VATs lobectomy [33].

The sample of subjects included in this study was representative of the general population undergoing lung resection, with similar sociodemographic characteristics [34,35]. In a similar way to our sample, the study by Ren D et al. [36], which observed the occurrence of ipsilateral shoulder pain after thoracoscopy, presented a sample with similar age, BMI, and duration of surgery.

Our results showed that the active range of motion of the shoulder complex was reduced in patients who had undergone pulmonary resection one year before. Consistent with our results, previous studies [10] observed a bilateral reduction in active shoulder range of motion after pulmonary resection. The study of Miranda APB et al. [8] also observed a bilateral reduction in shoulder range of motion in patients who underwent thoracotomy, which they attributed to the patient's position during surgery on the ipsilateral side, and to the pressure of the patient's weight on the contralateral side. However, they did not follow up on these musculoskeletal disorders and their consequent evolution in the long term.

Previous studies in similar populations show similar results to ours in algometry after medical treatment [37]. The study by Rodriguez-Torres J et al. [10] also observed similar results to ours, in which patients with lung cancer who received a lung resection presented a widespread hypersensitivity to mechanical pain at mid-term.

With regard to neurodynamic tests, we have not found studies that assess the mechanosensitivity of the neural tissue in this population, but studies in similar populations [38] also found results consistent with ours, showing a decrease in the ROM of these tests as a protective mechanism [38].

The fact that the algometric and neurodynamic pain tolerance results show statistically significant differences, with worse results in the lung resection group, may be due to problems with mechanosensitivity and/or central sensitivity [39]. Previous studies [40] have highlighted that acute thoracic pain after surgery could affect neuronal plasticity and be a good predictor of chronic pain.

In terms of upper extremity functional capacity, as assessed by the UULEX test, our results showed lower exercise capacity in the pulmonary resection group at one year. To the best of our knowledge, this is the first study to evaluate functionality in patients with pulmonary resection after one year, although previous studies [41] have found similar results in the first month after surgery. A decrease in functional capacity and muscle endurance after surgery has also been observed in similar populations, such as after breast cancer or cardiac surgeries [42,43]. However, these studies did not present long-term results.

The functional capacity assessment was carried out using the UULEX test and not a hand-held dynamometer, which is more widely used, since the UULEX is considered a test with better capacity and greater relevance for reflecting the individual's performance in activities of daily living [31]. Both tests show a moderate to high correlation, which is probably due to the fact that the muscle activity required to complete them is similar (mainly elbow and shoulder flexion) [44].

4.1. Limitations

Our study has several limitations to be mentioned. The sample size is limited because of the difficulty in recruiting subjects who met the selection criteria; however, previous studies have used similar sample sizes in this population [45]. In addition, in terms of study design, a prospective study with preoperative and postoperative evaluation may have been more rewarding, allowing each patient to be in his or her own control. However, the control group was carefully selected, matching age and sex with the group of patients evaluated and avoiding other pathologies, so as not to influence the results or introduce a possible source of bias. Finally, some characteristics of the study sample, including the age range and physical activity levels, could disturb the differences found between the groups. Future studies with multivariate regression analyses are necessary to observe the influence of these aspects on the upper limb musculoskeletal disorders presented by patients with lung cancer in the long term.

4.2. Clinical Implications

The study of these long-term alterations is an important factor to consider. Knowledge of the risk of long-term disability is one of the determining factors in the surgical decision [46]. Additionally, long-term upper limb impairment is a key factor in the patient's functionality, as it limits the activities of daily living [12], reducing the quality of life of these patients [47]. It is also important to define the possibility of presenting central and peripheral sensitization, as this implies greater difficulty in the rehabilitation approach [48]. For these reasons, the significance of this study in reducing the comorbidity of these patients, making easier their recovery after the intervention, and preventing disability one year after the surgery is highlighted.

Moreover, knowing musculoskeletal disorders related to upper limb disability after one-year lung cancer resection could also make the design of future rehabilitation interventions easier to manage the musculoskeletal disorders that disturb the quality of life of these patients in the long term.

5. Conclusions

Patients with lung cancer who suffer a pulmonary resection show upper limb musculoskeletal disorders and functional impairment after one-year lung resection, exposing the presence of a limited active shoulder range of motion, widespread hypersensitivity to mechanical pain, mechanosensitivity of the neural tissue, and low exercise capacity, which could be altering the functionality of the patients and their quality of life.

Future studies with a longer follow-up period could help to obtain more precise data on the chronic physical impairment suffered by these patients. Future research could also be proposed with interventions that approach the mentioned alterations, thus improving the quality of life of these patients.

Author Contributions: Conceptualization, M.C.V. and J.M.N.; methodology, J.M.N. and A.N.O.; software, A.H.C.; validation, F.Q.V. and A.C.M.; formal analysis, M.C.V. and A.H.C.; investigation, A.C.M.; resources, J.R.B.; data curation, F.Q.V. and A.N.O.; writing—original draft preparation, M.C.V. and J.M.N.; writing—review and editing, M.C.V. and A.H.C.; visualization, J.R.B.; supervision, M.C.V. and J.R.B.; project administration, J.M.N. and A.H.C. All authors have read and agreed to the published version of the manuscript.

Funding: This work was supported by the Spanish Ministry of Education, grant numbers [FPU:21/00451; FPU:22/01543].

Institutional Review Board Statement: The study was conducted according to the guidelines of the Declaration of Helsinki and approved by the Granada Provincial Research Ethics Committee (Granada, Spain) (FISIOLUNG; 12 March 2018).

Informed Consent Statement: Informed consent was obtained from all subjects involved in the study.

Data Availability Statement: Data is contained within the article.

Conflicts of Interest: The authors declare no conflict of interest.

References

1. Ginsberg, R.J.; Rubinstein, L.V. Randomized trial of lobectomy versus limited resection for T1 No non-small cell lung cancer. Lung Cancer Study group. *Ann. Thorac. Surg.* **1995**, *60*, 615–622. [CrossRef] [PubMed]
2. Abbas, E. Surgical Management of Lung Cancer: History, Evolution, and Modern Advances. *Curr. Oncol. Rep.* **2018**, *20*, 98. [CrossRef] [PubMed]
3. Ng, C.S.; Gonzalez-Rivas, D.; D'Amico, T.A.; Rocco, G. Uniportal VATS-a new era in lung cancer surgery. *J. Thorac. Dis.* **2015**, *7*, 1489–1491.
4. Salati, M.; Refai, M.; Pompili, C.; Xiume, F.; Sabbatini, A.; Brunelli, A. Major morbidity after lung resection: A comparison between the European Society of Thoracic Surgeons Database system and the Thoracic Morbidity and Mortality system. *J. Thorac. Dis.* **2013**, *5*, 217–222. [PubMed]

5. Pompili, C.; Brunelli, A. Quality of life after lung resection is not associated with functional objective measures. *Eur. Respir. J.* **2013**, *42*, 283–285. [CrossRef] [PubMed]
6. Bobčíková, K.; Macounová, P.; Bužgová, R.; Tomášková, H.; Staňková, A.; Janulková, T.; Mitták, M.; Mad'ar, M. An assessment of quality of life, health, and disability in patients undergoing lung resection. *KONTAKT J. Nurs. Soc. Sci. Relat. Health Illn.* **2023**, *25*, 307–313. [CrossRef]
7. Cykert, S.; Kissling, G.; Hansen, C.J. Patient preferences regarding possible outcomes of lung resection: What outcomes should preoperative evaluations target? *Chest* **2000**, *117*, 1551–1559. [CrossRef]
8. Miranda, A.P.B.; de Souza, H.C.D.; Santos, B.F.A. Bilateral shoulder dysfunction related to the lung resection area after thoracotomy. *Medicine* **2015**, *94*, e1927. [CrossRef]
9. Lowe, E. Shoulder Dysfunction After Lung Cancer Resection. *Rehabil. Oncol.* **2022**, *40*, E41–E44. [CrossRef]
10. Rodríguez-Torres, J.; Lucena-Aguilera, M.; Cabrera-Martos, I.; López-López, L.; Torres-Sánchez, I.; Valenza, M.C. Musculoskeletal Signs Associated with Shoulder Pain in Patients Undergoing Video-Assisted Thoracoscopic Surgery. *Pain Med.* **2019**, *20*, 1997–2003. [CrossRef]
11. Athanassiadi, K.; Kakaris, S.; Theakos, N.; Skottis, I. Muscle-sparing versus posterolateral thoracotomy: A prospective study. *Eur. J. Cardio-Thorac. Surg. Off. J. Eur. Assoc. Cardio-Thorac. Surg.* **2007**, *31*, 496–500. [CrossRef] [PubMed]
12. Triffitt, P.D. The relationship between motion of the shoulder and the stated ability to perform activities of daily living. *J. Bone Jt. Surg.* **1998**, *80*, 41–46. [CrossRef] [PubMed]
13. Bando, T.; Onishi, C.; Imai, Y. Postoperative discomfort and its influence on daily life in patients with lung cancer: A study concern-ing the period from hospital discharge to 6 months after surgery. *J. Jpn. Soc. Cancer Nurs.* **2015**, *29*, 18–22.
14. Ercegovac, M.; Subotic, D.; Zugic, V.; Jakovic, R.; Moskovljevic, D.; Bascarevic, S.; Mujovic, N. Postoperative complications do not influence the pattern of early lung function recovery after lung resection for lung cancer in patients at risk. *J. Cardiothorac. Surg.* **2014**, *9*, 92. [CrossRef] [PubMed]
15. Brunelli, A.; Pompili, C.; Koller, M. Changes in quality of life after pulmonary resection. *Thorac. Surg. Clin.* **2012**, *22*, 471–485. [CrossRef]
16. Landreneau, R.J.; Mack, M.J.; Hazelrigg, S.R.; Naunheim, K.; Dowling, R.D.; Ritter, P.R.N.; Magee, M.J.; Nunchuck, S.; Keenan, R.J.; Ferson, P.F. Prevalence of chronic pain after pulmonary resection by thoracotomy or video-assisted thoracic surgery. *J. Thorac. Cardiovasc. Surg.* **1994**, *107*, 1079–1086. [CrossRef] [PubMed]
17. Lin, S.M.; Yang, S.C.; Wu, T.I.; Wang, J.D.; Liu, L.F. Estimation of disability free life expectancy in non small cell lung cancer based on real world data. *Sci. Rep.* **2023**, *13*, 13318. [CrossRef] [PubMed]
18. Von Elm, E.; Altman, D.G.; Egger, M.; Pocock, S.J.; Gøtzsche, P.C.; Vandenbroucke, J.P.; STROBE Initiative. The Strengthening the Reporting of Observational Studies in Epidemiology (STROBE) Statement: Guidelines for reporting observational studies. *Int. J. Surg.* **2014**, *12*, 1495–1499. [CrossRef]
19. Birim, O.; Maat, A.P.; Kappetein, A.P.; van Meerbeeck, J.P.; Damhuis, R.A.; Bogers, A.J. Validation of the Charlson comorbidity index in patients with operated primary non-small cell lung cancer. *Eur. J. Cardio-Thoracic Surg.* **2003**, *23*, 30–34. [CrossRef]
20. Koegelenberg, C.F.; Swart, F.; Irusen, E.M. Guideline for office spirometry in adults, 2012. *S. Afr. Med. J.* **2012**, *103*, 52–62. [CrossRef]
21. Riddle, D.L.; Rothstein, J.M.; Lamb, R.L. Goniometric reliability in a clinical setting. Shoulder measurements. *Phys. Ther.* **1987**, *67*, 668–673. [CrossRef] [PubMed]
22. Correll, S.; Field, J.; Hutchinson, H.; Mickevicius, G.; Fitzsimmons, A.; Smoot, B. Reliability and validity of the halo digital goniometer for shoulder range of motion in healthy subjects. *Int. J. Sports Phys. Ther.* **2018**, *13*, 707–714. [CrossRef] [PubMed]
23. Wildgaard, K.; Ringsted, T.K.; Aasvang, E.K.; Ravn, J.; Werner, M.U.; Kehlet, H. Neurophysiological characterization of persistent postthoracotomy pain. *Clin. J. Pain* **2012**, *28*, 136–142. [CrossRef] [PubMed]
24. Chesterson, L.S.; Sim, J.; Wright, C.C.; Foster, N.E. Interrater reliability of algometry in measuring pressure pain thresholds in healthy humans, using multiple raters. *Clin. J. Pain* **2007**, *23*, 760–766. [CrossRef] [PubMed]
25. Jones, D.H.; Kilgour, R.D.; Comtois, A.S. Test-retest reliability of pressure pain threshold measurements of the upper limb and torso in young healthy women. *J. Pain* **2007**, *8*, 650–656. [CrossRef]
26. Blichfeldt-Eckhardt, M.R. From acute to chronic postsurgical pain: The significance of the acute pain response. *Dan. Med. J.* **2018**, *65*, B5326.
27. Staud, R.; Cannon, R.C.; Mauderli, A.P.; Robinson, M.E.; Price, D.D.; Vierck, C.J. Temporal summation of pain from mechanical stimulation of muscle tissue in normal controls and subjects with fibromyalgia syndrome. *Pain* **2003**, *102*, 87–95. [CrossRef] [PubMed]
28. Butler, D.S. *The Sensitive Nervous System*; Noigroup Publications: Adelaide, Australia, 2000.
29. Caro-Morán, E.; Díaz-Rodríguez, L.; Cantarero-Villanueva, I.; Galiano-Castillo, N.; Arroyo-Morales, M.; Fernández-Lao, C. Nerve pressure pain hypersensitivity and upper limb mechanosensitivity in breast cancer survivors: A case–control study. *Pain Med.* **2014**, *15*, 1715–1723. [CrossRef] [PubMed]
30. Norkin, C.C.; White, D.J. *Measurement of Joint Motion: A Guide to Goniometry*, 4th ed.; F.A. Davis: Philadelphia, PA, USA, 2009.
31. Takahashi, T.; Jenkins, S.C.; Strauss, G.R.; Watson, C.P.; Lake, F.R. A new unsupported upper limb exercise test for patients with chronic obstructive pulmonary disease. *J. Cardiopulm. Rehabil.* **2003**, *23*, 430–437. [CrossRef]
32. Borg, G. Ratings of perceived exertion and heart rates during short-term cycle exercise and their use in a new cycling strength test. *Int. J. Sports Med.* **1982**, *3*, 153–158. [CrossRef] [PubMed]

33. Farkas, A.; Csókási, T.; Fabó, C.; Szabó, Z.; Lantos, J.; Pécsy, B.; Lázár, G.; Rárosi, F.; Kecskés, L.; Furák, J. Chronic postoperative pain after non-intubated uniportal VATS lobectomy. *Front. Surg.* **2023**, *13*, 1282937. [CrossRef] [PubMed]
34. Linares-Moya, M.; Rodríguez-Torres, J.; Heredia-Ciuró, A.; Granados-Santiago, M.; López-López, L.; Quero-Valenzuela, F.; Valenza, M.C. Psychological distress prior to surgery is related to symptom burden and health status in lung cancer survivors. *Support. Care Cancer* **2022**, *30*, 1579–1586. [CrossRef] [PubMed]
35. Blichfeldt-Eckhardt, M.R.; Andersen, C.; Ørding, H.; Licht, P.B.; Toft, P. Shoulder pain after thoracic surgery: Type and time course, a prospective cohort study. *J. Cardiothorac. Vasc. Anesth.* **2017**, *31*, 147–151. [CrossRef] [PubMed]
36. Ren, D.; Zhang, B.; Xu, J.; Liu, R.; Wang, J.; Huo, H.; Zhang, H.; Zeng, J.; Wang, H.; Xu, X.; et al. Effect of Upper Arm Position Changes on the Occurrence of Ipsilateral Shoulder Pain After Single-Operator Port Thoracoscopy. *Front. Surg.* **2022**, *2*, 823259. [CrossRef] [PubMed]
37. Fernández-Lao, C.; Cantarero-Villanueva, I.; Fernández-de-las-Peñas, C.; Del-Moral-Ávila, R.; Menjón-Beltrán, S.; Arroyo-Morales, M. Widespread mechanical pain hypersensitivity as a sign of central sensitization after breast cancer surgery: Comparison between mastectomy and lumpectomy. *Pain Med.* **2011**, *12*, 72–78. [CrossRef] [PubMed]
38. Elvey, R.L. Physical evaluation of the peripheral nervous system in disorders of pain and dysfunction. *J. Hand Ther.* **1997**, *10*, 122–129. [CrossRef] [PubMed]
39. Arendt-Nielsen, L.; Laursen, R.J.; Drewes, A.M. Referred pain as an indicator for neural plasticity. *Prog. Brain Res.* **2000**, *129*, 343–356. [PubMed]
40. Blichfeldt-Eckhardt, M.R.; Andersen, C.; Ørding, H.; Licht, P.B.; Toft, P. From acute to chronic pain after thoracic surgery: The significance of different components of the acute pain response. *J. Pain Res.* **2018**, *16*, 1541–1548. [CrossRef] [PubMed]
41. Bobbio, A.; Chetta, A.; Carbognani, P.; Internullo, E.; Verduri, A.; Sansebastiano, G.; Rusca, M.; Olivieri, D. Changes in pulmonary function test and cardio-pulmonary exercise capacity in COPD patients after lobar pulmonary resection. *Eur. J. Cardiothorac. Surg.* **2005**, *28*, 754–758. [CrossRef]
42. Nouri, R.; Braumann, K.M.; ChamPiri, B.M.; Schröder, J.J.; Akochakian, M. Cancer Related Fatigue and Upper Limb Disabilities Cannot Improve after 6 Weeks Resistance Training with Thera-Band in Breast Cancer Survivors. *Int. J. Appl. Exerc. Physiol.* **2018**, *7*, 76–84. [CrossRef]
43. Izawa, K.; Kasahara, Y.; Hiraki, K.; Hirano, Y.; Watanabe, S. Relation between the disability of the arm, shoulder and hand score and muscle strength in post-cardiac surgery patients. *Diseases* **2017**, *5*, 31. [CrossRef] [PubMed]
44. Janaudis-Ferreira, T.; Hill, K.; Goldstein, R.S.; Wadell, K.; Brooks, D. Relationship and responsiveness of three upper-limb tests in patients with chronic obstructive pulmonary disease. *Physiother. Canada* **2013**, *65*, 40–43. [CrossRef] [PubMed]
45. Vagvolgyi, A.; Rozgonyi, Z.; Kerti, M.; Vadasz, P.; Varga, J. Effectiveness of perioperative pulmonary rehabilitation in thoracic surgery. *J. Thorac. Dis.* **2017**, *9*, 1584–1591. [CrossRef] [PubMed]
46. Choi, H.; Mazzone, P. Preoperative evaluation of the patient with lung cancer being considered for lung resection. *Curr. Opin. Anaesthesiol.* **2015**, *28*, 18–25. [CrossRef] [PubMed]
47. Assis, M.R.; Marx, A.G.; Magna, L.A.; Ferrigno, I.S. Late morbidity in upper limb function and quality of life in women after breast cancer surgery. *Braz. J. Phys. Ther.* **2013**, *17*, 236–243. [CrossRef]
48. Jull, G.; Sterling, M.; Kenardy, J.; Beller, E. Does the presence of sensory hypersensitivity influence outcomes of physical rehabilitation for chronic whiplash? A preliminary RCT. *Pain* **2007**, *129*, 28–34. [CrossRef]

cancers

MDPI

Article

LKB1 Loss Correlates with STING Loss and, in Cooperation with β-Catenin Membranous Loss, Indicates Poor Prognosis in Patients with Operable Non-Small Cell Lung Cancer

Eleni D. Lagoudaki [1,2,*], Anastasios V. Koutsopoulos [1,2], Maria Sfakianaki [3], Chara Papadaki [3], Georgios C. Manikis [4], Alexandra Voutsina [3], Maria Trypaki [3], Eleftheria Tsakalaki [3], Georgia Fiolitaki [3], Dora Hatzidaki [3], Emmanuel Yiachnakis [5], Dimitra Koumaki [6], Dimitrios Mavroudis [2,3,7], Maria Tzardi [1,2], Efstathios N. Stathopoulos [1,2], Kostas Marias [4], Vassilis Georgoulias [2,3,7] and John Souglakos [2,3,7]

1 Department of Pathology, University General Hospital of Heraklion, 71500 Heraklion, Greece; akoutsop@uoc.gr (A.V.K.); tzardi@med.uoc.gr (M.T.); stath@med.uoc.gr (E.N.S.)
2 School of Medicine, University of Crete, 70013 Heraklion, Greece; mavroudis@uoc.gr (D.M.); georgoul@uoc.gr (V.G.); j.souglakos@med.uoc.gr (J.S.)
3 Laboratory of Translational Oncology, School of Medicine, University of Crete, 70013 Heraklion, Greece; msfakianak@uoc.gr (M.S.); chapapadak@uoc.gr (C.P.); voutsina@med.uoc.gr (A.V.); chemp945@edu.chemistry.uoc.gr (M.T.); med4p1030249@med.uoc.gr (E.T.); fiolitakigeorgia@pagni.gr (G.F.); dorachat@med.uoc.gr (D.H.)
4 Foundation for Research and Technology Hellas (FORTH), 70013 Heraklion, Greece; gmanikis@ics.forth.gr (G.C.M.); kmarias@ics.forth.gr (K.M.)
5 Laboratory of Bio-Medical Data Analysis Digital Applications and Interdisciplinary Approaches, University of Crete, 71003 Heraklion, Greece; giahnaki@med.uoc.gr
6 Department of Dermatology, University General Hospital of Heraklion, Voutes, 71500 Heraklion, Greece; dkoumaki@pagni.gr
7 Department of Medical Oncology, University General Hospital of Heraklion, 71500 Heraklion, Greece
* Correspondence: elagoudakimd@gmail.com; Tel.: +30-2810394706

Simple Summary: Deleterious LKB1 inactivation in KRAS-driven lung adenocarcinomas (LUACs) has been studied thoroughly; however, LKB1 inactivation is not limited in adenocarcinomatous histology, nor in KRAS mutational status. We investigated LKB1 loss by IHC in 188 metastatic and 60 non-metastatic tumors from patients with operable non-small cell lung cancer (NSCLC) of various histologies and its correlation with cell cycle targets, EMT inducers, antitumor immunity response regulators, cell adhesion molecules and KRAS co-mutations. LKB1 loss was associated with STING loss irrespective of KRAS status both overall and in lung adenocarcinomas (LUACs) and, importantly, also in the metastatic setting. Concurrent LKB1 loss and β-catenin loss of membranous expression correlated with a significant decrease in median overall survival and increased risk of death. The expression status of LKB1 in association with STING and β-catenin membranous expression status could be used as stratification factors for patients with operable NSCLC in the procedure of precision medicine in lung cancer.

Abstract: To investigate the incidence and prognostically significant correlations and cooperations of LKB1 loss of expression in non-small cell lung cancer (NSCLC), surgical specimens from 188 metastatic and 60 non-metastatic operable stage I-IIIA NSCLC patients were analyzed to evaluate their expression of LKB1 and pAMPK proteins in relation to various processes. The investigated factors included antitumor immunity response regulators STING and PD-L1; pro-angiogenic, EMT and cell cycle targets, as well as metastasis-related (VEGFC, PDGFRα, PDGFRβ, p53, p16, Cyclin D1, ZEB1, CD24) targets; and cell adhesion (β-catenin) molecules. The protein expression levels were evaluated via immunohistochemistry; the RNA levels of LKB1 and NEDD9 were evaluated via PCR, while KRAS exon 2 and BRAF^{V600E} mutations were evaluated by Sanger sequencing. Overall, loss of LKB1 protein expression was observed in 21% (51/248) patients and correlated significantly with histotype ($p < 0.001$), KRAS mutations ($p < 0.001$), KC status (concomitant KRAS mutation and p16 downregulation) ($p < 0.001$), STING loss ($p < 0.001$), and high CD24 expression ($p < 0.001$). STING loss also correlated significantly with loss of LKB1 expression in the metastatic setting both overall

($p = 0.014$) and in lung adenocarcinomas (LUACs) ($p = 0.005$). Additionally, LKB1 loss correlated significantly with a lack of or low β-catenin membranous expression exclusively in LUACs, both independently of the metastatic status ($p = 0.019$) and in the metastatic setting ($p = 0.007$). Patients with tumors yielding LKB1 loss and concomitant nonexistent or low β-catenin membrane expression experienced significantly inferior median overall survival of 20.50 vs. 52.99 months; $p < 0.001$ as well as significantly greater risk of death (HR: 3.32, 95% c.i.: 1.71–6.43; $p < 0.001$). Our findings underscore the impact of the synergy of LKB1 with STING and β-catenin in NSCLC, in prognosis.

Keywords: NSCLC; LKB1; STING; PD-L1; β-catenin; pAMPK; KRAS; BRAF; VEGFC; PDGFRβ; ZEB-1; Cyclin D1; p16

1. Introduction

Lung cancer remains the leading cause of cancer-related death worldwide, estimated to be responsible for one in four deaths (25.3%) [1,2]. The stage at diagnosis determines treatment options and has the strongest influence on survival in NSCLC patients. Approximately half of the patients undergoing complete surgical resection for low-stage disease die from recurrent disease or distant metastases.

The STK11/LKB1 gene was identified when germline heterozygous mutations in the p13.3 region of chromosome 19 were revealed as the causal mutation in Peutz–Jeghers Syndrome (PJS), an autosomal dominant disorder characterized by the development of benign gastrointestinal hamartomas, and were associated with the early onset of cancer [3,4]. LKB1 gene codes for Liver Kinase B1 (LKB1) an evolutionarily conserved serine threonine kinase with manifold tasks and master upstream kinase of AMPK, a major regulator of energy sensing and cellular metabolism [5–7]. Moreover, LKB1 is a master kinase of at least 13 more AMPK-related kinases and is in a constitutively active state in growing cells [8].

The predisposition of patients with PJS to early onset tumors indicates that LKB1 inactivation is an important event in carcinogenesis. Genetic analysis acknowledged LKB1 as a critical tumor-suppressor gene that is frequently inactivated in a broad spectrum of human cancers. LKB1 inactivation takes place mostly through somatic alterations in the LKB1 gene, such as nonsense mutation, loss of heterozygosity, insertions, intragenic deletions, or chromosomal deletions, the majority of which affect the kinase domain, resulting in a loss of kinase activity, while others affect the production, stability, or localization of the protein [9–17]. Additionally, alterations in LKB1 expression can also occur as a result of non-mutational mechanisms [18] such as hyper-methylation of the promoter region [19,20], as well as at the post-translational level, at which they are induced by micro-RNAs [21].

In a study examining 4446 patients with various solid tumors, the rate of LKB1 alterations in the pan-cancer setting was 1.35%, the overwhelming majority (45%) of which were NSCLC-related [22]. Remarkably, LKB1 was found to be the third most commonly altered gene in LUACs, after TP53 and KRAS [23]. LKB1 inactivation occurs early in the development of lung cancer, as demonstrated by the loss of LKB1 protein expression in atypical adenomatous hyperplasia (AAH) [24] and in LUACs in early pathological stages (I and II) [25].

The most frequently LKB1 co-mutated genes are KRAS, TP53, BRAF, and CDKN2A(HD), with KRAS and TP53 co-mutation being present in about half of LKB1-altered cancers [23,26,27]. The prevalence of LKB1 alterations in LUACs is 8–21% [27–31], whereas in Lung Squamous Cell Carcinoma (LSCCs), LKB1 alterations are detected in 1.5–5% of patients [26,28]. Various studies have highlighted the role of LKB1 loss as an enhancer of cell growth, motility, invasion, and as a metastasis promoter.

In a seminal paper, Ji et al. used a mutant KRAS-driven model of mouse lung cancer to show that LKB1 inactivation stimulated the growth of tumors of various histotypes with vigorously strong shortened latency to growth and to metastasis development compared to the LKB1-wild-type (WT) counterpart. Furthermore, LKB1-deficient tumors yielded increased expression of genes involved in angiogenesis and cell migration, such as NEDD9 and CD24 [32].

In vitro studies revealed that LKB1 inactivation increased cell motility and invasiveness [16,33] and favored epithelial–mesenchymal transition in lung cancer cells through upregulation of Zinc-finger E-box-binding homeobox factor 1 (ZEB1), a transcriptional repressor for E-cadherin and an EMT inducer, thus enhancing metastatic potential [34,35].

Moreover, in recent years, increasing amounts of evidence have highlighted the role of LKB1 in modulating the tumor immune microenvironment. Skoulidis et al., focusing on KRAS mutant LUACs, revealed different co-mutational subsets of KRAS mutants with distinct biologic and vulnerabilities and immune profiles [36] and showed that KL tumors exhibited lower densities of CD3+ and CD8+ lymphocytes, but not FOXP3+ cells, and lacked PD-L1 expression in the tumor cells despite intermediate–high TMB [37].

Nearly half of the KRAS-mutant tumors harbor concomitant TP53 mutations, followed by LKB1 (18% to 28%) and KEAP1 (24%), while less than 5% of KRAS-mutant NSCLC patients have another oncogenic-driven co-mutation, such as BRAF, EGFR, PIK3CA, or MET amplification, with no concurrent ALK or ROS1 rearrangements described [27–29,36–38].

Considering all of the above factors, we performed a comprehensive retrospective study in a large series of patients with resectable (stage I-IIIA) NSCLC with the aim of performing an in situ immunohistochemical evaluation of the incidence of loss of LKB1 expression in surgical specimens of NSCLC patients with and without lymph node metastasis, including all of the various histotypes, in order to elucidate possible patterns of expression and characteristics of the LKBl-less phenotype and to identify potential correlations of prognostic significance.

Furthermore, we investigated the incidence and the characteristics of tumors characterized by concurrent KRAS mutations with loss of LKB1 expression (now referred to as KL), with p53 mutational immunohistochemical status (now referred to as KP), and with p16 downregulation (hereafter referred to as KC), the KRAS mutant and LKB1 intact combination, as well as triple mutants KRAS-p53-p16 (hereafter referred to as KPL), LKB-only mutants (hereafter referred to as L status), which are defined as tumors with LKB1 loss and no KRAS, p53, p16 co-mutations, and of KRAS-only tumors with no identifiable LKB1, p53, and p16 commutations (hereafter referred to as K status) and their impact on prognosis.

2. Materials and Methods

2.1. Patient Population/Study Design

To perform this retrospective translational research study, we searched the records of the Pathology department of the University General Hospital of Heraklion and retrieved the pathology reports of patients who underwent surgery, with curative intent, for NSCLC between 2007 and 2023. Successively, and after re-evaluating the slides of excised tumor tissue and excised lymph node specimens slides for each patient to determine (i) the histologic subtype according to the 2015 WHO classification [39] and (ii) the stage in accordance with the 8th American Joint Committee on Cancer Staging AJCC [40], we enrolled 188 treatment-naïve patients with operable, stage I-IIIA NSCLC harboring pathologically confirmed metastasis of regional and distant lymph nodes, whom we assigned to the experimental group. Meanwhile, 60 treatment-naive patients with pathologically confirmed tumor-free lymph nodes were assigned to the control group. Furthermore, patient selection for enrollment did not account for the histological type and mutational status of the tumor to ensure that the entire repertoire of histologies of NSCLCs and all the potential mutational cohorts were included.

The clinical data of the patients were collected from the medical records of the Department of Medical Oncology, University General Hospital of Heraklion. The study was conducted in accordance with the Declaration of Helsinki and Good Clinical Practice guidelines and after approval by the Ethics Committee of the Institution. Prior to surgery, all patients gave their informed written consent for the use of tumor samples for laboratory analysis. All laboratory analyses were performed blinded to clinical data.

2.2. Specimen's Characteristics and Assays

Four-micron-thick formalin-fixed, paraffin-embedded (FFPE) tissue sections were prepared on charged glass slides as per the standard protocols for IHC. Tissue sections were deparaffinized and peroxidase was quenched with methanol and 3% H2O2 for 15 min. Heat-induced epitope retrieval was performed by immersing the slides either in EDTA buffer at pH8 or in Citrate buffer at pH6, followed by two cycles of microwave treatment at 500 watts. After a thorough rinse with distilled water, primary antibodies were applied at validated dilutions and incubation times (Supplementary Table S1). UltravisionTM Quanto Detection System HRP (Thermo Scientific™, Waltham, MA, USA) was used to detect antibody binding, according to the manufacturer's recommendations. Slides were counterstained with hematoxylin PD-L1 and expression status was assessed using the VENTANA PD-L1 (SP142) assay (ROCHE; Basel, Switzerland).

Immunohistochemical evaluation of the LKB1 [37,41], pAMPK [42], STING [43], ZEB1 [34,35], p53 [44], Cyclin D1, p16 [45–47], PDGFRα, PDGFRβ [48], CD24 [49], VEGFC [50], and β-catenin [51] expression status was performed by two independent pathologists (E.L. and A.K.) based on previously published data. A detailed description of the methodology [Supplementary Table S1] and a table of the antibodies used [Supplementary Table S2] are provided. In all experiments, along with tumor tissue, matched adjacent normal lung tissue that was located at least 5 cm away from the tumor lesions was selected and evaluated. Regarding LKB1 immunohistochemical expression, the control lung tissue showed uniform LKB1 expression. LKB1 protein was present in all the epithelial cells lining the trachea and bronchus, except in goblet cells, whereas it was almost undetectable in the alveolar pneumocytes. LKB1 was highly expressed in the apical surface (i.e., cilia), which is consistent with LKB1's known roles in the establishment and maintenance of epithelial polarity.

Moreover, 4 µm thick serial sections of each FFPE block of tumor were cut, mounted on non-coated glass slides, and routinely stained with hematoxylin and eosin to perform tissue microdissection. An adequate number of tumor cells from each mounted tumor section was collected using a piezoelectric microdissector (MicroDissector; Eppendorf AG, Hamburg, Germany) and subsequently deposited in a pellet. mRNA transcript levels of LKB1 and NEDD9 were evaluated in all 248 specimens by real-time quantitative reverse transcription polymerase chain reaction. Mutations analysis, DNA extraction, KRAS (codons 12 and 13) and BRAFV600E mutation analysis (by Sanger sequencing) [Supplementary Material Table S3] were performed as previously reported [52–54].

2.2.1. IHC Evaluation of LKB1 Expression Status

It is necessary to comment on the strategy implemented for the IHC evaluation of LKB1 expression status. To overcome the fact that immunohistochemical staining of total LKB1 protein does not distinguish between functional and non-functional protein, we employed the use of phosphorylated AMPK at thr172 (pAMPKthr172) to validate our interpretation of the status of expression of LKB1, as it has been shown [5] that LKB1 and pAMPK (Thr172) are interrelated biomarkers that are useful for interrogating LKB1 status of expression in human lung tumors [55]. In fact, the overwhelming majority of the tumors presented almost overlapping areas of LKB1 and pAMPK immunohistochemical staining, with similar degrees of heterogeneous staining intensity ranging from none to strongly cytoplasmic (0–3). This heterogeneity could be interpreted biologically as a reflection of the stages of the evolutionary pattern of LKB1 loss as a tumor suppressor alongside tumor progression. The juxtaposition of the variable combinations of heterogenous staining intensities of LKB1 and pAMPK in the different areas of the tumor in each of the 248 tumor samples yielded a statistically significant association between the status of expression of the two markers, Kendall's tau 0.524, $p < 0.001$, convalidating our interpretation of LKB1 status expression Figure 1. Even so, it is noteworthy that using IHC to test for the loss of expression of a protein by IHC is definitely more challenging than confirming its presence. Interpreting LKB1 status of expression based on IHC is demanding, with pitfalls to overcome, such as the heterogeneous staining patterns, excessive background staining, and the ambiguous staining of internal positive controls. To date, notwithstanding several reports of LKB1 immunodetection in defined research settings, a widely adopted scoring methodology with optimal accuracy has yet to be selected.

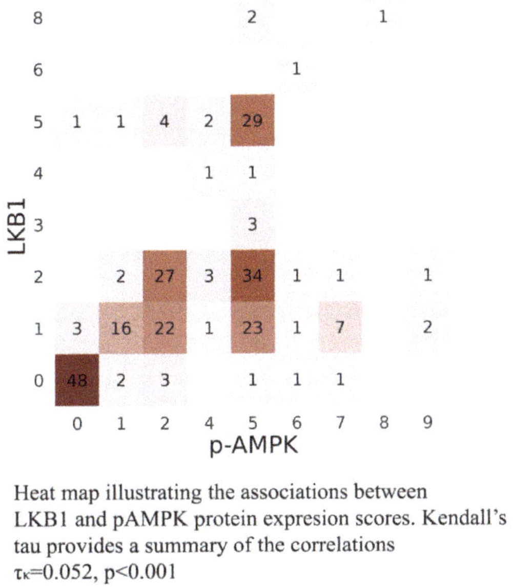

Figure 1. Heat map of LKB1-pAMPK. Combinations of intensities observed in the heterogeneous staining areas of the tumors observed in both LKB1 and pAMPK staining. In total, scores 0–9 were assigned to include as many of the multifaceted combinations of intensities as possible (0 = lost, 1 = low, 2 = moderate, 3 = strong staining present in different areas of the majority of the tumors). [0 = 0, 1 = 0-1, 2 = 0-1-2, 3 = 0-2-3, 4 = 0-2-3, 5 = 0-1-2-3, 6 = 1-2, 7 = 2, 8 = 1-2-3, 9 = 0-3].

2.2.2. Staging of Lymph Node Metastasis

Pathological lymph node staging was implemented according to the 8th edition of the AJCC [40]. Accordingly, regional (LN1) metastatic involvement is referred to as the metastatic infiltration of ipsilateral peribronchial and/or ipsilateral hilar lymph nodes as well as of intrapulmonary nodes, including involvement by direct extension. Distant (LN2) lymph node involvement refers to metastatic infiltration of ipsilateral mediastinal and/or subcarinal lymph node(s), and distant (LN3) involvement refers to the presence of metastasis in contralateral mediastinal, contralateral, hilar, ipsilateral or contralateral scalene, or supraclavicular lymph node(s) [39].

2.2.3. Statistical Considerations

This is a retrospective translational research study evaluating the expression of different proteins and genes in tumor cells from patients with resectable NSCLC. Due to the observational nature of the study, it was not possible to provide a specific hypothesis to define a sample size estimation. Statistical analysis was executed using R software version 4.3.0 (R core team, Vienna, Austria). Chi-square or Fisher's exact test was used to compare qualitative variables. Overall survival (OS) was calculated from the date of diagnosis of disease to the date of death from any cause. Median OS (mOS) was estimated using the Kaplan–Meier method (a two-sided log-rank test). A univariate Cox regression analysis, with hazard ratios and 95% CIs, was used to assess the association between each potential predictive factor and survival. These factors were then included in a multivariate Cox proportional hazards regression model with a stepwise procedure to evaluate the independent significance of different variables on survival. All results were considered statistically significant if $p < 0.05$ (two-sided test) level.

3. Results

3.1. Patients' Characteristics and Clinicopathological Features

The main demographic and clinical characteristics of the population of our study are summarized in Supplementary Table S4. The 248 patients were predominately males 89% ($n = 220$), <70 years of age, 73% ($n = 181$), 76% ($n = 188$) of which presented lymph node metastatic involvement. A total of 48% ($n = 120$) of the primary lung tumors were diagnosed as LUACs, 10 of which (4%) were pleomorphic LUACs; 49.2% ($n = 122$) were diagnosed as Lung Squamous cell carcinoma (LSCC), 3 of which were classified as pleomorphic LSCC (1.2%); 3 (1.2%) were diagnosed as Adenosquamous carcinomas; $n = 2$ (0.8%) as pleomorphic (spindle cell and large cell, one of each) carcinomas; and $n = 1$ case (0.4%) was diagnosed as large cell carcinoma. More than half, 61% ($n = 151$), of the tumors were poorly differentiated grade III tumors and 49% ($n = 121$) were of IIIA p-stage.

At the time of analysis and after a median follow-up of 25.7 months (min–max: 1.3–225.9 months); 156 (63%) disease relapses and 193 (77%) deaths were recorded.

3.2. Laboratory Analysis and Correlations

3.2.1. Overall Results of the Laboratory Analysis

The results of the laboratory analysis are presented in Supplementary Table S5. Immunohistochemical evaluation of LKB1, pAMPK, PD-L1, STING, p16, p53, CD24, Cyclin-D1, ZEB1, VEGFC, PDGFRα, PDGFRβ, and β-catenin protein expression was successfully performed in all 248 tumor specimens, as shown in Figures 2 and 3. Sequencing for LKB1 and NEDD9 RNA levels was also successfully implemented in all 248 specimens, whereas KRAS exon 2 and BRAF exon 15 mutation analysis was performed in 248 (100%) and 244 (98.3%) specimens, respectively.

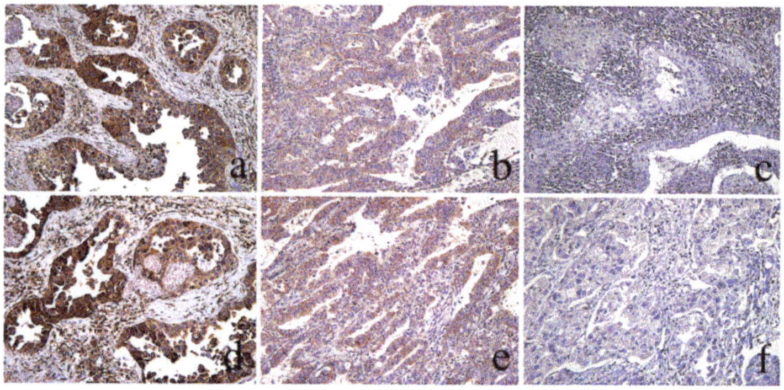

Figure 2. LKB1 and p-AMPK immunohistochemical evaluation. Top row: Three different NSCLC tumors immunohistochemically stained for LKB1. Bottom row: Three different NSCLC tumors immunohistochemically stained against p-AMPK. (**a**,**d**) The same area of a LUAC stained with LKB1 (**a**), and pAMPK (**b**) showing cytoplasmic staining of similar, moderate and strong (scores: 2–3), intensity, therefore evaluated as "intact". (**b**,**e**) Same area of a LUAC showing similar, very low (score: 1), staining intensity of LKB1 and pAMPK expression, evaluated as "intact". (**c**,**f**) The same area of a LSCC with complete absence, (score: 0), of staining for both LKB1 and pAMPK was evaluated as "lost"(score: 0); [(**a**–**e**) magnification ×100, (**f**) magnification ×200].

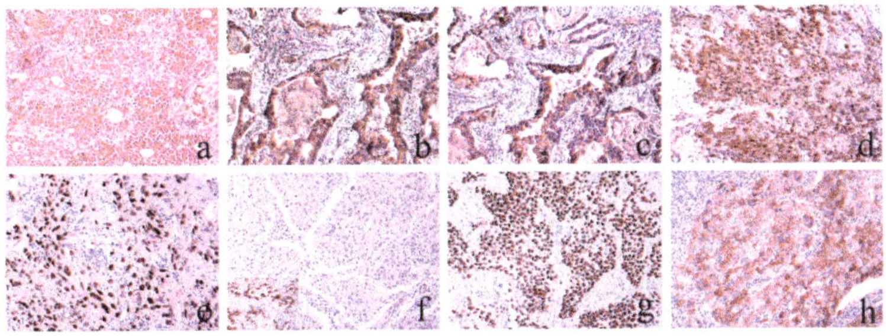

Figure 3. Representative sections of NSCLC tumors immunohistochemically stained for the assessment of VEGFC (**a**), PDGFRα (**b**), PDGFRβ (**c**), ZEB1 (**d**), Cyclin D1 (**e**), p16 (**f**), p53 (**g**), and CD24 (**h**) expression. For VEGFC, PDGFRα, and PDGFRβ, the cytoplasmic staining was evaluated, while for ZEB1, Cyclin D1, p16, and p53, nuclear staining was assessed. Ultimately, membranous staining was evaluated to determine the expression of CD24. Staining intensity was assessed by comparison using an accepted external/internal positive control [(**a–f**): magnification ×200]. (**f**) The f insert shows positive p16 nuclear expression [magnification ×400].

LKB1 loss was observed in 21% of specimens (51/248); p16 downregulation was detected in 71% (177/248); low or no PD-L1 expression was detected in 64% (159/248); Cyclin D1 overexpression was detected in 73% (182/248). High expression of PDGFRβ and PDGFRα in the tumor stroma was observed in 83% (205/248) and 74% (183/248), respectively. Ultimately, ZEB1 was highly expressed in 64% (158/248) of the tumors overall. Almost equal percentages of loss and intact expression were observed for STING, p53, VEGFC, CD24, PDGFRα, and PDGFRβ in tumor cells, for ZEB1 in the tumor stroma, as well as for LKB1 and NEDD9 RNA levels. KRAS mutations were detected in 15% (37/248) of the tumors and consisted of G12V (n = 9), G13D (n = 7), G23D (n = 6) G12S (n = 5), G12D (n = 5), G12C (n = 5), G12A (n = 2), G13R (n = 1), and double G12D + G23D (n = 1). BRAF mutations were harbored by 8.2% (20/248) of the tumors, consisting preponderantly of V600E (x17) and to a lesser extent in V600E + K601E (n = 2) and V600K (n = 1), as shown in Supplementary Table S6.

3.2.2. Pleomorphic vs. Non-Pleomorphic LUACs

Confronting non-pleomorphic with pleomorphic LUACs, we assessed statistically significant correlations related to the pleomorphic—dedifferentiated—histology [Supplementary Table S7]. Dedifferentiation in LUACs correlated with high PD-L1 expression ($p < 0.001$), with no/low β-catenin membranous staining ($p = 0.024$), with high ZEB1 expression in the tumor ($p = 0.017$), and with KC status ($p = 0.034$). Even though LKB1 loss characterized half,(50% (5/10)), of the pleomorphic LUACs in our study, vs. only one-third (33% (36/110)) of the non-pleomorphic LUACs yielding LKB1 loss, no statistical significance ($p = 0.3$) was established between dedifferentiation and LKB1 loss of expression. Similarly, although 40% (4/10) of the pleomorphic LUACs harbored KRAS mutations versus the 21% (23/110) KRAS mutations present in the non-pleomorphic group, again, no statistical significance was recognized. BRAF mutations were present in almost equal percentages in both pleomorphic and non-LUAC cohorts, 10% (10/110) in the non-pleomorphic LUACs vs. 9.8%, (1/10). Interestingly one-third, (30% (3/10)), of the pleomorphic LUACs harbored KL mutational status.

3.2.3. Pleomorphic vs. Non-Pleomorphic LSCCs

The only laboratory variable correlating with statistical significance with dedifferentiation in pleomorphic LSCCs was the high expression of PD-L1. Specifically, 100% (3/3) of the pleomorphic LSCCs yielded high expression of PD-L1 versus only 39% (47/119) of tumors in the non-pleomorphic cohort ($p = 0.05$) [Supplementary Table S8], as shown in Figure 4. Loss of LKB1 expression did not correlate with dedifferentiated LSCCs, as none

(0%) of the three (3/3) pleomorphic LSCCs in our group presented LKB1 loss compared to 5.9% (7/119) non-pleomorphic LSCCs with loss of LKB1 expression ($p > 0.9$). Notably, in contrast to the pleomorphic LUACs, no statistically significant correlation was shown between pleomorphic LSCCs and no/low β-catenin membranous staining.

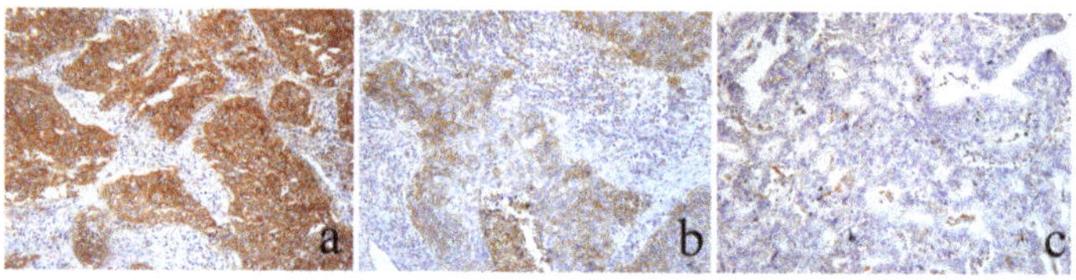

Figure 4. PD-L1 immunohistochemical staining. (**a**) Area of a LUAC of solid predominant histological pattern showing strong membranous PD-L1 staining in 100% of the tumor cells, therefore scored as "high positive"; (**b**) Area from a LUAC showing focally moderate-weak membrane staining in 15% of the tumor cells, scored as "low positive"; (**c**) Area from a LUAC with complete absence of PD-L1 staining 0%, in the presence of internal positive control (immune cells), scored as "negative". [(**a**,**b**): magnification ×100, (**c**): magnification ×200].

3.3. *Characterization of NSCLC Tumors with the LKB1-Less Phenotype*

3.3.1. Correlation of LKB1 Loss of Expression with Patients Clinical Characteristics and Tumor Histotype

Loss of LKB1 expression correlated significantly with age, as 82% (42/51), of the tumors with LKB1 loss were obtained from patients under the age of 70 ($p = 0.091$), and of male gender, 78% (40/51), ($p = 0.009$) [Supplementary Table S9]. Furthermore, almost half (47% (24/51)) of the tumors with LKB1 loss were p-stage IIIA, while 24% (12/51) were p-stage IIB, and only 16% (8/51) were p-stage IIA. More than half (67% (34/51)) were poorly differentiated grade 3 tumors, and 66% (27/120) of the LUACs (both non-pleomorphic and pleomorphic) had a solid predominant histological pattern. Even though the clear majority (80% (41/51)) of the tumors characterized by loss of LKB1 expression presented concomitant lymph node metastasis LKB1 loss did not show a statistically significant correlation with lymph node metastatic status. Metastatic lymph node dissemination involved mostly regional, LN1, lymph node stations (this was true of 47% (24/51)), but also implicated the coexistence of both regional and distant (LN1 and LN2) lymph nodes, while only 2% (1/51) involved LN3 lymph node stations [Supplementary Table S13].

As already mentioned above, loss of LKB1 expression was observed in all distinctive tumor histotypes, although as expected, the overwhelming majority of the tumors exhibiting loss of LKB1 expression were LUACs, of which 71% (36/51) were non-pleomorphic and 9.8% (5/51) pleomorphic. LKB1 loss was also observed in 14% (7/51) of the LSCCs, all of which were non-pleomorphic LSCCs. Furthermore, loss of LKB1 expression characterized also 33% (1/3) of the adenosquamous carcinomas, and in addition, the pleomorphic large cell carcinoma (100% (1/1)), the pleomorphic spindle cell carcinoma (100% (1/1)), and the large cell carcinoma included in our study (100% (1/1)) ($p < 0.001$).

Interestingly, high percentages of LKB1 loss of expression was observed and characterized the less-differentiated tumor histotypes. Specifically, half (50% (3/6)) of the pleomorphic LUACs yielded loss of LKB1 expression (vs. 32.7% (36/117) LKB1 loss in the non-pleomorphic LUACs). Likewise, the total (100% (1/1)) pleomorphic large cell carcinoma, (1/1) large cell carcinoma, and also 1 of the 3 adenosquamous carcinomas showed loss of LKB1 expression. Instead, none of the three pleomorphic LSCCs yielded LKB1 loss (0% (0/3)).

3.3.2. Overall Number of Tumors with LKB1 Loss: Correlations with the Examined Laboratory Variables

Overall, loss of LKB1 expression was in absolute agreement with pAMPK loss of expression 100% (51/51) ($p < 0.001$) and yielded a statistically significant correlation with

STING loss, since 71% (36/51) of the overall tumors exhibiting LKB1 loss presented concomitant loss of STING expression vs. 44% (87/197) STING loss in the LKB1-intact tumors ($p < 0.001$) [Supplementary Table S10], Figure 5.

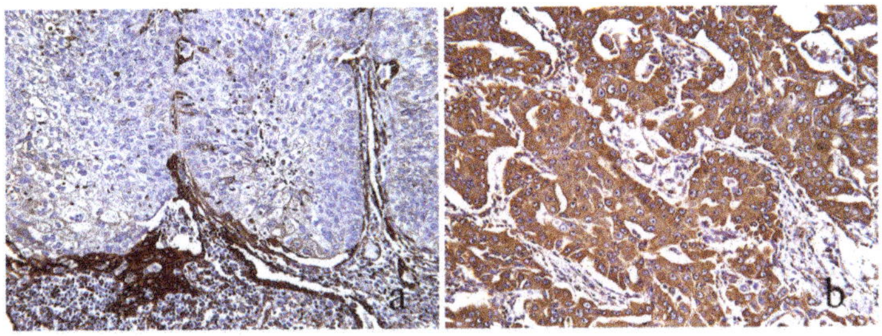

Figure 5. STING immunohistochemical staining. (**a**) An area of a LSCC showing complete loss of STING expression in the presence of positively stained stromal cells and immune cells as internal positive controls. (**b**) An area of a LUAC exhibiting "high", score: 3, cytoplasmic staining intensity of STING in 100% of the tumor cells. [(**a**,**b**): magnification ×200].

As expected, LKB1 loss correlated with KRAS mutations, which were harbored by one-third (31% (16/51)) of the tumors with loss of LKB1 expression vs. 11% (21/197) of KRAS mutations present in the LKB1-intact tumors ($p < 0.001$). Significant correlation was also observed, with low LKB1 RNA levels as the clear majority: 69% (35/51) of the tumors that were evaluated by immunohistochemistry to exhibit loss of LKB1 expression were found to also entertain low levels of LKB1 RNA, 69% (35/51), versus the 45% (89/197) LKB1-intact tumors exhibiting low RNA levels in ($p = 0.003$). Moreover, LKB1 loss correlated significantly with high CD24 expression, with 71% (36/51) of the LKB1 loss tumors yielding high CD24 expression vs. the 45% (99/197) that yielded high CD24 expression in LKB1-intact tumors ($p = 0.009$). Similarly, LKB1 loss correlated significantly with the KC co-mutational status, since 24% (12/51) of KC tumors exhibited LKB1 loss versus the 9% (4/6) of KCs that yielded intact LKB1 expression; ($p < 0.001$). BRAF mutations were observed in 14% (7/51) of the tumors with LKB1 loss vs. 6.5% (13/197) in tumors with LKB1-intact expression ($p = 0.15$). No statistically significant correlations were observed among the KP cohort, as only one of the fourteen tumors co-occurred with LKB1 loss ($p = 0.3$). Interestingly, the single tumor in our study with KPL triple co-mutation presented LKB1 loss by definition, so this did not have statistical significance. Additionally, even though the majority of the tumors showing LKB1 loss were characterized by no/low PD-L1 expression —73% (37/51) vs. 62% (122/197) in LKB1-intact tumors—this did not have statistical significance ($p = 0.2$). Ultimately, no statistically significant correlation was observed between LKB1 status and the β-catenin status of membranous expression ($p > 0.9$).

3.3.3. LUACs with LKB1 Loss: Correlations with the Examined Laboratory Variables

Likewise, in LUACs, LKB1 loss correlated with statistical significance with pAMPK ($p < 0.001$) and STING ($p < 0.001$) loss, as well as with KC co-mutational status ($p = 0.004$). Interestingly, contrary to the overall findings in LUACs, LKB1 loss correlated significantly with no/low β-catenin membranous expression ($p = 0.019$), as shown in Figure 6. Meanwhile, the overall correlation observed between LKB1 loss and CD24 was not shown in LUACs, as almost equal percentages of high CD24 expression were observed in LUACs with intact (76%) and tumors showing loss of LKB1 expression (71%) ($p = 0.5$). KRAS mutations were harbored by 37% (15/41) of LUACs showing LKB1 loss vs. 15% (12/79) in the LKB1-intact cohort ($p = 0.008$). BRAF mutations were detected in 15% (6/41) of LUACs with LKB1 loss vs. 6.4% (5/79) in the LUACs with intact LKB1 expression ($p = 0.2$). LKB1 loss correlated significantly with low LKB1 RNA levels ($p = 0.047$) and PD-L1 expression in LUACs did not correlate with the status of LKB1 expression ($p = 0.3$) [Supplementary Table S11].

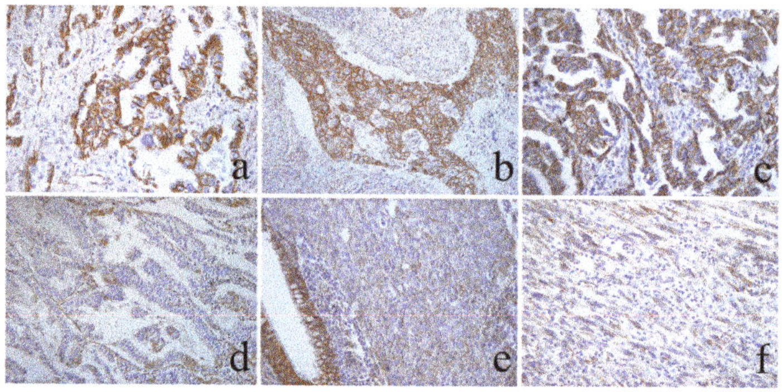

Figure 6. Immunohistochemical evaluation of β-catenin membranous expression. (**a**) Area of a LUAC showing strong complete β-catenin membranous staining in 95% of the tumor cells, scored as 3: "high". (**b**) Area of an LSCC showing heterogeneous β-catenin membranous expression. There is coexistence of areas of tumor cells that exhibit strong and complete membranous staining (peripheric zones) and areas with tumor cells showing moderate–weak β-catenin membranous expression (centrally). The latter is observed in 60% of the tumor cells, and therefore is scored as 2: "moderate". Distinct, patchy foci of single cells and small groups of cells with vanishing or lost membranous expression are also present. (**c**) Area of a LUAC with complete membranous staining preservation of moderate–strong intensity in >70% of cells, scored as 3: "high". (**d**) An area of a LUAC showing vanishing β-catenin membranous expression with only small patchy foci observed in 5% of the tumor cells, retaining a membranous expression score of 1: "low". (**e**) Area from a grade 3 LUAC with a solid predominant histological pattern showing complete loss of membrane staining of β-catenin, in the presence of the intact membrane staining of the by standing bronchial epithelium as internal positive control. (**f**) Dedifferentiated area morphology of a pleomorphic LUAC with sarcomatous spindle cell exhibiting complete absence of β-catenin membranous expression and consequently scored 0: "lost". Magnification ×100.

3.3.4. LUACs with LKB1 Loss—Correlations with Clinicopathological Characteristics

Of the 41 total LUACs with LKB1, more than half (66% (27/41)) were characterized by a predominantly solid histological pattern, 20% (8/41) by acinar, and 9.8% (4/41) presented with a predominantly papillary pattern Meanwhile, 12% (5/41) of the total LUACs with LKB1 loss were pleomorphic LUACs. More than three-quarters were accompanied by lymph node metastases, which similar to overall showed a lack of correlation with the status of LKB1 expression [Supplementary Table S12].

3.3.5. LSCCs with LKB1 Loss—Correlations with the Examined Laboratory Variables

Of the 122 LSCCs involved in our study, only 5.77% (7/122) yielded LKB1 loss. The only statistically significant correlation detected in the LSCCs with LKB1 loss was loss of p-AMPK expression, which was observed in 100% the LSCCs (7/7), ($p < 0.001$). Even though the overwhelming majority of LSCCs tumors were characterized by concomitant loss of LKB1 and STING expression (86% (6/7) versus 51% (59/115) STING loss in LKB1-intact LSCCs tumors) this correlation did not gain statical significance ($p = 0.12$), most likely due to the very small number of tumors representative of this category ($n = 7$). Notably, 0% of the seven (0/7) LSCCs showing LKB1 loss harbored KRAS mutations compared to the 7% (8/119) of KRAS mutant tumors in the LSCCs with intact LKB1 expression. Instead, BRAF mutations were detected in 14%, (1/7) of the LSCCs with LKB1 loss versus 7.1% (8/115) in the LSCCs with LKB1 intact expression ($p = 0.4$), the total exclusively harbored by non-pleomorphic LSCCs. PD-L1 expression did not correlate with LKB1 status, as almost equal percentages of LKB1 loss were observed in both LSCCs with loss and IN LSCCs with intact LKB1 expression. Likewise, PD-L1 expression was similar in pleomorphic and non-pleomorphic LSCCs.

3.3.6. LSCCs with LKB1 Loss—Correlation with Clinicopathological Characteristics

A total of 86% (6/7) of the LSCCs with LKB1 loss presented concomitant lymph node metastasis. Most of these (71% (5/7)) involved regional lymph nodes, whereas 14% (1/7) involved both regional and distant (LN1 and LN2) lymph node stations. Interestingly, the majority (71% (5/7)) were p-stage I–II, although poorly differentiated grade 3 tumors, and most of the patients (71% (5/7) were <70 years of age. None of the LSCCs with LKB1 loss were pleomorphic.

3.4. Correlation of LKB1 Loss and Lymph Node Metastatic Status

3.4.1. Metastatic NSCLCs with LKB1 Loss vs. Metastatic NSCLC with LKB1 Intact in Relation to the Examined Laboratory Variables

Overall, 41/188 patients with lymph node metastases yielded tumors with concomitant loss of LKB1 expression. Importantly, in metastatic tumors, loss of LKB1 protein expression was found to correlate significantly with concurrent loss of STING, ($p = 0.014$) and p-AMPK expression; with KRAS mutations, 39% (13/147 vs. 19/147); with KC status, 29% (12/41), ($p < 0.001$); with low levels of LKB1 RNA ($p = 0.008$); and with high CD24 expression ($p = 0.025$). No statistically significant correlations were observed between metastatic tumors with LKB1 loss and β-catenin membranous expression status, or with PD-L1 expression. BRAF mutations were harbored by (12%) 5/41 vs. (7.7%) 11/147 of the metastatic tumors with intact LKB1 expression. The majority (71% (29/41)) of the 41 metastatic tumors showing LKB1 loss were non-pleomorphic LUACs, while 9.8% (4/41) were pleomorphic LUACs, and 15% (6/41) were LSCCs [Supplementary Table S13].

3.4.2. Metastatic LUACs with LKB1 Loss vs. Metastatic LUACs with LKB1 Intact in Relation to the Examined Laboratory Variables

More than three-quarters (80.5% (33/41)) of the metastatic tumors with LKB1 loss were LUACs. Similarly, in metastatic LUACs, LKB1 loss correlated significantly with STING loss ($p = 0.005$), with p-AMPK loss ($p < 0.001$), with KRAS mutations 45% (15/33) [vs. 20% (11/56) in the metastatic LUACs with intact LKB1 expression] ($p = 0.010$), and with KC status ($p = 0.009$), while in contrast to overall findings in metastatic LUACs showing LKB1 loss, a significant correlation was observed with no/low β-catenin membranous expression ($p = 0.007$). No statistically significant correlation with PD-L1 expression was observed. BRAF mutations were detected in 22% (4/33) vs. 7.3% (4/56) in the metastatic LUACs with intact LKB1 expression [Supplementary Table S14].

3.4.3. Metastatic LSCCs with LKB1 Loss vs. Metastatic LSCCs with LKB1 Intact in Relation to the Examined Laboratory Variables

Even though of the seven total metastatic LSCCs, six yielded concomitant LKB1 loss, 86% (6/7), the only statistically significant correlation observed was with pAMPK loss ($p < 0.001$). Interestingly, even though STING loss was observed in 83% (5/6) of the metastatic LSCCs with LKB1 loss vs. 57% (51/89) in the metastatic LSCCs with intact LKB1expression, this did not gain statistical significance ($p = 0.4$) most likely attributable to the rarity of LSCCs showing LKB1 loss of expression ($n = 7$) [Supplementary Table S15].

3.5. KRAS Co-Mutational Cohorts—Incidence

KL co-mutation characterized 6.5% (16/248) of the NSCLC tumors included in our study, KC status 8.5% (21/248), KRAS mutant and LKB1 intact status 8.46% (21/248), KP status 5.6% (14/248), L status 2.4%, K status 1.6% (4/248), and finally, the triple-mutated KPL status only 0.4% of the tumors (1/248) [Supplementary Tables S16 and S17].

3.5.1. Clinicopathologic and Laboratory Outline of KRAS Co-Mutational Cohorts

- KL cohort ($n = 16$): The preponderance of the tumors with KL co-mutational status were characterized by p16 downregulation, 75% (12/16) and by a "wild type" p53 immunohistochemical pattern of expression, 94% (15/16). Moreover, 94% (15/16), showed high expression of PDGFRβ, 88% (14/16) exhibited the presence of PDGFRa, and 81% (13/16) showed similar expression in the tumor stroma, while high CD24 expression in the tumor was observed in 63% of cases (10/16). Furthermore, more than half (69% (11/16)) showed no/low β-catenin membranous expression. Similar percentages of STING loss and intact expression were observed: 56% (10/16) and 44% (7/10), respectively. Ultimately, BRAF commutation was detected in 6.3% of the tumors in this cohort (1/16).
  Overall, 75% (12/16) of the patients with KL tumors were males, and 94% (15/16) were aged <70 years. Interestingly, the KL tumor cohort did not include LSCCs and consisted almost exclusively of non-pleomorphic and pleomorphic LUACs, [75% (12/16) and 19% (3/16), respectively], with solid, 60% (9/16), and acinar, 27% (4/16) as the predominant histological patterns. Though the tumors showed various grades of differentiation, more than half (56% (9/16)) were p-stage III–IV.
- KC ($n = 21$): KC tumors yielded almost equal percentages of lost and intact LKB1 expression: 57% (12/21) vs. 43% (9/21), respectively, even though, curiously, more than three-quarters (81% (17/81)) of the tumors showed low LKB1 RNA levels. All of them (100% (21/21)) exhibited p16 downregulation. High expression of PDGFRβ and PDFGRα in the tumor stroma characterized 90% (19/21) and 86% (18/21) of the tumors, respectively. High CD24 expression was observed in 71% (15/21) and Cyclin D1 overexpression was observed in 86% (18/21). No/low β-catenin membranous expression was shown in 57% (8/21). Interestingly, 10% of the tumors with KC co-mutation (2/21) presented concomitant BRAF mutations. More than half of the KC status tumors (62% (13/21)) were p-stage IIIA, grade 3 poorly differentiated tumors, with 57% (12/21) exhibiting a size of >5 cm. Meanwhile, 57% (14/21) of KC tumors were LUACs, 62% (13/21) were non-pleomorphic, and 19% (4/21) were pleomorphic, including an invasive mucinous histological pattern (5.9%). The cohort also included LSCCs (14% (3/21)) and one (1/21) adenosquamous carcinoma ($p > 0.002$).

The laboratory and clinical characteristics of KRAS mutant and LKB1 intact, KP, L, KPL are described in detail in Supplementary Tables S16 and S17.

3.5.2. KRAS Co-Mutational Cohorts—Correlation with Lymph Node Metastatic Status

Notably, all mono-, bi-, and tri-mutational cohorts yielded significant percentages of lymph node metastasis, 90% (75/83), with statistically significant correlations between the mutational cohorts ($p = 0.032$).

KL and KC bi-mutational status correlated significantly with lymph node metastasis, as all (16/16) of the KL tumors and all but one (20/21) KC tumors were associated with lymph node metastasis 8.5% (16/188) and 10% (20/188) vs. 0% (0/60) and 1.7% (1/188) ($p = 0.015$) and ($p = 0.03$), respectively. On the contrary, KP status did not show a correlation with lymph node metastasis ($p = 0.2$). Specifically, KL and KPL cohorts yielded the highest percentage (100%) of concomitant lymph node metastasis (16/16 and 1/1, respectively) with none of the tumors in any cohort having intact lymph nodes, LN0. Additionally, 95% (20/21) of the KC, 93% (13/14) of the KP, and 90% (19/21) of the KRAS mutant and LKB1-intact tumors presented lymph node metastasis. The lowest percentages of lymph node metastasis were observed in the mono-mutational cohorts L and K with 75% (3/4) and 50% (3/6), respectively. In particular, 100% of the KPL (1/1) cohort, almost half of the KL and KC cohorts (44% (7/16) and 43% (9/21), respectively), one-third of the KP and KRAS mutant LKB1-intact cohorts (29% (4/14) and (6/21), respectively), and one-quarter of the K cohort (25% (1/4)) yielded metastasis in both regional and distant mediastinal (LN1 and LN2) lymph nodes. On the contrary, only half (50% (3/6)) of the tumors in the L cohort presented metastatic involvement, which was associated with exclusively regional LN1 lymph nodes. Interestingly, the only mutational subgroup presenting with LN3 involvement (supraclavicular lymph node in our case) was KL. KL yielded superior aggressiveness, with no tumors of LN0 status, exhibiting LN3 metastatic involvement besides the highest percentage of combined LN1+ LN2 involvement 44% (7/16).

3.6. Survival Analysis

3.6.1. Overall Survival Analysis—mOS

The univariate analysis in the overall cohort revealed that patients with tumors yielding loss of STING expression experienced significantly shorter median overall survival (mOS) compared to patients with tumors showing intact STING expression: 19.68 vs. 36.53 months; $p = 0.004$, as shown in Figure 7 [Supplementary Table S18].

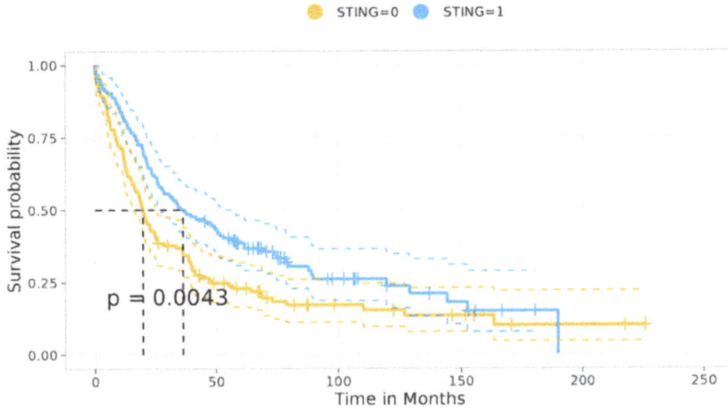

Figure 7. Overall—STING status of expression in relation to median overall survival.

Likewise, patients with tumors showing p53 mutational immunohistochemical expression status had significantly inferior mOS compared to patients with p53 intact expression: 19.83 vs. 34.76 months; $p = 0.029$. Similarly, patients with tumors harboring KRAS mutations had inferior mOS compared to KRAS wild-type tumors: 19.88 vs. 28.25 months; $p = 0.037$. Also, tumors with high PDGFRβ expression were associated with a distinct decrease in mOS compared to tumors with low PDGFRβ expression, with survival rates of 20.42 vs. 36.34 months; $p < 0.001$. Additionally, patients with tumors yielding no/low β-catenin membranous expression were associated with a clear decrease in mOS compared to tumors with intermediate/high β-catenin membranous expression: 20.70 vs. 36.40 months; $p = 0.003$. Furthermore, a clear decrease in mOS was observed in patients with tumors exhibiting high ZEB1 expression compared to that of patients with tumors with low ZEB1 expression: 21.45 vs. 37.29 months; $p = 0.045$. Ultimately, as expected, patients with metastatic involvement of regional and/or distal lymph nodes experienced a significant decrease in mOS compared to patients with intact lymph nodes: 21.29 vs. 46.75 months; $p < 0.001$. A trend of decreased mOS was observed in relation to Cyclin D1 overexpression and normal expression, with mOS of 20.09 vs. 33.23; $p = 0.056$, while high PDGFRβ expression in the tumor stroma resulted in survival rates of 24.90 vs. 48.36 months; $p = 0.068$. LKB1 loss vs. intact status did not show a significant correlation with mOS ($p > 0.9$)

3.6.2. Overall Survival Analysis—Hazard Ratio Univariate Analysis

Univariate analysis revealed that patients with tumors showing intact STING expression experienced a lower risk of death (HR: 0.66, 95% c.i.: 0.50–0.88; $p = 0.005$). On the contrary, patients with tumors yielding high PDGFRb expression (HR: 1.71, 95% c.i.: 1.28–2.28; $p < 0.001$), patients with metastasis to regional and distant lymph nodes (HR: 1.83, 95% c.i.: 1.27–2.64; $p = 0.001$), patients with tumors showing no/low β-catenin membranous expression (HR: 1.53, 95% c.i.: 1.15–2.03; $p = 0.004$), patients with KRAS mutations (HR: 1.50,

95% c.i.: 1.02–2.21; $p = 0.039$), patients with high ZEB1 expression in the tumor (HR: 1.36, 95% c.i.: 1.01–1.84; $p = 0.046$), with Cyclin D1 overexpression (HR: 0.74, 95% c.i.: 0.54–1.01; $p = 0.057$), as well as patients with tumors exhibiting p53 mutational immunohistochemical expression status (HR: 1.37, 95% c.i.: 1.03–1.83; $p = 0.030$) were at significantly higher risk of death.

3.6.3. Overall Survival Analysis—Multivariate Analysis

Furthermore, in multivariate analysis, STING intact expression emerged as an independent prognostic factor for increased survival with a significantly decreased risk of death (HR: 0.61, 95% c.i.: 0.45–0.82; $p < 0.001$). Instead, high PDGFRβ expression in the tumor and KRAS mutations emerged as independent prognostic factors for increased risk of death: (HR:1.62, c.i. 1.16–2.24; $p = 0.004$) and (HR: 1.81, 95% c.i.: 1.20–2.72; $p = 0.005$), respectively.

Loss of β-catenin membranous expression and p53 mutational expression status yielded a trend of correlation to a higher risk of death; (HR: 1.29, c.i. 0.96–1.74; $p = 0.094$) and (HR: 1.29, c.i. 0.96–1.74; $p = 0.091$). Metastasis to regional and/or mediastinal lymph nodes as well as high ZEB1 expression in the tumor did not reveal as independent prognostic for higher risk of death (HR: 1.15, c.i. 0.73–1.82; $p = 0.539$) and (HR: 1.06, c.i. 0.76–1.48; $p = 0.539$), respectively—Figure 8.

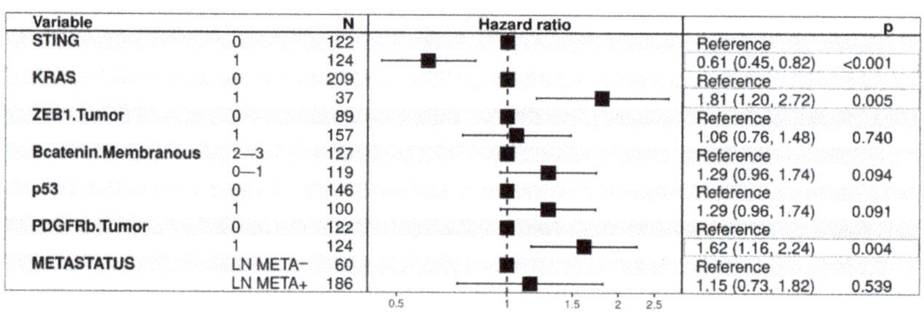

Figure 8. Overall multivariate analysis —Hazard Ratio.

3.6.4. Tumors with LKB1 Loss of Expression—Median Overall Surviival

The univariate analysis in the cohort of tumors with LKB1 loss revealed that patients with tumors yielding concomitant LKB1 loss and no/low β-catenin membranous expression experienced significantly decreased median survival mOS compared to tumors showing LKB1 loss and intact β-catenin membranous expression: 20.50 vs. 52.99 months; $p < 0.001$. All other comparisons did not reveal any significant correlations between the expression of the various proteins, RNA protein levels, or the presence of KRAS, and BRAF mutations with mOS (all long-rank $p > 0.05$), Figure 9. Supplementary Table S19.

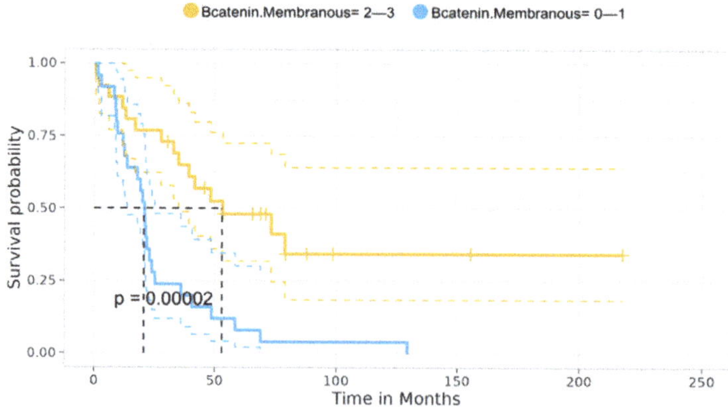

Figure 9. LKB1 loss tumors correlation with β-catenin membranous status of expression—mOS.

3.6.5. Tumors with LKB1 loss —Univariate Analysis Hazard Ratio

Importantly, the hazard ratio analysis revealed that patients with concurrent LKB1 loss and no/low β-catenin membranous expression experienced a significantly increased risk of death (HR: 3.32, 95% c.i.: 1.71–6.43; p =0.00002) Figure 10.

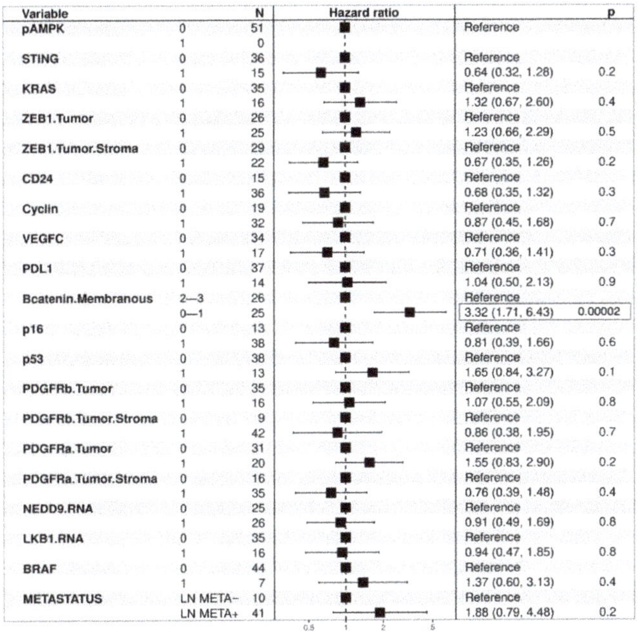

Figure 10. LKB1 loss tumors correlations—Hazard ratio.

3.6.6. KL Tumors Cohort Survival Analysis—mOS Univariate Analysis

KL tumors—univariate analysis of the KL cohort revealed that patients with KL tumors yielding concomitant loss of STING expression experienced significantly shorter median overall survival (mOS) compared to patients with KL status tumors showing intact STING expression, 18.73 vs. 52.99 months; p = 0.011 Figure 11.

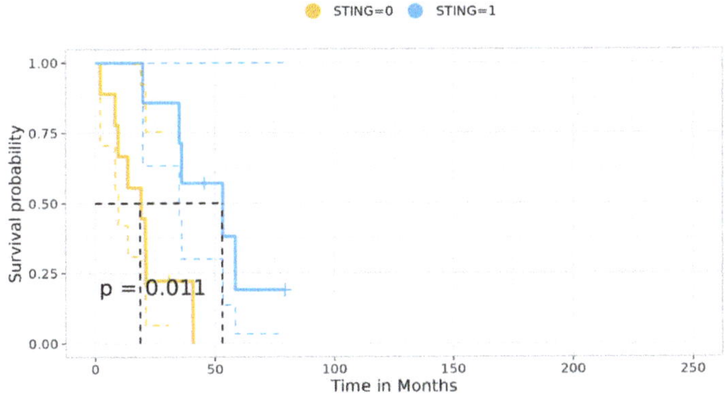

Figure 11. KL status tumors correlation with STING expression status—median overall survival.

Likewise, patients harboring the KL status and concomitant no/low β-catenin membranous expression showed a trend correlating with decreased mOS vs. patients of KL status with retained, medium–high β-catenin membranous expression: 20.07 vs. 52.99; $p = 0.069$, Supplementary Table S20.

3.6.7. KL Tumors—Univariate Analysis, Hazard Ratio

Furthermore, patients with KL mutational status and concurrent intact STING expression experienced a significant decrease in the risk of death (HR: 0.12, 95% ci: 0.05–0.76; $p = 0.02$). Inversely, patients with KL tumors yielding no/low β-catenin membranous expression showed a trend of increased risk of death (HR: 3.18, 95% ci: 0.86–110.78; $p = 0.08$), as shown in Figure 12.

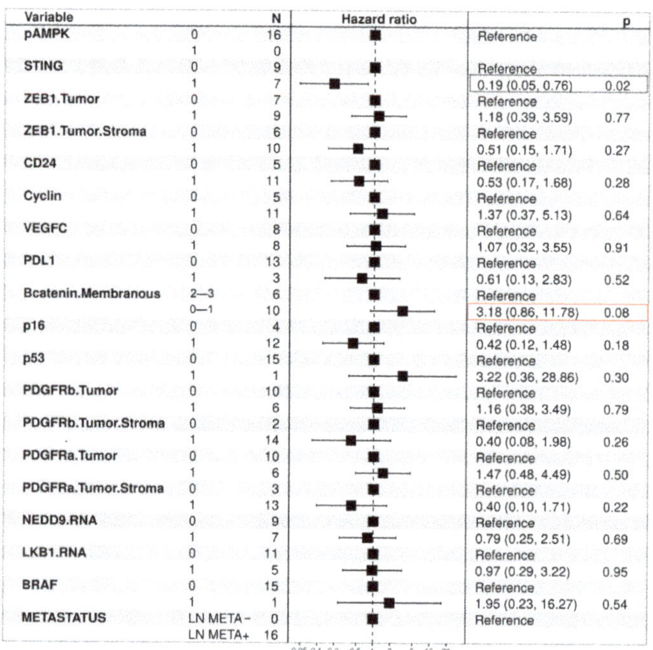

Figure 12. Tumors with the KL co-mutation—Hazard ratio.

4. Discussion

In this study, we performed an in situ immunohistochemical investigation of the status of LKB1 expression in all NSCLC histotypes, beyond and within *KRAS* mutational status, so as to investigate the LKB1-less phenotype and its possible correlations, as well as the impact of LKB1 status, the emergence of significant correlations, and tumor patients' prognosis. Furthermore, we aimed to explore the prevalence and the clinical and laboratory characteristics of defined KRAS co-mutational groups, as well as their prognostic impact in patients with operable non-small cell lung cancer (NSCLC).

Loss of LKB1 protein expression was observed in 21% of the overall examined tumors and correlated significantly with histotype ($p < 0.001$). Specifically, loss of LKB1 expression was observed with variable incidences in all the represented distinctive histotypes in our study, except the three pleomorphic LSCCs and the spindle cell pleomorphic carcinoma, which showed intact LKB1 expression.

Overall, tumors exhibiting loss of LKB1 expression were poorly differentiated grade 3 tumors, and were mainly observed in patients of male gender under 70 years of age. Metastatic lymph node dissemination involved mostly regional (LN1) lymph node stations, 47% (24/51), but also implicated both regional and distant (LN1 and LN2) lymph nodes.

Overall, LKB1 loss showed a significant correlation with p-AMPK loss, with KRAS mutations, with low LKB1 RNA levels, with high expression of CD24, with Cyclin-D1 overexpression, and with the KC mutational status, both overall and in LUACs.

The statistically significant correlation between LKB1 loss and the loss of STING expression documented overall ($p < 0.001$), and in LUACs ($p < 0.001$) was also observed in the metastatic tumors, with overall LKB1 loss of ($p = 0.014$), while that in LUACs was ($p = 0.005$).

No statistically significant correlation was established with LSCCs, most likely due to the small number of LSCCs in the LKB1 loss group due to the rarity of tumors representative of this category in our study ($n = 7$).

LKB1 loss showed a significant correlation with β-catenin no/low membranous expression, exclusively in LUACs, overall ($p = 0.019$) and, importantly, in the metastatic setting ($p = 0.005$). Furthermore, no/low β-catenin membranous staining was shown to characterize dedifferentiated—pleomorphic—LUACs ($p = 0.024$).

No significant correlation was observed between LKB1 loss and PD-L1 expression status, overall, in LUACs or LSCCs.

Remarkably, moderate–high PD-L1 expression (scores 2, 3) was observed to correlate with dedifferentiation, as high percentages of PD-L1 expression characterized the overwhelming majority of pleomorphic LUACs and LSCCs, as well as the histologically dedifferentiated pleomorphic tumors (spindle and large cell carcinomas) along with no/low β-catenin membranous expression. The high levels of PD-L1 expression could be related to the significant amount of inflammatory infiltrate that was prevalent in the pleomorphic lung carcinomas.

In contrast, high percentages (ε 50%) of no/low PD-L1 expression characterized all members of the KRAS co-mutational cohorts, with tumors harboring the triple-mutated KPL status showing the highest percentage (100% (1/1)), followed by tumors with KL status (81% (13/16)), KP and KC status tumors (71% (10/14 and 15/21, respectively)), and, ultimately, KRAS mut and LKB1-intact tumors, 67% (14/21).

Interestingly, the obligatory mono-mutational cohorts K and L showed the lowest percentages of no/low PD-L1 expression, at 50% (2/4 and 3/6, respectively), which was hypothesized to be due to the lower mutational load.

Additionally, even though LKB1 loss, per se, did not correlate with lymph node metastasis, when it co-occurred with KRAS mutations (KL) or as a component of KPL status, 100% of the KL and KPL (16/16 and 1/1) tumors showed lymph node metastasis versus only half (50% (3/6)) of the mono-mutational L cohort (LKB1 loss only, KRAS: wild type, p53: wild type, p16: not downregulated) with lymph node metastasis ($p = 0.032$).

Even though the loss of LKB1 expression, did not necessarily affect survival, patients with concomitant LKB1 loss and no/low β-catenin membranous expression experienced significantly inferior median overall survival of 20.50 vs. 52.99 months; $p < 0.001$, as well as significantly greater risk of death (HR: 3.32, 95% c.i.: 1.71–6.43; $p < 0.001$). This was observed in patients with tumors yielding LKB1 loss and intact, intermediate–high β-catenin membranous expression.

Notably, LKB1 loss in co-occurrence with KRAS mutation was the only KRAS co-mutation to implicate the LN3 lymph node station. Conversely, only half (50% (3/6)) of the tumors belonging to the mono-mutational (L) cohort presented lymph node metastasis. The survival analysis of the KL cohort revealed that patients with tumors yielding concomitant loss of STING expression experienced significantly shorter median overall survival (mOS) compared to patients with tumors showing intact STING expression (18.73 vs. 52.99 months; $p = 0.011$), while patients with tumors harboring the KL status and concomitant no/low β-catenin membranous expression showed a trend correlating with decreased mOS vs. patients of KL status with retained intermediate–high β-catenin membranous expression (20.07 vs. 52.99; $p = 0.069$). Ultimately, patients with tumors harboring KL mutational status and concurrent intact STING expression experienced a significant decrease in the risk of death (HR: 0.12, 95% ci: 0.05–0.76; $p = 0.02$), while patients with tumors yielding no/lower membranous expression of β-catenin showed a trend correlated with an increased risk of death (HR: 3.18, 95% ci: 0.86–110.78; $p = 0.08$).

Our results highlight the significant correlation between LKB1 loss and STING loss and are in accordance with the findings of Kitajima et al. [56]. In this seminal study, it was shown that LKB1 loss results in marked silencing of STING, which is mediated—at least in part—by hyperactivation of DNMT1 and EZH2 activity related to elevated S-adenylmethionine levels and reinforced by DNMT1 upregulation. The authors, after identifying KL-specific downregulation of genes involved in dsDNA sensing—especially TMEM173/STING, which was also reduced in LKB1-mutant KRAS wild-type NSCLC cell lines—performed IHC to validate their findings and analyzed tumor cell-specific STING protein levels across a panel of 64 patient-derived NSCLC samples enriched for KRAS-mutated status. The results revealed that LKB1 loss was robustly associated with either a complete absence of or a significant reduction in STING levels in tumor cells. Importantly, the authors found that STING silencing was associated with LKB1 loss also in KRAS WT lung cancers, and was especially robust when combined with elevated DNMT1 levels, suggesting that this mechanism is not purely limited to the KL cellular state.

Furthermore in our study we show that concurrent LKB1 loss and STING loss of expression correlates with statistical significance with lymph node metastasis in both overall NSCLC tumors but also in the LUACs cohort.

As already described, we observed very high percentages of no/low levels of PD-L1 expression in all KRAS mutational cohorts, with the KL presenting the highest percentages. This finding is also in agreement with [37,56], stating that defective dsDNA sensing links LKB1 loss with low PD-L1 levels. Thus, silencing of STING in KL cells directly contributes to impaired intratumoral T-cell recruitment and low PD-L1 expression.

Furthermore, also in the setting of KRAS-LKB1 co-mutation, we show that patients with KL tumors yielding concomitant loss of STING expression experienced significantly shorter median overall survival (mOS) compared to patients with KL status tumors showing intact STING expression, while patients with KL tumors and concurrent intact STING expression experienced a significant decrease in the risk of death. In multivariate analysis, STING intact expression emerged as an independent prognostic factor for increased survival. Instead, loss of β-catenin membranous expression status yielded a trend correlating with a higher risk of death.

An important finding of our study was the correlation of LKB1 loss with no/low β-catenin membranous expression observed in LUACs, both metastatic and non-metastatic. This correlation yielded significant implications in prognosis, as the survival analysis revealed that patients with concurrent LKB1 loss and no/low β-catenin membranous expression showed significant decreases in mOS and showed a higher risk of death (HR) compared to patients with LKB1 loss tumors and intact β-catenin membranous expression.

Our results are in accordance with data from a recent paper investigating the contribution of four missense LKB1 somatic mutations in the biology of the tumor. The researchers showed that LKB1R87K and, to a lesser extent, LKB1D194Y mutant isoform induced cell motility, promoting cytoskeleton regulation and β-catenin degradation and loss at the cell junctions in the 3D cultures [16].

β-catenin implements its structural function as a member of the catenins—proteins that link the key molecule of Ca^{2+}-dependent cell adhesion E-cadherin to cytoskeletal structures [57,58]. Several studies have highlighted the role of LKB1 metastasis, adhesion, and motility [33]. It has been shown that LKB1 serves as a focal adhesion kinase (FAK) repressor, where LKB1 depletion causes rapid focal adhesion site turnover [59] loss in cell polarity and motility through the regulation of PAK115 and the modulation of the phosphorylation status of FAK and CDC42 activation [60] and the contribution of LKB1 loss to the induction of epithelial–mesenchymal transition (EMT) and metastasis [33,34].

Although the results of the current study should be validated in the future, we consider that they are robust and in accordance with the literature. The weaknesses of the study are the retrospective nature of the analysis, the lack of a validation group, and the different management of patients after the surgical resection, since some of them have received adjuvant chemo- and/or radiotherapy while others have not. For this reason, an analysis of the Disease-Free Survival (DFS) was not performed, since this could be misleading. Furthermore, patients' samples were collected retrospectively even after 10 years, and several therapeutic improvements have been made during this period.

These results require further investigation in prospective studies. Despite this, the presented data provide a better understanding of the deregulations of key pathways downstream of LKB1 and of its substrates, which can expose weak points of LKB1 mutant tumors that may be therapeutically exploited to facilitate our understanding of the natural history of the disease. Immunohistochemical screening on FFPE tissue of both total LKB1 protein and AMPKthr172 as clinical biomarkers may provide an effective alternative approach to costly whole-gene or DNA-based sequencing, as it has the potential to capture most mechanisms conferring protein instability, loss-of-function mutations, and deletions, suggesting that protein degradation can be used as a means to identify the loss of LKB1 in cancer.

5. Conclusions

In summary, the results of the present study provide insights into the NSCLC tumors with the LKB1-less phenotype and KRAS co-mutations. Investigating the loss of LKB1 expression may have significant "theranostic" implications in the management of patients with operable NSCLC, and the investigation of LKB1 loss could be a step forward in the procedure of precision medicine in lung cancer. The expression status of LKB1 in association with STING and β-catenin membranous expression status could be used as stratification factors for patients with operable NSCLC.

Supplementary Materials: The following supporting information can be downloaded at: https://www.mdpi.com/article/10.3390/cancers16101818/s1.

Author Contributions: Conceptualization, E.D.L., A.V.K., M.S., C.P., J.S. and A.V.; methodology, E.D.L., M.T. (Maria Trypaki), E.T. and G.F.; software, E.D.L., G.C.M., K.M., E.Y. and D.H.; validation, E.D.L. and A.V.K.; formal analysis, E.D.L., A.V.K. and J.S.; resources, V.G., J.S., D.M. and M.T. (Maria Tzardi); data curation, E.D.L., A.V.K. and J.S.; writing—original draft preparation, E.D.L. and A.V.K.; writing—review and editing, E.D.L. and D.K.; visualization, E.D.L., A.V.K. and J.S.; supervision, E.D.L., V.G., J.S., E.N.S. and A.V.K.; project administration, E.D.L., A.V.K. and J.S.; funding acquisition, J.S. and V.G. All authors have read and agreed to the published version of the manuscript.

Funding: This study was partially supported by grants from the Cretan Association for Biomedical Research (CABR), the Hellenic Oncology Research Group (HORG), and the Hellenic Society of Medical Oncology (HeSMO). Grant funds from CABR, HORG, and HESMO were used to purchase all the required immunohistochemistry and RT-PCR products/reagents. The aforementioned associations had no involvement in the study design, data collection, analysis and interpretation of the data, the writing, or the decision to submit the article for publication.

Institutional Review Board Statement: The study was conducted in accordance with the Declaration of Helsinki and approved by the Institutional Review Board of the University Hospital of Heraklion, Heraklion, Greece (reference number: 4630/30-04-2010, approval date 28-06-2010).

Informed Consent Statement: Informed consent was obtained from all subjects involved in the study.

Data Availability Statement: The data that support the findings of this study are available from the corresponding author, E.L., upon reasonable request.

Acknowledgments: We would like to acknowledge CABR, HORG, and HeSMO, since without their financial support this work would have not been realized. We feel grateful to all the personnel of the Translational Oncology Laboratory of Heraklion Medical School, for their various contributions to this project, and to Mesdame Maria Klinaki for her technical assistance. Finally, we feel much obliged to Evangelia Tzouanaki for her valuable assistance in the collection of patients' clinical data.

Conflicts of Interest: The authors declare no conflicts of interest.

References

1. U.S. National Institutes of Health; National Cancer Institute. SEER Cancer Statistics Review. Available online: https://seer.cancer.gov/csr/ (accessed on 15 January 2024).
2. Global Cancer Observatory, Larc. Available online: https://Gco.Iarc.Fr/Today/Data/Factsheets/Cancers/15-Lung-Fact-Sheet.Pdf (accessed on 20 January 2024).
3. Hemminki, A.; Markie, D.; Tomlinson, I.; Avizienyte, E.; Roth, S.; Loukola, A.; Bignell, G.; Warren, W.; Aminoff, M.; Höglund, P.; et al. A Serine/Threonine Kinase Gene Defective in Peutz–Jeghers Syndrome. *Nature* **1998**, *391*, 184–187. [CrossRef]
4. Hemminki, A.; Tomlinson, I.; Markie, D.; Järvinen, H.; Sistonen, P.; Björkqvist, A.-M.; Knuutila, S.; Salovaara, R.; Bodmer, W.; Shibata, D.; et al. Localization of a Susceptibility Locus for Peutz-Jeghers Syndrome to 19p Using Comparative Genomic Hybridization and Targeted Linkage Analysis. *Nat. Genet.* **1997**, *15*, 87–90. [CrossRef]
5. Wingo, S.N.; Gallardo, T.D.; Akbay, E.A.; Liang, M.-C.; Contreras, C.M.; Boren, T.; Shimamura, T.; Miller, D.S.; Sharpless, N.E.; Bardeesy, N.; et al. Somatic LKB1 Mutations Promote Cervical Cancer Progression. *PLoS ONE* **2009**, *4*, e5137. [CrossRef]
6. Sanchez-Cespedes, M.; Parrella, P.; Esteller, M.; Nomoto, S.; Trink, B.; Engles, J.M.; Westra, W.H.; Herman, J.G.; Sidransky, D. Inactivation of LKB1/STK11 Is a Common Event in Adenocarcinomas of the Lung. *Cancer Res.* **2002**, *62*, 3659–3662.
7. Hezel, A.F.; Gurumurthy, S.; Granot, Z.; Swisa, A.; Chu, G.C.; Bailey, G.; Dor, Y.; Bardeesy, N.; Depinho, R.A. Pancreatic LKB1 Deletion Leads to Acinar Polarity Defects and Cystic Neoplasms. *Mol. Cell. Biol.* **2008**, *28*, 2414–2425. [CrossRef]
8. Lizcano, J.M.; Göransson, O.; Toth, R.; Deak, M.; Morrice, N.A.; Boudeau, J.; Hawley, S.A.; Udd, L.; Mäkelä, T.P.; Hardie, D.G.; et al. LKB1 Is a Master Kinase That Activates 13 Kinases of the AMPK Subfamily, Including MARK/PAR-1. *EMBO J.* **2004**, *23*, 833–843. [CrossRef]
9. Zheng, F.; Yuan, X.; Chen, E.; Ye, Y.; Li, X.; Dai, Y. Methylation of STK11 Promoter Is a Risk Factor for Tumor Stage and Survival in Clear Cell Renal Cell Carcinoma. *Oncol. Lett.* **2017**, *14*, 3065–3070. [CrossRef]
10. Gill, R.K.; Yang, S.-H.; Meerzaman, D.; Mechanic, L.E.; Bowman, E.D.; Jeon, H.-S.; Roy Chowdhuri, S.; Shakoori, A.; Dracheva, T.; Hong, K.-M.; et al. Frequent Homozygous Deletion of the LKB1/STK11 Gene in Non-Small Cell Lung Cancer. *Oncogene* **2011**, *30*, 3784–3791. [CrossRef]
11. Lee, S.M.; Choi, J.E.; Na, Y.K.; Lee, E.J.; Lee, W.K.; Choi, Y.Y.; Yoon, G.S.; Jeon, H.-S.; Kim, D.S.; Park, J.Y. Genetic and Epigenetic Alterations of the LKB1 Gene and Their Associations with Mutations in TP53 and EGFR Pathway Genes in Korean Non-Small Cell Lung Cancers. *Lung Cancer* **2013**, *81*, 194–199. [CrossRef]
12. Tanwar, P.S.; Mohapatra, G.; Chiang, S.; Engler, D.A.; Zhang, L.; Kaneko-Tarui, T.; Ohguchi, Y.; Birrer, M.J.; Teixeira, J.M. Loss of LKB1 and PTEN Tumor Suppressor Genes in the Ovarian Surface Epithelium Induces Papillary Serous Ovarian Cancer. *Carcinogenesis* **2014**, *35*, 546–553. [CrossRef]
13. Li, J.; Liu, J.; Li, P.; Mao, X.; Li, W.; Yang, J.; Liu, P. Loss of LKB1 Disrupts Breast Epithelial Cell Polarity and Promotes Breast Cancer Metastasis and Invasion. *J. Exp. Clin. Cancer Res.* **2014**, *33*, 70. [CrossRef]
14. Yang, J.-Y.; Jiang, S.-H.; Liu, D.-J.; Yang, X.-M.; Huo, Y.-M.; Li, J.; Hua, R.; Zhang, Z.-G.; Sun, Y.-W. Decreased LKB1 Predicts Poor Prognosis in Pancreatic Ductal Adenocarcinoma. *Sci. Rep.* **2015**, *5*, 10575. [CrossRef]
15. Zhang, W.; Yin, L.; Song, G.; Han, X.; Yin, Z.; Luo, D. LKB1 Loss Cooperating with BRAF V600E Promotes Melanoma Cell Invasion and Migration by Up-Regulation MMP-2 via PI3K/Akt/mTOR Pathway. *Oncotarget* **2017**, *8*, 113847–113857. [CrossRef]
16. Granado-Martínez, P.; Garcia-Ortega, S.; González-Sánchez, E.; McGrail, K.; Selgas, R.; Grueso, J.; Gil, R.; Naldaiz-Gastesi, N.; Rhodes, A.C.; Hernandez-Losa, J.; et al. STK11 (LKB1) Missense Somatic Mutant Isoforms Promote Tumor Growth, Motility and Inflammation. *Commun. Biol.* **2020**, *3*, 366. [CrossRef]
17. Borzi, C.; Galli, G.; Ganzinelli, M.; Signorelli, D.; Vernieri, C.; Garassino, M.C.; Sozzi, G.; Moro, M. Beyond LKB1 Mutations in Non-Small Cell Lung Cancer: Defining LKB1less Phenotype to Optimize Patient Selection and Treatment. *Pharmaceuticals* **2020**, *13*, 385. [CrossRef]
18. Trojan, J.; Brieger, A.; Raedle, J.; Esteller, M.; Zeuzem, S. 5′-CpG Island Methylation of the LKB1/STK11 Promoter and Allelic Loss at Chromosome 19p13.3 in Sporadic Colorectal Cancer. *Gut* **2000**, *47*, 272–276. [CrossRef]
19. Zhang, W.; Li, X.; Song, G.; Luo, D. Prognostic Significance of LKB1 Promoter Methylation in Cutaneous Malignant Melanoma. *Oncol. Lett.* **2017**, *14*, 2075–2080. [CrossRef]
20. Lao, G.; Liu, P.; Wu, Q.; Zhang, W.; Liu, Y.; Yang, L.; Ma, C. Mir-155 Promotes Cervical Cancer Cell Proliferation through Suppression of Its Target Gene LKB1. *Tumour Biol.* **2014**, *35*, 11933–11938. [CrossRef]
21. Figueroa-González, G.; Carrillo-Hernández, J.F.; Perez-Rodriguez, I.; Cantú de León, D.; Campos-Parra, A.D.; Martínez-Gutiérrez, A.D.; Coronel-Hernández, J.; García-Castillo, V.; López-Camarillo, C.; Peralta-Zaragoza, O.; et al. Negative Regulation of Serine Threonine Kinase 11 (STK11) through miR-100 in Head and Neck Cancer. *Genes* **2020**, *11*, 1058. [CrossRef] [PubMed]
22. Krishnamurthy, N.; Goodman, A.M.; Barkauskas, D.A.; Kurzrock, R. STK11 Alterations in the Pan-Cancer Setting: Prognostic and Therapeutic Implications. *Eur. J. Cancer* **2021**, *148*, 215–229. [CrossRef] [PubMed]
23. Clinical Lung Cancer Genome Project (CLCGP); Network Genomic Medicine (NGM) A Genomics-Based Classification of Human Lung Tumors. *Sci. Transl. Med.* **2013**, *5*, 209ra153. [CrossRef]
24. Ghaffar, H.; Sahin, F.; Sanchez-Cepedes, M.; Su, G.H.; Zahurak, M.; Sidransky, D.; Westra, W.H. LKB1 Protein Expression in the Evolution of Glandular Neoplasia of the Lung. *Clin. Cancer Res.* **2003**, *9*, 2998–3003. [PubMed]
25. Matsumoto, S.; Iwakawa, R.; Takahashi, K.; Kohno, T.; Nakanishi, Y.; Matsuno, Y.; Suzuki, K.; Nakamoto, M.; Shimizu, E.; Minna, J.D.; et al. Prevalence and Specificity of LKB1 Genetic Alterations in Lung Cancers. *Oncogene* **2007**, *26*, 5911–5918. [CrossRef]

26. Shire, N.J.; Klein, A.B.; Golozar, A.; Collins, J.M.; Fraeman, K.H.; Nordstrom, B.L.; McEwen, R.; Hembrough, T.; Rizvi, N.A. STK11 (LKB1) Mutations in Metastatic NSCLC: Prognostic Value in the Real World. *PLoS ONE* **2020**, *15*, e0238358. [CrossRef] [PubMed]
27. Facchinetti, F.; Bluthgen, M.V.; Tergemina-Clain, G.; Faivre, L.; Pignon, J.-P.; Planchard, D.; Remon, J.; Soria, J.-C.; Lacroix, L.; Besse, B. LKB1/STK11 Mutations in Non-Small Cell Lung Cancer Patients: Descriptive Analysis and Prognostic Value. *Lung Cancer* **2017**, *112*, 62–68. [CrossRef]
28. El Osta, B.; Behera, M.; Kim, S.; Berry, L.D.; Sica, G.; Pillai, R.N.; Owonikoko, T.K.; Kris, M.G.; Johnson, B.E.; Kwiatkowski, D.J.; et al. Characteristics and Outcomes of Patients With Metastatic KRAS-Mutant Lung Adenocarcinomas: The Lung Cancer Mutation Consortium Experience. *J. Thorac. Oncol.* **2019**, *14*, 876–889. [CrossRef]
29. La Fleur, L.; Falk-Sörqvist, E.; Smeds, P.; Berglund, A.; Sundström, M.; Mattsson, J.S.; Brandén, E.; Koyi, H.; Isaksson, J.; Brunnström, H.; et al. Mutation Patterns in a Population-Based Non-Small Cell Lung Cancer Cohort and Prognostic Impact of Concomitant Mutations in KRAS and TP53 or STK11. *Lung Cancer* **2019**, *130*, 50–58. [CrossRef]
30. Li, Z.; Ding, B.; Xu, J.; Mao, K.; Zhang, P.; Xue, Q. Relevance of STK11 Mutations Regarding Immune Cell Infiltration, Drug Sensitivity, and Cellular Processes in Lung Adenocarcinoma. *Front. Oncol.* **2020**, *10*, 580027. [CrossRef]
31. Schabath, M.B.; Welsh, E.A.; Fulp, W.J.; Chen, L.; Teer, J.K.; Thompson, Z.J.; Engel, B.E.; Xie, M.; Berglund, A.E.; Creelan, B.C.; et al. Differential Association of STK11 and TP53 with KRAS Mutation-Associated Gene Expression, Proliferation and Immune Surveillance in Lung Adenocarcinoma. *Oncogene* **2016**, *35*, 3209–3216. [CrossRef]
32. Ji, H.; Ramsey, M.R.; Hayes, D.N.; Fan, C.; McNamara, K.; Kozlowski, P.; Torrice, C.; Wu, M.C.; Shimamura, T.; Perera, S.A.; et al. LKB1 Modulates Lung Cancer Differentiation and Metastasis. *Nature* **2007**, *448*, 807–810. [CrossRef]
33. Zhang, S.; Schafer-Hales, K.; Khuri, F.R.; Zhou, W.; Vertino, P.M.; Marcus, A.I. The Tumor Suppressor LKB1 Regulates Lung Cancer Cell Polarity by Mediating Cdc42 Recruitment and Activity. *Cancer Res.* **2008**, *68*, 740–748. [CrossRef]
34. Roy, B.C.; Kohno, T.; Iwakawa, R.; Moriguchi, T.; Kiyono, T.; Morishita, K.; Sanchez-Cespedes, M.; Akiyama, T.; Yokota, J. Involvement of LKB1 in Epithelial-Mesenchymal Transition (EMT) of Human Lung Cancer Cells. *Lung Cancer* **2010**, *70*, 136–145. [CrossRef]
35. Yao, Y.-H.; Cui, Y.; Qiu, X.-N.; Zhang, L.-Z.; Zhang, W.; Li, H.; Yu, J.-M. Attenuated LKB1-SIK1 Signaling Promotes Epithelial-Mesenchymal Transition and Radioresistance of Non-Small Cell Lung Cancer Cells. *Chin. J. Cancer* **2016**, *35*, 50. [CrossRef]
36. Skoulidis, F.; Byers, L.A.; Diao, L.; Papadimitrakopoulou, V.A.; Tong, P.; Izzo, J.; Behrens, C.; Kadara, H.; Parra, E.R.; Canales, J.R.; et al. Co-Occurring Genomic Alterations Define Major Subsets of KRAS-Mutant Lung Adenocarcinoma with Distinct Biology, Immune Profiles, and Therapeutic Vulnerabilities. *Cancer Discov.* **2015**, *5*, 860–877. [CrossRef]
37. Skoulidis, F.; Goldberg, M.E.; Greenawalt, D.M.; Hellmann, M.D.; Awad, M.M.; Gainor, J.F.; Schrock, A.B.; Hartmaier, R.J.; Trabucco, S.E.; Gay, L.; et al. STK11/LKB1 Mutations and PD-1 Inhibitor Resistance in KRAS-Mutant Lung Adenocarcinoma. *Cancer Discov.* **2018**, *8*, 822–835. [CrossRef]
38. Arbour, K.C.; Jordan, E.; Kim, H.R.; Dienstag, J.; Yu, H.A.; Sanchez-Vega, F.; Lito, P.; Berger, M.; Solit, D.B.; Hellmann, M.; et al. Effects of Co-Occurring Genomic Alterations on Outcomes in Patients with KRAS-Mutant Non-Small Cell Lung Cancer. *Clin. Cancer Res.* **2018**, *24*, 334–340. [CrossRef]
39. WHO Classification of Tumours Editorial Board. Thoracic Tumours. In *WHO Classification of Tumors Series*, 5th ed.; IARC Scientific Publications: Lyon, France, 2012; Volume 5.
40. Amin, M.B.; Greene, F.L.; Edge, S.B.; Compton, C.C.; Gershenwald, J.E.; Brookland, R.K.; Meyer, L.; Gress, D.M.; Byrd, D.R.; Winchester, D.P. The Eighth Edition AJCC Cancer Staging Manual: Continuing to Build a Bridge from a Population-Based to a More "Personalized" Approach to Cancer Staging. *CA Cancer J. Clin.* **2017**, *67*, 93–99. [CrossRef]
41. Calles, A.; Sholl, L.M.; Rodig, S.J.; Pelton, A.K.; Hornick, J.L.; Butaney, M.; Lydon, C.; Dahlberg, S.E.; Oxnard, G.R.; Jackman, D.M.; et al. Immunohistochemical Loss of LKB1 Is a Biomarker for More Aggressive Biology in KRAS-Mutant Lung Adenocarcinoma. *Clin. Cancer Res.* **2015**, *21*, 2851–2860. [CrossRef]
42. William, W.N.; Kim, J.-S.; Liu, D.D.; Solis, L.; Behrens, C.; Lee, J.J.; Lippman, S.M.; Kim, E.S.; Hong, W.K.; Wistuba, I.I.; et al. The Impact of Phosphorylated AMP-Activated Protein Kinase Expression on Lung Cancer Survival. *Ann. Oncol.* **2012**, *23*, 78–85. [CrossRef]
43. Lohinai, Z.; Dora, D.; Caldwell, C.; Rivard, C.J.; Suda, K.; Yu, H.; Rivalland, G.; Ellison, K.; Rozeboom, L.; Dziadziuszko, R.; et al. Loss of STING Expression Is Prognostic in Non-Small Cell Lung Cancer. *J. Surg. Oncol.* **2022**, *125*, 1042–1052. [CrossRef]
44. Olivares-Hernández, A.; Del Barco Morillo, E.; Miramontes-González, J.P.; Figuero-Pérez, L.; Pérez-Belmonte, L.; Martín-Vallejo, J.; Martín-Gómez, T.; Escala-Cornejo, R.; Vidal-Tocino, R.; Hernández, L.B.; et al. Immunohistochemical Assessment of the P53 Protein as a Predictor of Non-Small Cell Lung Cancer Response to Immunotherapy. *Front. Biosci. (Landmark Ed.)* **2022**, *27*, 88. [CrossRef] [PubMed]
45. Brambilla, E.; Moro, D.; Gazzeri, S.; Brambilla, C. Alterations of Expression of Rb, P16(INK4A) and Cyclin D1 in Non-Small Cell Lung Carcinoma and Their Clinical Significance. *J. Pathol.* **1999**, *188*, 351–360. [CrossRef]
46. Filipits, M.; Pirker, R.; Dunant, A.; Lantuejoul, S.; Schmid, K.; Huynh, A.; Haddad, V.; André, F.; Stahel, R.; Pignon, J.-P.; et al. Cell Cycle Regulators and Outcome of Adjuvant Cisplatin-Based Chemotherapy in Completely Resected Non-Small-Cell Lung Cancer: The International Adjuvant Lung Cancer Trial Biologic Program. *J. Clin. Oncol.* **2007**, *25*, 2735–2740. [CrossRef]
47. Gazzeri, S.; Gouyer, V.; Vour'ch, C.; Brambilla, C.; Brambilla, E. Mechanisms of p16INK4A Inactivation in Non Small-Cell Lung Cancers. *Oncogene* **1998**, *16*, 497–504. [CrossRef]

48. Donnem, T.; Al-Saad, S.; Al-Shibli, K.; Andersen, S.; Busund, L.-T.; Bremnes, R.M. Prognostic Impact of Platelet-Derived Growth Factors in Non-Small Cell Lung Cancer Tumor and Stromal Cells. *J. Thorac. Oncol.* **2008**, *3*, 963–970. [CrossRef]
49. Kristiansen, G.; Schlüns, K.; Yongwei, Y.; Denkert, C.; Dietel, M.; Petersen, I. CD24 Is an Independent Prognostic Marker of Survival in Nonsmall Cell Lung Cancer Patients. *Br. J. Cancer* **2003**, *88*, 231–236. [CrossRef]
50. Pajares, M.J.; Agorreta, J.; Larrayoz, M.; Vesin, A.; Ezponda, T.; Zudaire, I.; Torre, W.; Lozano, M.D.; Brambilla, E.; Brambilla, C.; et al. Expression of Tumor-Derived Vascular Endothelial Growth Factor and Its Receptors Is Associated with Outcome in Early Squamous Cell Carcinoma of the Lung. *J. Clin. Oncol.* **2012**, *30*, 1129–1136. [CrossRef]
51. Hommura, F.; Furuuchi, K.; Yamazaki, K.; Ogura, S.; Kinoshita, I.; Shimizu, M.; Moriuchi, T.; Katoh, H.; Nishimura, M.; Dosaka-Akita, H. Increased Expression of Beta-Catenin Predicts Better Prognosis in Nonsmall Cell Lung Carcinomas. *Cancer* **2002**, *94*, 752–758. [CrossRef]
52. Koumaki, D.; Kostakis, G.; Koumaki, V.; Papadogeorgakis, N.; Makris, M.; Katoulis, A.; Kamakari, S.; Koutsodontis, G.; Perisanidis, C.; Lambadiari, V.; et al. Novel Mutations of the HRAS Gene and Absence of Hotspot Mutations of the BRAF Genes in Oral Squamous Cell Carcinoma in a Greek Population. *Oncol. Rep.* **2012**, *27*, 1555–1560. [CrossRef]
53. Kalikaki, A.; Koutsopoulos, A.; Trypaki, M.; Souglakos, J.; Stathopoulos, E.; Georgoulias, V.; Mavroudis, D.; Voutsina, A. Comparison of EGFR and K-RAS Gene Status between Primary Tumours and Corresponding Metastases in NSCLC. *Br. J. Cancer* **2008**, *99*, 923–929. [CrossRef]
54. Saridaki, Z.; Tzardi, M.; Sfakianaki, M.; Papadaki, C.; Voutsina, A.; Kalykaki, A.; Messaritakis, I.; Mpananis, K.; Mavroudis, D.; Stathopoulos, E.; et al. BRAFV600E Mutation Analysis in Patients with Metastatic Colorectal Cancer (mCRC) in Daily Clinical Practice: Correlations with Clinical Characteristics, and Its Impact on Patients' Outcome. *PLoS ONE* **2013**, *8*, e84604. [CrossRef] [PubMed]
55. Nagata, D.; Mogi, M.; Walsh, K. AMP-Activated Protein Kinase (AMPK) Signaling in Endothelial Cells Is Essential for Angiogenesis in Response to Hypoxic Stress. *J. Biol. Chem.* **2003**, *278*, 31000–31006. [CrossRef] [PubMed]
56. Kitajima, S.; Ivanova, E.; Guo, S.; Yoshida, R.; Campisi, M.; Sundararaman, S.K.; Tange, S.; Mitsuishi, Y.; Thai, T.C.; Masuda, S.; et al. Suppression of STING Associated with LKB1 Loss in KRAS-Driven Lung Cancer. *Cancer Discov.* **2019**, *9*, 34–45. [CrossRef]
57. Kline, E.R.; Shupe, J.; Gilbert-Ross, M.; Zhou, W.; Marcus, A.I. LKB1 Represses Focal Adhesion Kinase (FAK) Signaling via a FAK-LKB1 Complex to Regulate FAK Site Maturation and Directional Persistence. *J. Biol. Chem.* **2013**, *288*, 17663–17674. [CrossRef] [PubMed]
58. Ozawa, M.; Baribault, H.; Kemler, R. The Cytoplasmic Domain of the Cell Adhesion Molecule Uvomorulin Associates with Three Independent Proteins Structurally Related in Different Species. *EMBO J.* **1989**, *8*, 1711–1717. [CrossRef]
59. Konen, J.; Wilkinson, S.; Lee, B.; Fu, H.; Zhou, W.; Jiang, Y.; Marcus, A.I. LKB1 Kinase-Dependent and -Independent Defects Disrupt Polarity and Adhesion Signaling to Drive Collagen Remodeling during Invasion. *Mol. Biol. Cell* **2016**, *27*, 1069–1084. [CrossRef]
60. Park, S.Y.; Guo, X. Adaptor Protein Complexes and Intracellular Transport. *Biosci. Rep.* **2014**, *34*, e00123. [CrossRef]

cancers

MDPI

Article

Pulmonary Metastasectomy for Adrenocortical Carcinoma—Not If, but When †

Shamus R. Carr [1,*], Frank Villa Hernandez [2], Diana Grace Varghese [3], Hyoyoung Choo-Wosoba [4], Seth M. Steinberg [4], Martha E. Teke [2], Jaydira Del Rivero [3], David S. Schrump [1] and Chuong D. Hoang [1,*]

1 Thoracic Surgery Branch, Center for Cancer Research, National Cancer Institute, National Institutes of Health, Bethesda, MD 20892, USA; schrumpd@mail.nih.gov

2 Surgical Oncology Program, Center for Cancer Research, National Cancer Institute, National Institutes of Health, Bethesda, MD 20892, USA; frank.villahernandez@nih.gov (F.V.H.); martha.teke@utsouthwestern.edu (M.E.T.)

3 Developmental Therapeutics Branch, National Cancer Institute, National Institutes of Health, Bethesda, MD 20892, USA; diana.varghese@nih.gov (D.G.V.)

4 Biostatistics and Data Management Section, Center for Cancer Research, National Cancer Institute, National Institutes of Health, Bethesda, MD 20892, USA

* Correspondence: shamus.carr@nih.gov (S.R.C.); chuong.hoang@nih.gov (C.D.H.)

† This was orally presented at the Southern Thoracic Surgical Association 70th Annual Meeting in Orlando, Florida from 2–5 November 2023.

Simple Summary: Adrenocortical carcinoma is a rare tumor with a very high propensity to metastasize to the lungs. There are limited systemic options once it does metastasize. Pulmonary metastasectomy has been utilized in these patients as part of a treatment paradigm. However, there is little information available to help guide patient selection for pulmonary metastasectomy. Herein, our experience treating adrenocortical patients with only lung metastases was reviewed to try and identify associations between different variables (e.g., number of metastases, time to resection) and outcomes. The results demonstrated that, unlike other malignancies, the total number of nodules should not preclude patients who have adequate pulmonary reserve. Additionally, the time from original surgery to the development of lung metastases may have prognostic implications. Future work should focus on identifying genetic markers associated with outcomes that can be used independently or in combination with other clinical variables.

Abstract: Background: Adrenocortical carcinoma (ACC) commonly metastasizes to the lungs, and pulmonary metastasectomy (PM) is utilized due to limited systemic options. Methods: All ACC patients with initially only lung metastases (LM) from a single institution constituted this observational case series. Kaplan-Meier and Cox proportional hazard analyses evaluated the association with potential prognostic factors and outcomes. Overall survival (OS) was calculated from the date of the PM or, in those patients who did not undergo surgery, from the development of LM. Results: A total of 75 ACC patients over a 45-year period met the criteria; 52 underwent PM, and 23 did not. The patients undergoing PM had a median OS of 3.1 years (95% CI: 2.4, 4.7 years) with the 5- and 10-year OS being 35.5% and 32.8%, respectively. The total resected LM did not impact the OS nor the DFS. The patients who developed LM after 11 months from the initial ACC resection had an improved OS (4.2 years; 95% CI: 3.2, NR; $p = 0.0096$) compared to those developing metastases earlier (2.4 years; 95% CI: 1.6, 2.8). Patients who underwent PM within 11 months of adrenalectomy demonstrated a reduced OS (2.2 years; 95% CI: 1.0, 2.7) compared to those after 11 months (3.6 years, 95% CI: 2.6, NR; $p = 0.0045$). PM may provide benefit to those patients with LM at presentation (HR: 0.5; $p = 0.2827$), with the time to first PM as a time-varying covariate. Conclusions: PM appears to have a role in ACC patients. The number of nodules should not be an exclusion factor. Patients developing LM within a year of primary tumor resection may benefit from waiting before further surgeries, which may provide additional insight into who may benefit from PM.

Keywords: adrenocortical cancer; pulmonary metastasectomy; survival; observational case series

1. Introduction

Despite initial questions about the utility of pulmonary metastasectomy (PM) as part of the treatment paradigm of lung metastases [1], this treatment option has been routinely recommended for decades [2–5]. Recently, the role of PM, specifically in colorectal cancer (CRC), has again been questioned [6,7]. However, in the treatment of CRC there exist systemic therapies that appear to rival PM in terms of overall survival (OS). While many other cancers develop lung metastases, extrapolating treatment strategies across tumor types should be avoided.

Adrenocortical carcinoma (ACC) is a rare disease where a large proportion of patients will develop recurrence or metastatic disease, with the lungs being the most common metastatic site (40–80%) [8,9]. This is compounded by few efficacious systemic therapy options for metastatic disease [10–13]. Some early studies suggested that PM could be considered an effective treatment option for patients with isolated lung metastases from ACC [14]. Further single-arm retrospective studies supported this claim, but none provide any insight into variables that affect outcomes when considering PM [15–17]. Repeat PM in ACC cases is lauded to benefit OS, but there are few studies with very few patients [18–21]. Thus, whether a true benefit exists remains unclear.

In 2011, our group published a review of twenty-six ACC patients who only had lung metastases and underwent PM [16]. At the time, it was one of the most comprehensive reviews of PM for ACC. We re-examined these patients, along with all new patients through 2022 to determine if our prior conclusions remained valid and if further insights could be gained regarding the management of these patients.

2. Methods

2.1. Data Collection

An observational case series review identified all patients diagnosed with ACC at the National Cancer Institute, Bethesda, Maryland, between 1977 and 2022 who had either (1) only lung metastases at the time of ACC diagnosis or (2) developed lung metastases as the initial site of recurrence. Patients whose first site of metastases was outside the lung were excluded. Medical records were reviewed and analyzed for patient demographics (Table 1), date of diagnosis and primary ACC resection, date of initial identification of lung metastases, date of PM, number of nodules resected, functional status of primary ACC tumor, date of recurrence, date(s) of re-recurrence or re-operative surgery, complications and length of stay after re-operative surgery, neoadjuvant and adjuvant chemotherapy for either primary ACC or lung metastases, overall survival (OS), disease-free survival (DFS), and progression-free survival (PFS). All the patients were enrolled in various Institutional Review Board-approved investigational protocols from either the National Institutes of Diabetes and Digestive and Kidney Disease (NIDDK) or the National Cancer Institute (NCI). Written informed consent was obtained prior to any interventions, as per protocol for participation in these clinical studies. The sharing of deidentified data can be considered after contact with the corresponding author.

Table 1. Patient demographics.

Variable	No. (%)
Feature:	
Sex, M/F	16/59
Age at primary adrenalectomy, non-PM group, median, years (range)	50 (27–59)
Age at primary adrenalectomy, PM group, median, years (range)	41 (9–68)
Age at first PM, median, years (range)	45 (9–72)
Number of lung metastases, median (range)	8 (1–75)
Pulmonary Metastasectomy:	

Table 1. *Cont.*

Variable	No. (%)
Yes	52 (69)
1–2 PMs	33 (63)
3–5 PMs	16 (31)
5–7 PMs	3 (6)
No	23 (31)
Hormonal Status at Presentation:	
Functional	41 (55)
Hypercortisolism	26 (63)
Hyperaldosteronism	8 (20)
Virilization	5 (12)
Feminization	2 (5)
Nonfunctional	31 (41)
Unknown	3 (4)
Systemic Therapy:	
Yes	71 (95)
No	4 (5)
Systemic Therapy PM Group:	
Induction Chemotherapy	5 (10)
Adjuvant Chemotherapy	46 (88)
Systemic Therapy Non-PM Group:	
Yes	23 (100)

2.2. Statistical Analysis

The OS for those patients who underwent PM was defined as the time until death or until the last follow-up after the first PM. The DFS and PFS were similarly defined as the length of time with no evidence of metastases after the first resection without a subsequent resection, or the length of time with evidence of metastases after the first resection without a subsequent resection, respectively. For the patients who underwent planned staged bilateral PM, the date of the second operation was used as the starting point for these calculations. In those who did not undergo PM, the starting point for OS was the initial identification of lung metastases.

Among all the patients, our analyses were based on quartiles of time between the initial ACC diagnosis and the initial lung metastases, which were defined as follows: Q1 $\leq$ 4.5 days; Q2 > 4.5 days and $\leq$326 days; Q3 > 326 days and $\leq$940 days; and Q4 > 940 days. Some analyses included only patients who underwent PM and were categorized into four equal-sized groups by quartiles of days between ACC diagnosis and the first pulmonary metastasis resection. These quartiles were defined as follows: Q1 $\leq$ 327.5 days; Q2 > 327.5 days and $\leq$947.5 days; Q3 > 947.5 days and $\leq$1875.5 days; and Q4 > 1875.5 days. Also, among those who underwent PM, an analysis of the total number of metastases resected was carried out, evaluated in four groups determined to make the sample sizes for each group as equal as possible. The following groups were defined: Q1 = 1; Q2 = 2 or 3; Q3 $\geq$ 4 and $\leq$10; and Q4 $\geq$ 11.

Kaplan-Meier (K-M) plots with medians and numbers at risk were provided. Survival probabilities with 95% confidence intervals (CIs) were provided at specific time points of corresponding outcomes as well. The *p*-values corresponding to K–M plots were exact, based on 100,000 random permutations.

In our analyses of the effect of a first PM following the diagnosis of lung metastases among all the patients, Cox proportional hazards modeling was used to estimate the hazard ratio (HR) of this factor, which was treated as a time-varying covariate, and determine the corresponding 95% CI for the HR. A similar analysis was carried out to ascertain the impact of a second metastatic resection among those who had an initial pulmonary resection.

It should be noted that all the statistical results for the analyses should be interpreted as exploratory, including interpreting p-values in this context. In analyses where the quartiles were combined after examining the initial results, the p-value reported was adjusted by multiplying by three to account for the implicit multiple comparisons resulting from reducing the categories from four to two groups (e.g., obtaining 0.0045 = 0.0015 (raw p-value) × 3). A statistical analysis was performed using SAS version 9.4 for Windows (Cary, NC, USA) and R version 4.1.1.

3. Results

A total of 80 patients were identified between 1977 and 2022. Fifty-two patients underwent at least one PM as part of their treatment. The remaining 28 patients did not undergo PM, 5 of whom were excluded due to a lack of information or failure to meet the inclusion criteria. The 23 patients who did not undergo PM did so for two main reasons: patient choice or poor pulmonary status. This resulted in a total of seventy-five patients, of which all but four received standard-of-care chemotherapy. Of these patients, 20 were part of the analysis from our institution published in 2011 [16]. The majority of operations consisted in open thoracotomy with a Perelman technique to preserve lung parenchyma [22]. However, VATSs (video-assisted thoracic surgery) with stapled wedge resections were also employed at the discretion of the surgeon (Figure S1).

3.1. All Patients

Overall survival was evaluated in all 75 patients using the time interval between the primary ACC diagnosis and the initial development of lung metastases as a time-varying covariate. There was a potential difference in the OS between the four quartiles: Q1 ≤ 4.5 days; Q2 > 4.5 days and ≤326 days; Q3 > 326 days and ≤940 days; and Q4 > 940 days (Figure 1a, $p = 0.0309$). It was noted that the OS probabilities in Q1 and Q2 seemed similar, with respect to the median OS, while Q3 and Q4 appeared to have similar but higher median OS times (Table 2). The re-categorization into two groups of Q1–Q2 and Q3–Q4 is shown in the K–M plots (Figure 1b, $p = 0.0096$). It is noticeable that the overall survival distributions are different between these re-categorized two groups, with corresponding small p-values ($p = 0.0096$).

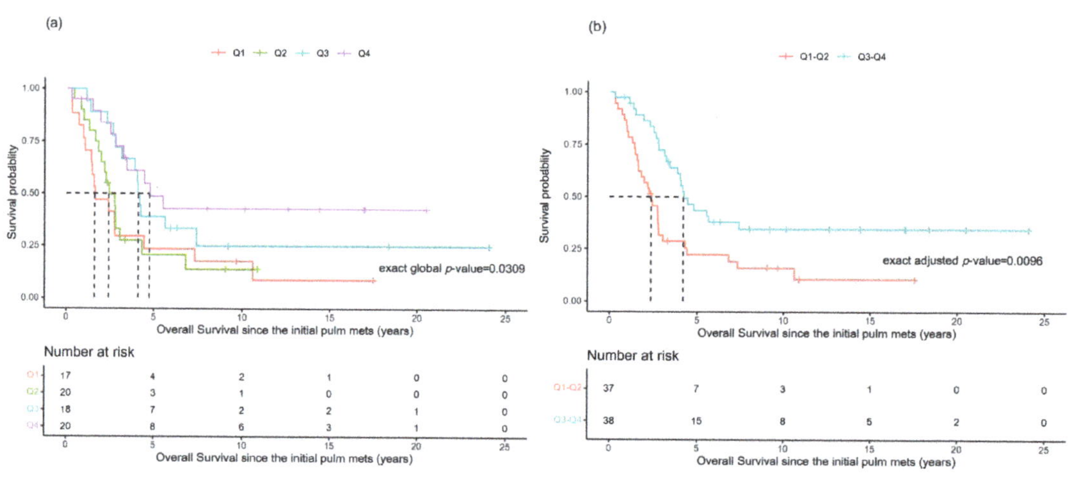

Figure 1. Overall survival based upon the time to the initial identification of lung metastases. Kaplan-Meier plots for the overall survival (OS) of patients based upon the time between the primary ACC diagnosis and the initial identification of lung metastases ($Time_{diag-initPM}$) grouped by quartiles (**a**) or re-categorized as Q1–Q2 versus Q3–Q4 (**b**).

Table 2. Overall survival (OS) from ACC diagnosis until development of lung metastases.

	Median (95% CI)						*p*-Value [a]	
	Q1	**Q2**	**Q3**	**Q4**	**Q1–Q2**	**Q3–Q4**	**Global** [b]	**As Grouped** [c]
OS (years)	1.6 (0.9, 4.4)	2.4 (1.6, 3.0)	4.1 (2.8, 7.4)	4.8 (2.8, -)	2.4 (1.6, 2.8)	4.2 (3.2, -)	0.031	0.0096 (0.0032)

[a] an exact log rank *p*-value is derived from 100,000 random permutations. [b] a global test-based *p*-value is based on a test for the null hypothesis of equal survival distributions among all four groups. [c] a Bonferroni-based adjusted *p*-value with raw *p*-value in parentheses. Quartiles defined as follows: Q1 $\leq$ 4.5 days; Q2 > 4.5 days and $\leq$326 days; Q3 > 326 days and $\leq$940 days; and Q4 > 940 days.

Additionally, a Cox proportional hazard analysis was performed to assess if there was any statistical difference in the hazard rates for the OS associated with the time-varying covariate of the first PM within each of the quartiles as defined by time from ACC diagnosis to the appearance of lung metastases. No statistically meaningful associations were found; there was no noticeable difference in the HR based on the patients with and without a first metastasis resection for any subgroup (Table 3). It could be noted that, in the 17 patients included in Q1, there was a potential effect of the benefit of an initial metastasis resection among those having initial pulmonary metastases at the same time as their primary ACC diagnosis (HR = 0.50; $p = 0.28$). This observation is based on a limited number of patients and would need to be interpreted cautiously.

Table 3. Hazard ratios if pulmonary metastasectomy was performed based upon the time patients took to develop lung metastases.

Quartiles Subgroups	N [a]	N_{yes} [b]	N_{no} [c]	HR [d]	*p*-Value [e]
Q1	17	7	10	0.50	0.2827
Q2	20	13	7	1.36	0.5588
Q3	18	16	2	1.33	0.7287
Q4	20	16	4	0.99	0.9838
Q1–Q2	37	20	17	0.90	0.7899
Q3–Q4	38	32	6	1.20	0.7212

Q1: $Time_{diag-initPM} \leq 4.5$ days; Q2: 4.5 days < $Time_{diag-initPM} \leq 326$ days; Q3: 326 days < $Time_{diag-initPM} \leq$ 940.50 days; and Q4: $Time_{diag-initPM} > 940.50$ days. [a] the number of patients used within the subgroup. [b] the number of patients undertaking their first metastasis resection at the end of the study. [c] the number of patients not undertaking their first metastasis resection at the end of the study the number of patients not undertaking the first metastasis resection at the end of the study. [d] estimated hazard ratio derived from a Cox proportional hazard model with the first metastasis resection indicator as a time-varying covariate within the subgroup. [e] *p*-value derived from a Cox proportional hazard model with the first metastasis resection indicator as a time-varying covariate within the subgroup.

3.2. Patients Undergoing PM

Analyses restricted to the 52 patients undergoing PM demonstrated a median OS of 3.1 years (95% CI: 2.4, 4.7 years) from the time of PM (Table 4). The survival probability decreased quite rapidly and then stabilized, resulting in OS at 5 and 10 years after PM of 35.5% and 32.8%, respectively. The median DFS and PFS after PM were 1.5 years and 3 months, respectively.

When grouped in quartiles according to the time between the primary ACC resection and the first pulmonary metastasis resection, the survival distributions of the OS appeared to be potentially different among the four groups (Figure 2a), with Q1 seemingly having a much shorter OS, as there were no survivors after 5 years, compared with the other groups. Thus, re-categorizing into two groups, Q1 versus Q2–Q4 (Figure 2b), demonstrated a significant survival difference ($p = 0.0045$). The median OS for Q1 was 2.2 years (95% CI: 1.0, 2.7), and for Q2–Q4 it was 3.6 years (95% CI: 2.6, NR).

Table 4. Survival analysis summary of only patients undergoing pulmonary metastasectomy.

Outcome	Median (95% CI)	Survival Probability (95% CI)	
OS	3.1 years (2.4, 4.7)	5 years 35.5% (22.3%, 49.0%)	10 years 32.8% (19.8%, 46.4%)
DFS	1.5 years (0.7, 2.2)	1 year 57.1% (33.8%, 74.9%)	2 years 33.3% (14.9%, 53.1%)
PFS	3.0 months (1.9, 9.9)	6 months 39.7% (22.5%, 56.5%)	12 months 27.8% (12.9%, 44.9%)

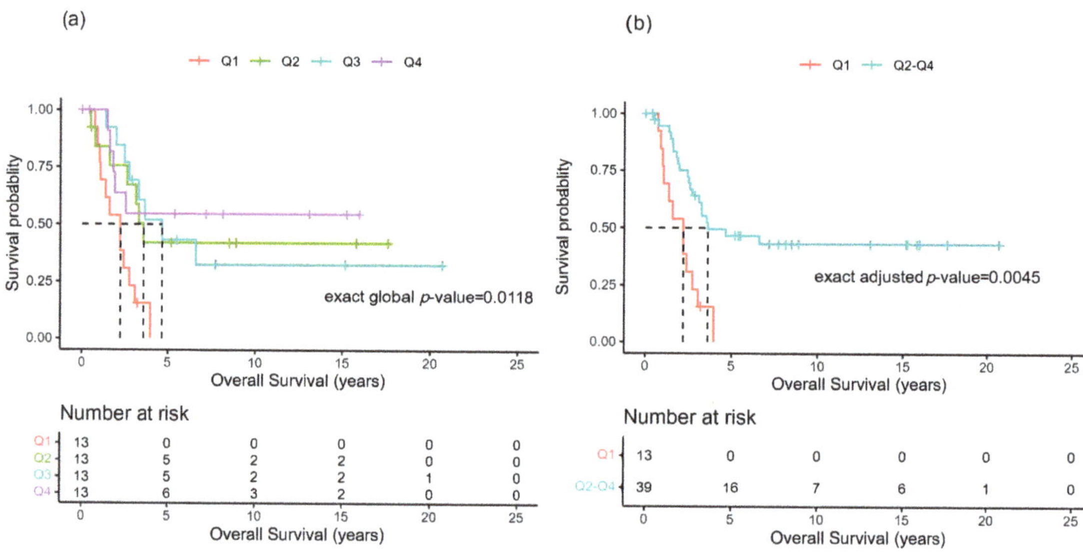

Figure 2. Overall survival after pulmonary metastasectomy. Kaplan-Meier plots for the overall survival (OS) of patients undergoing pulmonary metastasectomy grouped by quartiles of the time interval between the primary resection of ACC and the initial PM resection ($Time_{resc-initPM}$) (**a**) or re-categorized as Q1 versus Q2–Q4 (**b**).

The median number of PM resected per patient was eight (range 1–75). The grouping of the patients into four groups of approximately equal sample sizes revealed that there was no difference in the OS (Figure 3; $p = 0.71$), DFS ($p = 0.18$), or PFS ($p = 0.19$). Lastly, the patients undergoing PM were analyzed based upon the functional status of the primary tumor. These results do not demonstrate any recognizable differences in the distributions of the OS, DFI, or PFS, reflected by corresponding large p-values between those with and without functional ACC tumors.

Cox proportional hazard model analysis was used to test whether the OS differed according to whether the patients did or did not experience an additional metastasis resection. This factor was considered as a time-varying covariate in the model since subsequent resections may take place at various times after pulmonary metastasis diagnosis. The test resulted in a hazard ratio of about 0.66, with a corresponding p-value of 0.27. This implied that the hazard rate in the patients with a subsequent metastasis resection was about 34% lower on average than in the patients with only a primary PM. However, this magnitude of the difference in hazard rates might not indicate much of an effect, with a relatively large p-value (>0.2).

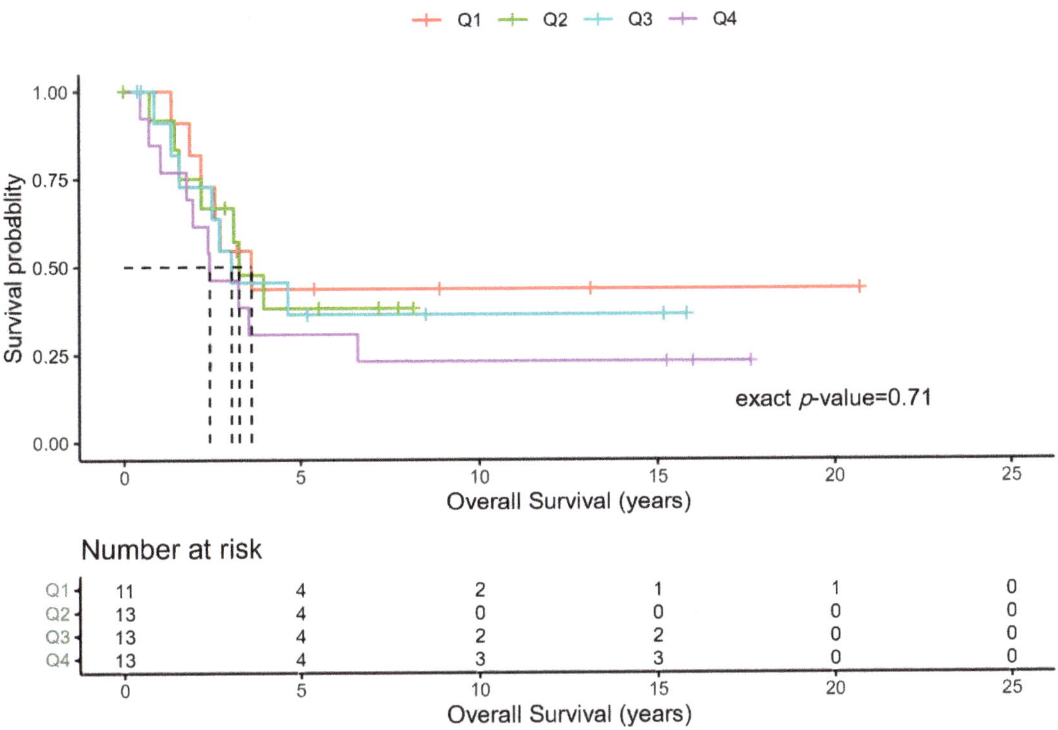

Figure 3. Overall survival by total number of resected lung metastases. Kaplan-Meier plots of the overall survival for the total number of initial lung metastases resected grouped by quartiles (N_{initPM}).

4. Comment

It is not uncommon for ACC to initially present with distant metastatic disease to the lungs. In addition, 40–80% of patients with ACC who do not have stage IV disease at presentation will develop pulmonary metastases [8,9]. Compounding the situation are limited efficacious options for systemic treatment [13,23]. Systemic therapy consists of either mitotane alone or in combination with other cytotoxic therapies [11,13,24,25]. Nevertheless, response rates are poor. These factors combined have propelled the consideration of surgical resection (PM and repeat PM) as part of the treatment paradigm for ACC when pulmonary metastatic disease is identified, despite limited evidence in the literature [14,16–18,24,26].

Understanding the actual survival and recurrence rates of patients with metastatic ACC is complex. Nearly all publications include heterogenous grouping of patients with the two most common sites of metastases: lung and liver. In these studies, the reported median survival after undergoing resection of metastatic disease is between 14 and 30 months [16–18,26]. A disease-free interval (DFI) of less than 12 months is associated with poor survival [17]. Another factor that negatively affects outcome includes the development of abdominal metastases [9]. Therefore, in order to better understand and more optimally guide the management of ACC patients with lung metastases, it is important to look solely at a homogenous population of patients with metastatic or recurrent disease confined to the lungs in the absence of extrathoracic recurrence. Findings gleaned from this selective cohort may enhance our understanding of what treatment options should be offered to patients.

We analyzed our 45-year single-institution experience to identify factors for improved patient selection and outcomes (OS). Our 2011 data suggested potential benefits of PM in well-chosen patients [16]. This was based on 26 patients, including 6 with concurrent extrapulmonary disease during PM. Neither adjuvant nor neoadjuvant chemotherapy were associated with an improved OS. Limited by the sample size and a quarter of patients having extrathoracic metastases, more definitive conclusions could not be drawn. Yet, the 5-year actuarial survival of 41% was consistent with the 35.5% that we now report.

Disease-free interval has been shown in many histologies as an influential factor associated with outcomes [5,27]; ACC is no different. However, non-ACC histologies with improved outcomes are usually associated with a DFI greater than 2 years. Our results (Figure 2) and others demonstrate that a DFI of at least 11 months in ACC is associated with an improved OS [17]. However, this study included patients with local and distant recurrence. Our results imply that those patients with only lung metastases who undergo an initial PM within 11 months of their primary ACC tumor resection are expected to have about a 1.4 year shorter median OS than those who undergo PM after 11 months. This does not mean that delaying PM improves the OS but may indicate that a delay before PM provides improved identification of either lung metastases or local recurrence. This period of observation indirectly acts as a surrogate evaluation of an individual tumor biology, allowing improved selection of patients in whom PM will be of benefit. In other words, are the initially seen lung metastases the complete picture or just the "tip of the iceberg"?

Yet, careful consideration of patients who have metastatic disease at the initial presentation of their primary tumor compared to those who develop lung metastases within 11 months does show a difference. In fact, patients with lung metastases at the time of initial presentation of their ACC tumor who undergo PM have a 50% lower hazard ratio compared with the patients who did not (Table 3). However, the p-value is relatively large, and there is a relatively large standard error for the HR estimate of 0.5. Further scrutiny of the results in Table 3 could be interpreted as not having a survival advantage to patients who undergo PM, regardless of the timing. However, the actual OS (Table 4) demonstrates a 5-year survival of 35.5% where it plateaus and remains essentially unchanged for up to 10 years (32.8%) in those undergoing PM in our study of patients accrued over 45 years. Yet, due to the small number of patients in various groups who did not undergo any resection due to an implicit selection bias for surgery, definitive conclusions with respect to recommendations about who should and should not undergo PM are still lacking and require further study to include a genetic evaluation of both the primary tumor and lung metastases.

When considering PM, it is generally accepted that the total number of lung lesions is prognostic and indirectly associated with the outcomes, but this has not been explored previously in ACC. Most histologies find that a number greater than four pulmonary lesions tends to be associated with poor survival and that PM should not be recommended in these patients [5,28]. One possible exception may be in patients with primary sarcoma with 10 or more metastases among who there was an OS at 5 and 10 years of 26% and 17%, respectively [3]. Thus, ACC seems to be similar to sarcoma lung metastases in this regard. While the median number of metastatic lung nodules resected in our study was eight, the range was from one to seventy-five. When separating the patients into equal quartiles, there was no meaningful difference in the OS for patients with a single metastatic lung lesion or those with more than eleven lung metastases (Figure 3). Therefore, it appears that, if a patient has an adequate pulmonary reserve, the total number of lung lesions should not preclude PM.

Although this analysis provides an updated comprehensive evaluation of the role of PM in one of the largest single institutional experiences of patients with only pulmonary metastases from ACC, our analysis suffers from some key limitations. The retrospective nature of this study over 45 years and the limited sample size within groups continue to affect our findings. However, the majority of the patients in our study were treated in the past 15 years (Supplemental Figure S1), thus providing a contemporary perspective. While technology and surgical approaches have advanced during the time of this study, these likely had a limited impact on the outcomes. An important factor associated with long-term survival is the ability to resect all disease, whether by VATS or open-chest techniques. The other important factor is the inherent biology of the individual tumor, which is under investigation. Additionally, referral bias to our institution and implicit selection bias for surgery may also limit some of our conclusions.

5. Conclusions

ACC with lung metastases poses challenges due to limited systemic options and the absence of a genetic signature for guiding PM recommendations. It appears that there is a role for PM in ACC patients with isolated lung metastases based upon 5- and 10-year OS rates of 35.5% and 32.8%, respectively. The development of lung metastases after resection of the primary ACC tumor, especially in the first year, is associated with worse overall outcomes despite PM. A prudent strategy of careful surveillance may provide insight into individual tumor biology and help delineate those patients who would benefit from surgery. PM potentially extends a patient's OS when lung metastases appear more than a year after the primary ACC resection. The total number of nodules should not sway patient selection. For stage IV cases with only lung metastases at diagnosis, the role of PM is uncertain due to insufficient data. Future work should explore genetic and sequencing analyses to enhance treatment strategies.

Supplementary Materials: The following supporting information can be downloaded at https://www.mdpi.com/article/10.3390/cancers16040702/s1, Figure S1: Pulmonary Metastasectomies by Year.

Author Contributions: Conceptualization, S.R.C., F.V.H. and M.E.T.; methodology, S.R.C., J.D.R. and C.D.H.; software, H.C.-W. and S.M.S.; validation, H.C.-W. and S.M.S.; formal analysis, S.R.C., H.C.-W., C.D.H. and D.S.S.; investigation, F.V.H., D.G.V. and M.E.T.; resources, S.R.C., C.D.H. and D.S.S.; data curation, F.V.H., D.G.V., M.E.T. and S.R.C.; writing—original draft preparation, S.R.C.; writing—review and editing, J.D.R., D.S.S. and C.D.H.; visualization, S.R.C. and H.C.-W.; supervision, D.S.S. and S.M.S.; project administration, J.D.R. and C.D.H.; funding acquisition, C.D.H. and D.S.S. All authors have read and agreed to the published version of the manuscript.

Funding: This research was supported in part by the Intramural Research Program of the NIH (SRC), the NIH Intramural Grants (D.S.S.—ZIA BC 011115; C.D.H.—ZIA BC 011657), and the Stephen J. Solarz Memorial Fund Foundation for the National Institutes of Health.

Institutional Review Board Statement: All the patients were enrolled in the Institutional Review Board-approved investigational protocol NIH IRB: 06C0014. This is a continually reviewed and renewed protocol with most recent approval: 23 June 2020.

Informed Consent Statement: Written informed consent was obtained prior to any interventions, as per protocol for participation in these clinical studies.

Data Availability Statement: Data are contained within the article and supplementary materials.

Conflicts of Interest: The authors declare no conflicts of interest.

Abbreviations

ACC	adrenocortical carcinoma
CI	confidence interval
CRC	colorectal carcinoma
DFI	disease-free interval
DFS	disease-free survival
HR	hazard ratio
K-M	Kaplan-Meier
LM	lung metastases
NCI	National Cancer Institute
NIDDK	National Institutes of Diabetes and Digestive and Kidney Disease

OS	overall survival
PFS	progression-free survival
PM	pulmonary metastasectomy
Q1	first quartile
Q2	second quartile
Q3	third quartile
Q4	fourth quartile
VATS	video-assisted thoracoscopic surgery

References

1. Aberg, T.; Malmberg, K.A.; Nilsson, B.; Nöu, E. The Effect of Metastasectomy: Fact or Fiction? *Ann. Thorac. Surg.* **1980**, *30*, 378–384. [CrossRef]
2. Erhunmwunsee, L.; D'Amico, T.A. Surgical Management of Pulmonary Metastases. *Ann. Thorac. Surg.* **2009**, *88*, 2052–2060. [CrossRef] [PubMed]
3. Pastorino, U.; Buyse, M.; Friedel, G.; Ginsberg, R.J.; Girard, P.; Goldstraw, P.; Johnston, M.; McCormack, P.; Pass, H.; Putnam, J.B. Long-Term Results of Lung Metastasectomy: Prognostic Analyses Based on 5206 Cases. *J. Thorac. Cardiovasc. Surg.* **1997**, *113*, 37–49. [CrossRef]
4. Migliore, M.; Jakovic, R.; Hensens, A.; Klepetko, W. Extending Surgery for Pulmonary Metastasectomy: What Are the Limits? *J. Thorac. Oncol.* **2010**, *5* (Suppl. S2), S155–S160. [CrossRef] [PubMed]
5. Onaitis, M.W.; Petersen, R.P.; Haney, J.C.; Saltz, L.; Park, B.; Flores, R.; Rizk, N.; Bains, M.S.; Dycoco, J.; D'Amico, T.A.; et al. Prognostic Factors for Recurrence after Pulmonary Resection of Colorectal Cancer Metastases. *Ann. Thorac. Surg.* **2009**, *87*, 1684–1688. [CrossRef]
6. Treasure, T.; Farewell, V.; Macbeth, F.; Batchelor, T.; Milošević, M.; King, J.; Zheng, Y.; Leonard, P.; Williams, N.R.; Brew-Graves, C.; et al. The Pulmonary Metastasectomy in Colorectal Cancer Cohort Study: Analysis of Case Selection, Risk Factors and Survival in a Prospective Observational Study of 512 Patients. *Color. Dis.* **2021**, *23*, 1793–1803. [CrossRef] [PubMed]
7. Milosevic, M.; Edwards, J.; Tsang, D.; Dunning, J.; Shackcloth, M.; Batchelor, T.; Coonar, A.; Hasan, J.; Davidson, B.; Marchbank, A.; et al. Pulmonary Metastasectomy in Colorectal Cancer: Updated Analysis of 93 Randomized Patients—Control Survival Is Much Better than Previously Assumed. *Color. Dis.* **2020**, *22*, 1314–1324. [CrossRef]
8. Terzolo, M.; Berruti, A. Adjunctive Treatment of Adrenocortical Carcinoma. *Curr. Opin. Endocrinol. Diabetes Obes.* **2008**, *15*, 221–226. [CrossRef]
9. Glenn, J.A.; Else, T.; Hughes, D.T.; Cohen, M.S.; Jolly, S.; Giordano, T.J.; Worden, F.P.; Gauger, P.G.; Hammer, G.D.; Miller, B.S. Longitudinal Patterns of Recurrence in Patients with Adrenocortical Carcinoma. *Surgery* **2019**, *165*, 186–195. [CrossRef]
10. Kimpel, O.; Bedrose, S.; Megerle, F.; Berruti, A.; Terzolo, M.; Kroiss, M.; Mai, K.; Dekkers, O.M.; Habra, M.A.; Fassnacht, M. Adjuvant Platinum-Based Chemotherapy in Radically Resected Adrenocortical Carcinoma: A Cohort Study. *Br. J. Cancer* **2021**, *125*, 1233–1238. [CrossRef]
11. Megerle, F.; Kroiss, M.; Hahner, S.; Fassnacht, M. Advanced Adrenocortical Carcinoma—What to Do When First-Line Therapy Fails? *Exp. Clin. Endocr. Diab.* **2018**, *127*, 109–116. [CrossRef]
12. Megerle, F.; Herrmann, W.; Schloetelburg, W.; Ronchi, C.L.; Pulzer, A.; Quinkler, M.; Beuschlein, F.; Hahner, S.; Kroiss, M.; Fassnacht, M.; et al. Mitotane Monotherapy in Patients with Advanced Adrenocortical Carcinoma. *J. Clin. Endocrinol. Metab.* **2017**, *103*, 1686–1695. [CrossRef]
13. Fassnacht, M.; Terzolo, M.; Allolio, B.; Baudin, E.; Haak, H.; Berruti, A.; Welin, S.; Schade-Brittinger, C.; Lacroix, A.; Jarzab, B.; et al. Combination Chemotherapy in Advanced Adrenocortical Carcinoma. *N. Engl. J. Med.* **2012**, *366*, 2189–2197. [CrossRef] [PubMed]
14. Quiros, R.M.; Scott, W.J. Surgical Treatment of Metastatic Disease to the Lung. *Semin. Oncol.* **2008**, *35*, 134–146. [CrossRef]
15. Icard, P.; Goudet, P.; Charpenay, C.; Andreassian, B.; Carnaille, B.; Chapuis, Y.; Cougard, P.; Henry, J.-F.; Proye, C. Adrenocortical Carcinomas: Surgical Trends and Results of a 253-Patient Series from the French Association of Endocrine Surgeons Study Group. *World J. Surg.* **2001**, *25*, 891–897. [CrossRef] [PubMed]
16. Kemp, C.D.; Ripley, R.T.; Mathur, A.; Steinberg, S.M.; Nguyen, D.M.; Fojo, T.; Schrump, D.S. Pulmonary Resection for Metastatic Adrenocortical Carcinoma: The National Cancer Institute Experience. *Ann. Thorac. Surg.* **2011**, *92*, 1195–1200. [CrossRef] [PubMed]
17. Datrice, N.M.; Langan, R.C.; Ripley, R.T.; Kemp, C.D.; Steinberg, S.M.; Wood, B.J.; Libutti, S.K.; Fojo, T.; Schrump, D.S.; Avital, I. Operative Management for Recurrent and Metastatic Adrenocortical Carcinoma. *J. Surg. Oncol.* **2012**, *105*, 709–713. [CrossRef] [PubMed]
18. Schulick, R.D.; Brennan, M.F. Long-Term Survival after Complete Resection and Repeat Resection in Patients with Adrenocortical Carcinoma. *Ann. Surg. Oncol.* **1999**, *6*, 719–726. [CrossRef] [PubMed]
19. Jensen, J.C.; Pass, H.I.; Sindelar, W.F.; Norton, J.A. Recurrent or Metastatic Disease in Select Patients with Adrenocortical Carcinoma: Aggressive Resection vs Chemotherapy. *Arch. Surg.* **1991**, *126*, 457–461. [CrossRef]

20. Grubbs, E.G.; Callender, G.G.; Xing, Y.; Perrier, N.D.; Evans, D.B.; Phan, A.T.; Lee, J.E. Recurrence of Adrenal Cortical Carcinoma Following Resection: Surgery Alone Can Achieve Results Equal to Surgery Plus Mitotane. *Ann. Surg. Oncol.* **2010**, *17*, 263–270. [CrossRef]
21. op den Winkel, J.; Pfannschmidt, J.; Muley, T.; Grünewald, C.; Dienemann, H.; Fassnacht, M.; Allolio, B. Metastatic Adrenocortical Carcinoma: Results of 56 Pulmonary Metastasectomies in 24 Patients. *Ann. Thorac. Surg.* **2011**, *92*, 1965–1970. [CrossRef]
22. Cooper, J.D.; Perelman, M.; Todd, T.R.; Ginsberg, R.J.; Patterson, G.A.; Pearson, F.G. Precision Cautery Excision of Pulmonary Lesions. *Ann. Thorac. Surg.* **1986**, *41*, 51–53. [CrossRef]
23. Schulick, R.D.; Brennan, M.F. Adrenocortical Carcinoma. *World J. Urol.* **1999**, *17*, 26–34. [CrossRef]
24. Owen, D.H.; Patel, S.; Wei, L.; Phay, J.E.; Shirley, L.A.; Kirschner, L.S.; Schmidt, C.; Abdel-Misih, S.; Brock, P.; Shah, M.H.; et al. Metastatic Adrenocortical Carcinoma: A Single Institutional Experience. *Hormones Cancer* **2019**, *10*, 161–167. [CrossRef] [PubMed]
25. Haak, H.; Hermans, J.; van de Velde, C.; Lentjes, E.; Goslings, B.; Fleuren, G.-J.; Krans, H. Optimal Treatment of Adrenocortical Carcinoma with Mitotane: Results in a Consecutive Series of 96 Patients. *Br. J. Cancer* **1994**, *69*, 947–951. [CrossRef] [PubMed]
26. Dy, B.M.; Strajina, V.; Cayo, A.K.; Richards, M.L.; Farley, D.R.; Grant, C.S.; Harmsen, W.S.; Evans, D.B.; Grubbs, E.G.; Bible, K.C.; et al. Surgical Resection of Synchronously Metastatic Adrenocortical Cancer. *Ann. Surg. Oncol.* **2015**, *22*, 146–151. [CrossRef] [PubMed]
27. Smith, R.; Pak, Y.; Kraybill, W.; Kane, J.M. Factors Associated with Actual Long-Term Survival Following Soft Tissue Sarcoma Pulmonary Metastasectomy. *Eur. J. Surg. Oncol.* **2009**, *35*, 356–361. [CrossRef] [PubMed]
28. Younes, R.N.; Fares, A.L.; Gross, J.L. Pulmonary Metastasectomy: A Multivariate Analysis of 440 Patients Undergoing Complete Resection. *Interact. Cardiovasc. Thorac. Surg.* **2012**, *14*, 156–161. [CrossRef] [PubMed]

cancers

MDPI

Article

Influencing Factors on the Quality of Lymph Node Dissection for Stage IA Non-Small Cell Lung Cancer: A Retrospective Nationwide Cohort Study

Piotr Gabryel [1,*,†], Piotr Skrzypczak [1,†], Magdalena Roszak [2], Alessio Campisi [3], Dominika Zielińska [1], Maciej Bryl [1], Katarzyna Stencel [1] and Cezary Piwkowski [1]

1 Department of Thoracic Surgery, Poznan University of Medical Sciences, Szamarzewskiego 62 Street, 60-569 Poznan, Poland
2 Department of Computer Science and Statistics, Poznan University of Medical Sciences, Rokietnicka 7 Street, 60-806 Poznan, Poland
3 Department of Thoracic Surgery, University and Hospital Trust–Ospedale Borgo Trento, Piazzale Aristide Stefani 1, 37126 Verona, Italy
* Correspondence: pgabryel@ump.edu.pl or piotrgabryel@gmail.com; Tel.: +48-60-344-4042
† These authors contributed equally to this work.

Simple Summary: The excision of the lymph nodes, known as lymphadenectomy, is an essential part of surgical operation for lung cancer. This nationwide study was conducted to identify factors influencing the quality of lymphadenectomy. We included 4271 patients who underwent a minimally invasive surgical operation for early-stage lung cancer. Our findings indicate that the requirements for lymphadenectomy were satisfied in 27.9% of patients. Statistical analysis revealed that patients who underwent positron emission tomography–computed tomography before surgery, patients with larger tumors, and those operated on by experienced surgeons had a higher accuracy of lymphadenectomy. Additionally, the study revealed a declining trend in the quality of lymphadenectomy over time. Importantly, more extensive lymph node excision did not correlate with elevated complication rates or in-hospital mortality. In light of these findings, it is imperative to implement actions aimed at enhancing the quality of lymphadenectomy for lung cancer.

Abstract: Lymphadenectomy is an essential part of complete surgical operation for non-small cell lung cancer (NSCLC). This retrospective, multicenter cohort study aimed to identify factors that influence the lymphadenectomy quality. Data were obtained from the Polish Lung Cancer Study Group Database. The primary endpoint was lobe-specific mediastinal lymph node dissection (L-SMLND). The study included 4271 patients who underwent VATS lobectomy for stage IA NSCLC, operated between 2007 and 2022. L-SMLND was performed in 1190 patients (27.9%). The remaining 3081 patients (72.1%) did not meet the L-SMLND criteria. Multivariate logistic regression analysis showed that patients with PET-CT (OR 3.238, 95% CI: 2.315 to 4.529; $p < 0.001$), with larger tumors (pT1a vs. pT1b vs. pT1c) (OR 1.292; 95% CI: 1.009 to 1.653; $p = 0.042$), and those operated on by experienced surgeons (OR 1.959, 95% CI: 1.432 to 2.679; $p < 0.001$) had a higher probability of undergoing L-SMLND. The quality of lymphadenectomy decreased over time (OR 0.647, 95% CI: 0.474 to 0.884; $p = 0.006$). An analysis of propensity-matched groups showed that more extensive lymph node dissection was not related to in-hospital mortality, complication rates, and hospitalization duration. Actions are needed to improve the quality of lymphadenectomy for NSCLC.

Keywords: lung cancer; early-stage; surgery; thoracoscopy; VATS; minimally invasive surgery; lobectomy; lymphadenectomy; mediastinal lymph node dissection; quality

1. Introduction

According to the World Health Organization data, lung cancer is currently one of the most common malignancies and the leading cause of cancer-related death worldwide [1].

It is typically diagnosed at an advanced stage and, in most cases, surgical treatment is not feasible [2]. Consequently, substantial efforts have been made in recent years to improve lung cancer detection and treatment. The introduction of low-dose chest computed tomography screening has increased the detection rate of early-stage lung cancer, enabling more frequent qualification for surgical treatment and reducing lung cancer mortality [3,4]. Video-assisted thoracoscopic surgery (VATS) has improved both the early- and long-term outcomes of surgical operations, compared to open approaches [5–7]. Robotic-assisted surgery may yield even better outcomes, including more accurate lymphadenectomy and lower conversion rates compared to VATS [8,9], but the high cost of the procedure may impede its widespread implementation [10]. Concerning the type of anatomical resection, lobectomy has been considered the standard of care for early-stage non-small cell lung cancer (NSCLC) since the study by Ginsberg et al. [11]. Recent trials have demonstrated comparable outcomes of segmentectomy for peripheral IA1 and IA2 NSCLC [12,13]. However, segmentectomy is a complex procedure suitable only for small, intrasegmental tumors, and may be associated with increased local recurrence rate [14,15]. Due to the limitations of robotic surgery and segmentectomy, VATS lobectomy will likely continue to be the procedure of choice for the majority of the early-stage NSCLC patients worldwide.

In addition to lung anatomical resection, mediastinal lymph node dissection (MLND) is essential for achieving complete NSCLC resection. The International Association for the Study of Lung Cancer (IASLC) guidelines recommend one of two types of MLND, either systematic (SMLND) or lobe-specific (L-SMLND) [16]. However, there is no consensus on whether one type of MLND is superior to the other [17]. While SMLND is believed to be more accurate in detecting mediastinal lymph node metastases [18], Deng et al. demonstrated that stage cIA NSCLC most often metastasize to the lymph nodes specific for a given lobe of the lung [19]. Shapiro et. al. found that in patients with cN0/N1 NSCLC, pN2 metastases followed the lobe-specific pattern and the recurrence rate was similar after L-SMLND and SMLND [20]. Moreover, recent meta-analyses demonstrated that L-SMLND, compared to SMLND, can be associated with a lower incidence of postoperative complications, such as chylothorax and arrhythmia, comparable recurrence-free survival and favorable overall survival [21,22]. These findings support the role of L-SMLND for the treatment of selected patients with early-stage NSCLC.

Despite the evidence, intraoperative nodal assessment very often falls short of recommendations [23]. In a study by Ray et al., only 18% of patients operated on for early-stage NSCLC had any type of MLND, and 6% had nodal sampling. The remaining 75% of patients had an intraoperative nodal assessment that met neither standard. Moreover, the authors found that MLND was associated with superior survival compared to less comprehensive nodal staging [24]. These findings were supported by the recent study that demonstrated that among patients after VATS lobectomy for stage IA NSCLC, only 28.8% met the criteria for L-SMLND. More importantly, the study also found that L-SMLND was related to higher 5-year survival rates compared to patients with less comprehensive nodal assessment [25].

The reasons for poor-quality lymph node assessment for early-stage NSCLC are not well understood. Some studies found that demographic factors, comorbidities, cancer stage, type of surgery, and the type of surgical equipment may influence MLND [26–28]. These studies, however, included heterogenous populations of patients operated on at all stages of lung cancer, with both minimally invasive and open approaches. Factors that could influence the quality of MLND during VATS lobectomy for early-stage NSCLC are poorly researched. As the quality of MLND significantly affects the long-term outcomes of lung cancer treatment, and the number of minimally invasive procedures for early-stage lung cancer is likely to increase, research in this area may be of great clinical importance. The objectives of this study were to evaluate the quality of MLND in patients undergoing VATS lobectomy for early-stage lung cancer, identify factors related to the quality of MLND, and to evaluate the impact of MLND on postoperative complications.

2. Materials and Methods

The Bioethics Committee of the Poznan University of Medical Sciences waived the need to obtain consent for the collection and analysis of the anonymized data, and for the publication of the results of this multicenter, retrospective, cohort study.

2.1. Diagnosis, Surgical Treatment, and Reporting of Treatment Results for Lung Cancer in Poland

Lung cancer in Poland is diagnosed by pulmonologists and thoracic surgeons, as part of outpatient, as well as in-hospital specialist medical care. The public healthcare system provides good access to lung cancer treatment. All decisions regarding oncological treatment, including non-surgical and surgical treatment, are made by multidisciplinary tumor boards. In Poland, approximately 4000 patients are operated on for lung cancer annually, constituting about 20% of all newly diagnosed cases of the disease [29]. Operations are carried out in 29 thoracic surgery centers covering the country's total population of 38 million people. Anatomical lung resection can only be performed by board-certified thoracic surgeons, or residents under the supervision of a thoracic surgeon. Data regarding surgical treatment are obligatorily entered by residents and consultants into the Polish Lung Cancer Study Group Database. The database includes data on patients' demographics, comorbidities, pulmonary function tests, radiological tests, invasive staging, surgical approach, type of operation, number of lymph nodes and lymph node stations removed, results of histopathological examination, postoperative complications, chest tube duration and postoperative hospital stay, neoadjuvant and adjuvant treatment, and follow-up. TNM stage is automatically calculated based on the entered data, and updated to the most recent version, in this case to the eighth edition, of the TNM classification.

2.2. Study Design

This retrospective, multicenter cohort study included patients who underwent VATS lobectomy for pathological stage IA lung cancer between 17 April 2007 and 14 October 2022. Data for the study were obtained from the Polish Lung Cancer Study Group Database. The study excluded patients after induction treatment (chemo-, immuno-, and/or radiotherapy), with an open approach, after sublobar resection, extended resection or pneumonectomy, with histology other than NSCLC (benign histology, metastases, or small-cell lung cancer), and with missing information on the surgical approach, dissected lymph nodes, histological type, or postoperative care.

For the purpose of the study, L-SMLND was defined according to the IASLC guidelines, and included the following nodal stations for each of type of lobectomy:

1. Right upper paratracheal (2R), right lower paratracheal (4R), and subcarinal (7) nodes for right upper and right middle lobectomy, and for right upper bilobectomy.
2. Right lower paratracheal (4R), subcarinal (7), and paraesophageal (8) or pulmonary ligament (9) nodes for right lower lobectomy.
3. Aorto-pulmonary window (5), paraaortic (6), and subcarinal (7) nodes for left upper lobectomy.
4. Subcarinal (7), paraesophageal (8), and pulmonary ligament (9) nodes for left lower lobectomy.
5. All right-sided stations (2R, 4R, 7, and 8 or 9) for right lower bilobectomy.

Systematic mediastinal nodal dissection included stations 2R, 4R, 7, 8, and 9 for the right-sided lobectomy and stations 5, 6, 7, 8, and 9 for the left-sided lobectomy.

The study cohort was divided into two groups. Patients were assigned to either the L-SMLND group, or to the non-L-SMLND group, depending on whether the IASLC criteria for lobe-specific mediastinal nodal dissection were met.

The primary endpoint of the study was the lobe-specific mediastinal lymph node dissection (L-SMLND). The study analyzed the relationship between preoperative and surgery-related variables, and the accuracy of the lymph node assessment. The secondary endpoints were postoperative complications and other variables related to the postoperative course.

2.3. Statistical Analyses

The analyzed data were expressed as mean ± standard deviation, median, minimum, maximum values, interquartile range (Q1 lower quartile, Q3 upper quartile), or percentage, as appropriate. The relationship between variables was analyzed using Spearman's rank correlation coefficient. The normality of distribution was tested using the Shapiro–Wilk test and equality of variances was checked using Levene's test. A comparison of two unpaired groups was performed using the unpaired t-test for data that followed a normal distribution and had homogeneity of variances or the Mann–Whitney U-test. Categorical data were analyzed using the $\chi 2$ test when the sample size was larger than 40 and all expected values were greater than ten; for other situations, the exact test of Fisher or $\chi 2$ test with Yate's correction was used. All results were considered significant at $p < 0.05$. Factors that obtained $p < 0.05$ in univariate analysis were then analyzed in logistic regression. Differences in perioperative outcomes between types of lymph node assessment were evaluated using a propensity-matched analysis of non-L-SMLND versus L-SMLND. Propensity scores were developed, defined as the probability of treatment assignment, conditional on age, sex, Charlson Comorbidity Index, Thoracic Revised Cardiac Risk Index, chronic obstructive, pulmonary disease, surgeon's experience, and type of lobectomy. All covariates were determined to be clinically relevant. Using a nearest neighbor matching algorithm without replacement with a caliper of 0.01, the most appropriately matched pairs were selected. Data manipulation and all calculations were performed in IBM® SPSS® Statistics version 27th (PS Imago Pro 8).

3. Results

The study comprised 4271 patients who underwent VATS lobectomy for stage IA non-small cell lung cancer and met all study criteria. The rates of postoperative complications and in-hospital mortality were 21.9% and 0.54%, respectively. The median postoperative chest tube duration was 3 days (IQR 2 to 4 days), and the hospital stay duration was 6 days (IQR 5 to 7 days).

Lobe-specific mediastinal lymph node dissection (L-SMLND) guidelines were met in 1190 patients (27.9%). The remaining 3081 patients (72.1%) did not meet L-SMLND criteria. Patients with L-SMLND had higher numbers of lymph nodes removed (median 12 vs. 8, $p < 0.001$) and lymph nodes stations dissected (median 6 vs. 4, $p < 0.001$).

Univariate analysis revealed that the L-SMLND criteria were more likely to be met in patients with a smoking history ($p < 0.001$), a higher body mass index ($p = 0.04$), chronic obstructive pulmonary disease ($p < 0.001$), and larger diameter tumors (T1a vs. T1b vs. T1c; $p < 0.001$). The quality of nodal assessment was also influenced by preoperative staging procedures—patients with preoperative positron emission tomography–computed tomography (PET-CT, $p < 0.001$) were more likely to meet L-SMLND criteria, while patients who had undergone endobronchial ultrasound-transbronchial needle aspiration (EBUS-TBNA, $p = 0.038$) were less likely. Mediastinoscopy was associated with a higher L-SMLND rate ($p = 0.023$), but the number of subjects with this procedure was low and the results should be interpreted with caution. L-SMLND was more frequently performed in patients undergoing right-sided lobectomy ($p < 0.001$) by surgeons with greater surgical experience, i.e., who performed more than 50 VATS lobectomies ($p = 0.003$). Interestingly, patients operated on more recently exhibited lower quality lymphadenectomy and were less likely to meet L-SMLND criteria. This relationship was evident both when the study period was chronologically divided into four periods of three years each ($p < 0.001$; Figure 1a) and when the study group was chronologically divided into four groups of equal sizes ($p < 0.001$; Figure 1b). The decreasing quality of lymphadenectomy was associated with the increasing number of surgeons performing VATS lobectomy (Figure 1c,d). The baseline, surgical, postoperative, and histopathological characteristics, along with the results of univariate analyses, are presented in Tables 1 and 2.

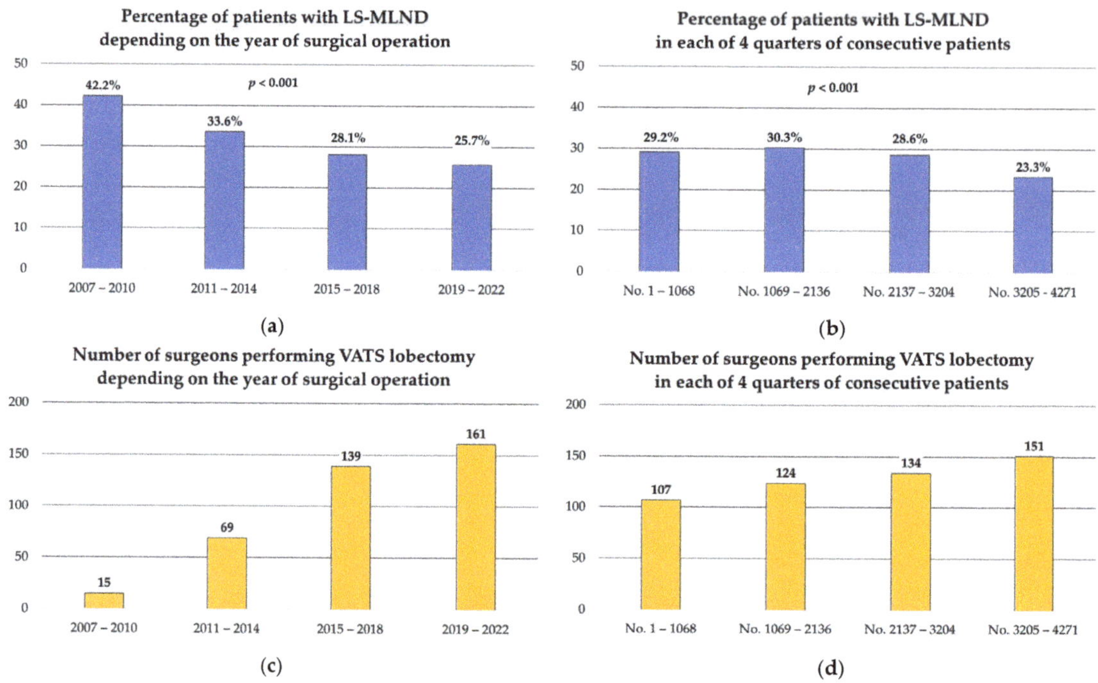

Figure 1. Changes in the accuracy of lymph nodes assessment and numbers of surgeons performing VATS lobectomy over time: (**a**) Percentage of patients with LS-MLND, depending on the year of surgical operation; (**b**) percentage of patients with LS-MLND in each of 4 quarters of consecutive patients; (**c**) number of surgeons performing VATS lobectomy, depending on the year of surgical operation; (**d**) number of surgeons performing VATS lobectomy in each of 4 quarters of consecutive patients.

The variables that demonstrated significance in the multivariate logistic regression analysis were PET-CT (OR, 3.238; 95% CI: 2.315 to 4.529; $p < 0.001$), pT (OR, 1.292; 95% CI: 1.009 to 1.653; $p = 0.042$), surgeon's experience (OR, 1.959; 95% CI: 1.432 to 2.679; $p < 0.001$), and period of surgery (OR, 0.647; 95% CI: 0.474 to 0.884; $p = 0.006$). Patients who underwent PET-CT, had larger tumors (pT1a vs. pT1b vs. pT1c), and were operated on by experienced thoracic surgeons exhibited a higher probability of meeting L-SMLND criteria. Conversely, the likelihood of meeting L-SMLND criteria decreased in patients operated on more recently. The results of the multivariate analysis are presented in Table 3.

Lastly, we assessed the relationship between the extent of lymph node dissection and postoperative course. To minimize bias, propensity score matching was performed, resulting in two groups with similar basic characteristics, each comprising 1184 patients (Supplementary Table S1). Analysis of propensity-matched groups showed that L-SMLND did not significantly influence the postoperative course and the complication rates. The chest tube duration was slightly longer in the non-L-SMLND group compared to the L-SMLND group (4 days, IQR 3 to 5 days vs. 3 days, IQR 2 to 5 days; $p < 0.001$). Other variables, including hospital stay duration, in-hospital death, and complication rates did not differ between the groups (Table 4).

Table 1. Univariable analysis of demographic and preoperative variables associated with compliance to the lobe-specific mediastinal lymphadenectomy guidelines.

	Lobe-Specific Lymph Node Dissection		p-Value
	Non L-SMLND (n = 3081)	**L-SMLND (n = 1190)**	
Age, years, mean (SD)	65.1 (SD: 8.1)	65.9 (SD: 7.8)	0.794
Male, n (%)	1408 (45.7)	568 (47.7)	0.233
Smoking history, n (%)	2052 (66.6)	934 (78.5)	<0.001 *
BMI, kg/m^2, mean (SD)	26.9 (SD: 4.9)	27.6 (SD: 5.1)	0.040 *
ppFEV1%, mean (SD)	89.0 (SD: 19.4)	88.6 (SD: 19.1)	0.631
Comorbidities, n (%)	2444 (79.3)	932 (78.3)	0.469
Chronic obstructive pulmonary disease	542 (17.6)	274 (23.0)	<0.001 *
Coronary arterial disease	433 (14.1)	158 (13.3)	0.510
Cerebrovascular disease	40 (1.3)	23 (1.9)	0.123
Peripheral arterial disease	103 (3.3)	53 (4.5)	0.083
Hypertension	1571 (51.0)	605 (50.8)	0.930
Diabetes mellitus	462 (15.0)	185 (15.5)	0.652
Chronic kidney disease	24 (0.8)	16 (1.3)	0.085
Other neoplasm	502 (16.3)	173 (14.5)	0.159
ThRCRI, n (%)			0.806
Group A (n = 3622)	2610 (84.7)	1012 (85.1)	
Group B (n = 644)	469 (15.2)	175 (14.7)	
Group C (n = 5)	2 (0.1)	3 (0.2)	
CCI, median (IQR)	3 (IQR, 2 to 4)	3 (IQR, 2 to 4)	0.587
Patients with PET-CT	972 (31.5)	521 (43.8)	<0.001 *
Patients with EBUS-TBNA	364 (11.8)	114 (9.6)	0.038 *
Patients with mediastinoscopy	25 (0.8)	19 (1.6)	0.023 *

L-SMLND = lobe-specific mediastinal lymph node dissection; SD = standard deviation; BMI = body mass index; ppFEV1% = predicted postoperative percentage of calculated forced expiratory volume in 1 s; ThRCRI = Thoracic Revised Cardiac Risk Index; IQR = interquartile range; CCI = Charlson comorbidity index; PET-CT = positron emission tomography–computed tomography; EBUS-TBNA = endobronchial ultrasound-transbronchial needle aspiration. * Statistically significant ($p < 0.05$).

Table 2. Univariable analysis of surgery-related and histopathological variables associated with compliance to the lobe-specific mediastinal lymphadenectomy guidelines.

	Lobe-Specific Lymph Node Dissection		p-Value
	Non L-SMLND (n = 3081)	**L-SMLND (n = 1190)**	
Side of surgery, n (%)			<0.001 *
Right (n = 2543)	1719 (67.6)	824 (32.4)	
Left (n = 1728)	1362 (78.8)	366 (21.2)	
Type of surgery, n (%)			<0.001 *
Right upper lobectomy (n = 1415)	946 (66.9)	469 (33.1)	
Right middle lobectomy (n = 361)	266 (73.7)	95 (26.3)	
Right lower lobectomy (n = 739)	485 (65.6)	254 (34.4)	
Right upper bilobectomy (n = 14)	9 (64.3)	5 (35.7)	
Right lower bilobectomy (n = 14)	13 (92.9)	1 (7.1)	
Left upper lobectomy (n = 1055)	767 (72.7)	288 (27.3)	
Left lower lobectomy (n = 673)	595 (88.4)	78 (11.6)	

Table 2. *Cont.*

	Lobe-Specific Lymph Node Dissection		p-Value
	Non L-SMLND (n = 3081)	**L-SMLND (n = 1190)**	
Surgeons' experience, n (%)			0.003 *
Initial 50 VATS lobectomies (n = 2523)	1863 (73.8)	660 (26.2)	
Later lobectomies (>50) (n = 1748)	1218 (69.7)	530 (30.3)	
Histology, n (%)			0.059
Adenocarcinoma (n = 2363)	1694 (71.7)	669 (28.3)	
Squamous cell carcinoma (n = 1036)	731 (70.6)	305 (29.4)	
Other types (n = 872)	656 (75.2)	216 (24.8)	
pT, n (%)			<0.001 *
pT 1a (n = 442)	336 (76.0)	106 (24.0)	
pT 1b (n = 2136)	1566 (73.3)	570 (26.7)	
pT 1c (n = 1691)	1177 (69.6)	514 (30.4)	
Number of lymph nodes stations removed, median (IQR)			
N1 stations	2 (IQR, 1 to 2)	2 (IQR, 1 to 2)	<0.001 *
N2 stations	2 (IQR, 1 to 3)	4 (IQR, 3 to 4)	<0.001 *
Total number of lymph nodes stations	4 (IQR, 3 to 5)	6 (IQR, 5 to 6)	<0.001 *
Number of lymph nodes removed, median (IQR)			
N1 lymph nodes	4 (IQR, 2 to 6)	4 (IQR, 2 to 7)	<0.001 *
N2 lymph nodes	4 (IQR, 2 to 6)	8 (IQR, 5 to 12)	<0.001 *
Total number of lymph nodes	8 (IQR, 5 to 12)	12 (IQR, 8 to 18)	<0.001 *

L-SMLND = lobe-specific mediastinal lymph node dissection; IQR = interquartile range. * Statistically significant ($p < 0.05$).

Table 3. Results of the multivariate analysis of variables related to the L-SMLND for stage IA NSCLC.

	Odds Ratio	95% Confidence Interval	p-Value
Smoking	1.265	0.897 to 1.784	0.181
BMI	1.030	0.999 to 1.063	0.058
COPD	1.252	0.863 to 1.817	0.237
PET-CT	3.238	2.315 to 4.529	<0.001 *
Mediastinoscopy	1.934	0.119 to 31.561	0.643
EBUS-TBNA	0.889	0.572 to 1.380	0.599
pT	1.292	1.009 to 1.653	0.042 *
Surgeon's experience	1.959	1.432 to 2.679	<0.001 *
No. of surgery (quarters)	0.647	0.474 to 0.884	0.006 *
Side of surgery	0.816	0.083 to 8.005	0.862
Right upper lobectomy	1.493	0.153 to 14.557	0.730
Right middle lobectomy	0.952	0.094 to 9.655	0.967
Right lower lobectomy	1.577	0.159 to 15.589	0.697
Right upper bilobectomy	3.570	0.128 to 99.477	0.453
Left upper lobectomy	1.306	0.133 to 12.856	0.819
Left lower lobectomy	0.422	0.041 to 4.333	0.468

BMI = body mass index; COPD = Chronic obstructive pulmonary disease; PET-CT = positron emission tomography–computed tomography; EBUS-TBNA = endobronchial ultrasound-transbronchial needle aspiration. * Statistically significant ($p < 0.05$).

Table 4. Propensity-matched analysis of non-L-SMLND versus L-SMLND: postoperative characteristics and complications data.

	Lobe-Specific Lymph Node Dissection		p-Value
	Non L-SMLND (n = 1184)	**L-SMLND (n = 1184)**	
Complications, n (%)	255 (21.5)	272 (23.5)	0.258
Prolonged air leak > 5 days	102 (8.6)	107 (9.0)	0.717
Residual air space	39 (3.3)	24 (2.0)	0.055
Re-drainage	35 (3.0)	25 (2.1)	0.191
Atrial arrythmia	39 (3.3)	31 (2.6)	0.332
Transfusion	37 (3.1)	43 (3.6)	0.495
Pneumonia	16 (1.4)	22 (1.9)	0.326
Bronchoscopy for atelectasis	7 (0.6)	14 (1.2)	0.125
Surgery for postoperative bleeding	9 (0.8)	12 (1.0)	0.511
Surgery for other postoperative complications	12 (1.0)	17 (1.4)	0.350
Delirium	5 (0.4)	6 (0.5)	0.762
Prolonged intubation	5 (0.4)	5 (0.4)	1.000
Bronchopleural fistula	1 (0.1)	1 (0.1)	1.000
Chylothorax	1 (0.1)	5 (0.4)	0.102
Recurrent laryngeal nerve palsy	1 (0.1)	2 (0.2)	0.563
Pulmonary embolism	1 (0.1)	4 (0.3)	0.179
Myocardial infarction	1 (0.1)	1 (0.1)	1.000
Cerebrovascular complications	1 (0.1)	4 (0.3)	0.179
Kidney failure	0	2 (0.2)	0.157
Other complications	22 (1.9)	25 (2.1)	0.658
Chest tube duration, days, median (IQR)	4 (IQR, 3 to 5)	3 (IQR, 2 to 5)	<0.001 *
Hospital stay, days, median (IQR)	6 (IQR, 4 to 7)	6 (IQR, 4 to 7)	0.870
In-hospital death	3 (0.3)	7 (0.6)	0.205

L-SMLND = lobe-specific mediastinal lymph node dissection; IQR = interquartile range. * Statistically significant ($p < 0.05$).

4. Discussion

Several studies have demonstrated that in many patients undergoing surgery for lung cancer, intraoperative lymph nodes assessment does not meet generally accepted guidelines. This study aimed to identify factors related to the quality of MLND in patients undergoing surgery for early-stage NSCLC. Analyzing all VATS lobectomies for stage IA NSCLC performed in one large European country from 2007 to 2022, we found that the L-SMLND criteria were met in 27.9% of patients. Patients with PET-CT, larger tumors (pT1a vs. pT1b vs. pT1c), and those operated on by experienced thoracic surgeons, were more likely to meet L-SMLND criteria. However, we observed an unfavorable trend of decreasing lymphadenectomy quality over the years. Furthermore, the study revealed that patients with L-SMLND had a higher numbers of mediastinal lymph nodes and lymph node stations removed. L-SMLND was not associated with postoperative complications rates, in-hospital mortality, or hospitalization duration.

The current guidelines advocate for mediastinal lymph node dissection for lung cancer surgery. This study has substantiated that various factors influence the MLND accuracy. Familiarity with these factors provides an opportunity to adapt surgical procedures in order to improve the quality of treatment.

PET-CT holds a pivotal role in clinical staging and is endorsed by multiple lung cancer diagnostic guidelines [30,31]. PET-CT facilitates identification of lymph nodes suspected of cancer metastases, enabling precise targeting of invasive pre- and intraoperative lymph node assessment [32]. Our study demonstrated higher accuracy of lymphadenectomy among patients who underwent PET-CT. These findings underscore the importance of PET-CT in the diagnosis and treatment of lung cancer. PET-CT should be performed in all patients before anatomical resection for lung cancer, unless there are absolute contraindications.

This study also found that L-SMLND rates were lower for smaller lung nodules. These findings align with those of Pawelczyk et al. and Edwards et al., demonstrating that the adequacy of intraoperative nodal staging for NSCLC was lower in patients with T1a tumors [33,34]. Small nodules seldom metastasize to lymph nodes, likely explaining why surgeons are less inclined to undertake more extensive lymphadenectomy in such cases. However, even cIA tumors may give lymph node metastases. Bott et al. reported an incidence of the N2 feature in patients with stage cI NSCLC of approximately 8.5%. Their study included patients operated from 1998 to 2010, in whom PET-CT examination was performed in only 12.5%. This was a limitation of the study that potentially contributed to a higher non-detection rate of nodal metastases preoperatively [35]. A recent study by Tsai et al. unveiled nodal upstaging in almost 8% of patients following VATS lobectomy with SMLND for cT1a-b NSCLC. Within this group, 82% of patients exhibited N2 metastases. All those patients had excellent preoperative nodal assessment, including PET-CT, and invasive mediastinal staging if mediastinal metastases were suspected [36]. These studies underscore the necessity for a comprehensive lymphadenectomy, even in patients with small nodules and good preoperative mediastinal staging. The significance of high-quality MLND and detection of nodal metastases is heightened in light of recent studies revealing promising results of adjuvant therapy after lung cancer surgery [37].

The surgeon's experience greatly influences the results of minimally invasive lung cancer surgery. Numerous studies have demonstrated that with an increasing number of VATS lobectomies performed by the surgeon, there is a reduction in operating time, intraoperative blood loss, frequency of conversion to thoracotomy, and incidence of postoperative complications [38]. Ongoing discussions within the thoracic surgery community revolve around determining the number of operations required to overcome the learning curve, with estimates ranging from 25 to over 200 operations [39]. For the purposes of this study, we adopted a value of 50 surgical procedures, well established in the literature [40–42]. Most studies on VATS lobectomy learning curve focused on early postoperative outcomes. The relationship between the learning curve and lymphadenectomy accuracy has been infrequently explored. This study demonstrated that surgeons with more experience in VATS lobectomy were more likely to perform L-SMLND. Additionally, patients with L-SMLND had a greater number of lymph nodes and lymph node stations removed. These findings align with those of Mazzella et al., who reported that less experienced surgeons more frequently performed lymph node sampling instead of lymphadenectomy, harvested fewer lymph nodes, and performed fewer radical resections [43]. Lymph node dissection plays a crucial role in the surgical treatment of lung cancer as it improves staging accuracy and influences postoperative oncological treatment. During the learning phase of VATS lobectomy, attention should be directed not only to the anatomical resection itself, but also to the meticulous execution of lymph node dissection.

A concerning observation was the deterioration in the quality of lymphadenectomy over the study period. In the initial phase, spanning from 2007 to 2010, the proportion of patients with L-SMLND stood at 42.2%, whereas in the most recent period (from 2019 to 2022) it declined to 25.7%. Upon dividing the cohort into four equal-sized groups, it was revealed that the incidence of L-SMLND in the oldest group was 29.2%, while in the most recent group it was 23.3%. These findings markedly differed from those previously published in the literature. Osarogiagbon et al. employed the number of removed lymph nodes as a proxy for lymphadenectomy quality in lung cancer surgery and found that it gradually increased over the span of 12 years covered by their study [44]. Krantz et al. used the criterion of 15 or more lymph nodes as an indicator of good-quality lymphadenectomy, showing a rising trend of likelihood of patients having more than 15 nodes assessed from the year 2004 to 2013 [45]. The improvement in the quality of lymphadenectomy over time was observed not only in patients undergoing lung cancer surgery, but also in those treated for extrapulmonary cancer, such as rectal cancer [46]. The reasons for the decline in the quality of lymphadenectomy over the years observed in our study remain unclear. One possible contributing factor could be the increasing number of surgeons performing

VATS lobectomy, necessitating the overcoming of the learning curve and resulting in a reduction in the number of operations per surgeon per year. Other potential factors include economic pressure to increase the number of daily operations, leading to attempts to shorten the operation time, or inaccuracies in reporting data on lymph nodes collection. Further research is essential to elucidate the underlying causes and enhance the quality of MLND.

Several other variables, such as BMI, smoking history, COPD, EBUS-TBNA, mediastinoscopy, side of surgery, and type of lobectomy were significant in univariate analysis. Some of these, as along with other factors, have been previously identified in other studies as being associated with the quality of intraoperative lymph node assessment [27,33–35,45]. However, these factors will not be discussed here, as they lost significance in the multivariate analysis.

In this study, we also demonstrated that more extensive lymphadenectomy was not associated with an increased risk of postoperative complications. Existing literature confirms that a more extensive lymph node dissection does not necessarily increase the risk of postoperative complications [47–49]. However, during lymph node dissection, damage may occur to crucial anatomical structures, such as the superior vena cava, esophagus, intermediate or main bronchi, recurrent laryngeal nerve, phrenic nerve, thoracic duct, or others. This may result in severe bleeding, esophageal fistula, bronchial fistula, vocal cord paralysis, diaphragmatic paralysis, or chylothorax. The incidence of these adverse events is very low, which may complicate statistical analyses and lead to drawing false conclusions based on obtained results [50]. These rare, severe complications should rather be assessed on a case-by-case basis. In-depth knowledge of anatomy, good surgical technique, careful use of surgical instruments, especially electrosurgical equipment, and appropriate exposure and identification of anatomical structures allow for the avoidance of intraoperative complications in most cases [51].

This study demonstrated, that the thoroughness of lymph node assessment was generally low. Improving the quality of lymphadenectomy during lung cancer surgery is crucial for accurate staging, planning of adjuvant treatment, and achieving the best possible long-term treatment results. There are several measures that can be implemented to improve the quality of lymphadenectomy for lung cancer surgery.

Firstly, the surgical team, including both the surgeon and the assistant, should be well trained and experienced in performing minimally invasive lung surgery. Surgeons should have in-depth knowledge of the anatomy of the mediastinum, which will enable the location of individual anatomical structures and lymph nodes and will facilitate complete and safe lymphadenectomy. Nowadays, thanks to the abundance of written materials, anatomical atlases and video materials, access to information on how to perform high-quality lymphadenectomy is virtually unlimited.

Secondly, surgeons should possess a very good understanding of the principles of oncological thoracic surgery and current guidelines for the treatment of lung cancer. Several lung cancer organizations, such as the International Association for the Study of Lung Cancer (IASLC) and the National Comprehensive Cancer Network (NCCN) provide recommendations on which nodal sites should be removed and what criteria should be met for complete resection [16,30,52]. Heightened awareness of recommended quality standards regarding the MLND has been shown to improve the quality of lymph node assessment [53].

Thirdly, the use of various intraoperative techniques may enhance the accuracy of lymphadenectomies. Osarogiagbon et al. developed a lymph node collection kit and demonstrated its effectiveness in improving nodal staging quality [54]. Subsequent studies have shown that the use of this kit enhances the thoroughness of lymphadenectomy and overall survival after lung cancer surgery [53,55]. Advanced electrosurgical devices may also facilitate tissue dissection and increase the thoroughness of lymphadenectomy [27,56,57].

Fourth, quality control of surgical procedures is essential. One of the methods for controlling quality involves the mandatory entry of surgical care data into dedicated databases. The Polish Lung Cancer Study Group Database contains detailed data on many aspects of lung cancer treatment, including number of lymph nodes removed for each nodal station. Data are reported separately by thoracic surgeons and pathologists, providing a comprehensive assessment of the quality of lymphadenectomy performed by surgeons in each department. Another example of quality control measures is the ESTS Quality Certification Program [58]. Data entered by individual centers into the ESTS Database are used to calculate a composite performance score. Sufficiently high score is one of the conditions for obtaining the prestigious ESTS Accreditation. One of the variables used to calculate the score is the percentage of patients operated on for primary neoplastic disease submitted to systematic lymph node dissection. This provides some degree of external control over the quality of lymphadenectomy at participating centers. The annual publication of data in the form of an ESTS Database Annual Report is an additional mode of assessing the activities of the departments [59]. However, there are many issues related to reporting of the surgical data, such as incorrect identification of the lymph node groups during removal, lymph node fragmentation, variations of nodal dissection techniques and extent, and difficulties in interpreting surgical reports by individuals entering data into databases [60,61]. Further efforts are needed to improve and standardize data collection and usage for the assessment of the quality of thoracic surgical procedures.

The introduction of direct quality control methods could address some of these problems. The assessment of thoracic surgery quality traditionally relies mainly on indirect methods, such as the analysis of early and long-term treatment outcomes and, less frequently, on the analysis of patients' quality of life. Methods for assessing the quality of lymphadenectomy, such as determining the number of lymph nodes and nodal stations, or meeting appropriate guidelines, are also indirect and do not allow for the evaluation of the surgical procedure's course. In a recent survey involving surgeons, urologists, gynecologists, and trainees, the majority of respondents agreed that the current methods of surgical reporting was insufficient to meet future quality requirements. The authors concluded that implementing intraoperative video or audio recording should be considered [62]. Recently, the Society of American Gastrointestinal and Endoscopic Surgeons (SAGES) issued recommendations on video data acquisition, storage, sharing, use, and governance [63]. Despite the widespread use of video materials in thoracic surgery, they have not yet been widely employed for quality control. These issues may be important and interesting for thoracic surgeons and should be the subject of further research.

Strengths and Limitations

The main strength of the study was the inclusion of all patients who underwent VATS lobectomy in one large European country. This allowed us to obtain a very large amount of data for analysis. By covering a large period of time, from 2007 to 2022, we were able to analyze the impact of the learning curve on the accuracy of lymphadenectomy and changes in accuracy over time. A great advantage was the good quality of data, especially regarding the surgical procedure and histopathological examination results. The multicenter nature of the study made it possible to reflect the variability of surgical proceedings between various departments.

The study also had several limitations. Most of these limitations were due to the fact that this was a retrospective, multicenter cohort study. First, although included in one database, data originated from multiple departments. Differences in patient populations, treatment protocols, and data collection methods across departments might have introduced confounders that affected the study results. Secondly, although the definitions of variables entered into the database were unambiguous, we cannot exclude unforeseen differences between departments. Those could have led to inconsistencies in the data that influenced the results. Thirdly, selection bias is a common limitation of retrospective studies. Given the results obtained, in this study, it may have concerned qualification for surgery by different surgeons depending on clinical stage, including the results of PET-CT scans. Moreover, retrospective studies do not allow establishment of causation. For this reason, the results of the study enable us to draw conclusions solely on the relationship between the variables and the quality of MLND, and not on causation. Finally, the study was conducted on patients operated on within one type of healthcare system. Generalizing the study results to patients operated on in other countries should take into account differences healthcare settings.

The quality of histopathological and surgical data was good, but there were some missing data in other areas. The database contains information on the fact of performing PET-CT, but not on maximal standardized uptake value of fluorodeoxyglucose in lymph nodes and tumor. Analyzing the relationship between those variables and the accuracy of lymph node assessment would be interesting and should be considered in further trials. Data on body weight and height have been entered into the database since 2019. For this reason, information on BMI was available only in one quarter of patients, and only those operated on recently. Although BMI is a risk factor for postoperative complications, we could not include this variable in propensity score matching. Other data not included in the database were the type of VATS approach (uniportal vs. multiportal), information on conversion to thoracotomy, and on lymph node fragmentation. It would also be interesting to assess the relationship between the expression of molecular biomarkers, and long-term outcomes and quality of lymphadenectomy. However, these data were incomplete, their accuracy varied significantly between centers, and we did not include them in the statistical analysis. All this information could be useful for the purposes of the current research, and its absence should also be considered a limitation of the study.

5. Conclusions

This study demonstrated that a significant number of patients operated on for early-stage NSCLC did not undergo a sufficiently thorough mediastinal lymph nodes dissection. A detailed lymphadenectomy allows a more accurate assessment of the NSCLC stage, a precise determination of the long-term prognosis, and the planning of adjuvant treatment. Therefore, it is imperative to take measures to improve the quality of mediastinal lymph nodes dissection.

All identified risk factors associated with less accurate lymphadenectomy, such as smaller nodule diameter, lack of PET-CT, and lower surgeon's experience, underscore the pivotal role of the surgeon in ensuring the quality of nodal assessment. There is concern about the declining quality of lymphadenectomy in recent years, particularly in the context of rapidly evolving adjuvant therapy.

Meanwhile, more extensive lymph node dissection does not appear to increase the incidence of complications. However, this should not diminish the surgeon's responsibility to exercise caution during surgery. It is essential to recognize that very rare, but serious complications, such as damage to the recurrent laryngeal nerve, phrenic nerve, esophagus, bronchi, or vessels, may not be captured in statistical analysis.

To address these concerns, it is crucial to implement actions focused on enhancing the accuracy of surgery, including lymphadenectomy, while maintaining or reducing the incidence of postoperative complications. This may include initiatives such as education and quality control of surgical operations.

Supplementary Materials: The following supporting information can be downloaded at: https://www.mdpi.com/article/10.3390/cancers16020346/s1, Table S1: Patient baseline characteristics of full sample and propensity-matched cohort.

Author Contributions: Conceptualization, P.G. and A.C.; Data curation, P.G. and P.S.; Formal analysis, P.S. and M.R.; Investigation, P.G., D.Z. and P.S.; Methodology, P.G.; Project administration, C.P.; Resources, P.G.; Software, P.S.; Supervision, M.B. and C.P.; Visualization, P.G.; Writing—original draft, P.G. and P.S.; Writing—review and editing, A.C., D.Z., M.B., K.S., M.R. and C.P. All authors have read and agreed to the published version of the manuscript.

Funding: This research received no external funding.

Institutional Review Board Statement: Ethical review and approval were waived study by the Bioethics Committee of the Poznan University of Medical Sciences for this retrospective, non-interventional study based on the analysis of the anonymized data.

Informed Consent Statement: Patient consent for collection, analysis, and publication of the retrospectively obtained and anonymized data for this non-interventional study was waived by the Bioethics Committee of the Poznan University of Medical Sciences.

Data Availability Statement: The data presented in this study are available on request from the corresponding author.

Acknowledgments: We would like to acknowledge the contribution of data for the Polish Lung Cancer Study Group Database from all the departments that were involved in this Database, including the following: Instytut Gruźlicy i Chorób Płuc w Warszawie; Narodowy Instytut Onkologii im. Marii Skłodowskiej—Curie w Warszawie; Uniwersytet Medyczny w Białymstoku; Gdański Uniwersytet Medyczny; Uniwersytet Medyczny w Lublinie; Dolnośląskie Centrum Chorób Płuc; Śląski Uniwersytet Medyczny; Uniwersytecki Szpital Kliniczny im. Wojskowej Akademii Medycznej w Łodzi; Kujawsko-Pomorskie Centrum Pulmonologii w Bydgoszczy; Centrum Pulmonologii i Torakochirurgii w Bystrej Śląskiej; Wojewódzki Szpital Specjalistyczny im. św. Rafała w Czerwonej Górze; Krakowski Szpital Specjalistyczny im. Jana Pawła II; Centrum Onkologii i Traumatologii im. Mikołaja Kopernika w Łodzi; Miejski Szpital Zespolony w Olsztynie; Mazowieckie Centrum Leczenia Chorób Płuc i Gruźlicy w Otwocku; Uniwersytet Medyczny w Poznaniu; Szpital Specjalistyczny w Prabutach; Uniwersytecki Szpital Kliniczny im. Fryderyka Chopina w Rzeszowie; Pomorski Uniwersytet Medyczny w Szczecinie; Szpital Uniwersytecki im. Karola Marcinkowskiego w Zielonej Górze; Szpital Specjalistyczny Chorób Płuc „Odrodzenie" im. Klary Jelskiej w Zakopanem; Centrum Onkologii im. prof. Franciszka Łukaszczyka w Bydgoszczy; 4 Szpital Wojskowy z Polikliniką we Wrocławiu; Świętokrzyskie Centrum Onkologii w Kielcach; Wojewódzki Zespół Zakładów Opieki Zdrowotnej, Centrum Leczenia Chorób Płuc i Rehabilitacji w Łodzi; Wojskowy Instytut Medyczny w Warszawie; Szpital Specjalistyczny im. Świętej Rodziny w Głogowie Mało-polskim; Uniwersytecki Szpital Kliniczny we Wrocławiu; Uniwersyteckie Centrum Kliniczne Warszawskiego Uniwersytetu Medycznego.

Conflicts of Interest: The authors declare no conflicts of interest.

References

1. Ferlay, J.; Ervik, M.; Lam, F.; Colombet, M.; Mery, L.; Piñeros, M. *Global Cancer Observatory: Cancer Today*; International Agency for Research on Cancer: Lyon, France, 2022.
2. Howlader, N. SEER Cancer Statistics Review, 1975–2011. Available online: https://seer.cancer.gov/archive/csr/1975_2014/ (accessed on 20 October 2023).
3. De Koning, H.J.; van der Aalst, C.M.; de Jong, P.A.; Scholten, E.T.; Nackaerts, K.; Heuvelmans, M.A.; Lammers, J.W.; Weenink, C.; Yousaf-Khan, U.; Horeweg, N.; et al. Reduced lung-cancer mortality with volume CT screening in a randomized trial. *N. Engl. J. Med.* **2020**, *382*, 503–513. [CrossRef]
4. Oudkerk, M.; Devaraj, A.; Vliegenthart, R.; Henzler, T.; Prosch, H.; Heussel, C.P.; Bastarrika, G.; Sverzellati, N.; Mascalchi, M.; Delorme, S.; et al. European position statement on lung cancer screening. *Lancet Oncol.* **2017**, *18*, e754–e766. [CrossRef] [PubMed]
5. Dziedzic, R.; Marjanski, T.; Binczyk, F.; Polanska, J.; Sawicka, W.; Rzyman, W. Favourable outcomes in patients with early-stage non-small-cell lung cancer operated on by video-assisted thoracoscopic surgery: A propensity score-matched analysis. *Eur. J. Cardiothorac. Surg.* **2018**, *54*, 547–553. [CrossRef] [PubMed]
6. Piwkowski, C.; Gabryel, P.; Campisi, A.; Orłowski, T.M.; Zieliński, M.; Rzyman, W.; Kowalewski, J.; Czyżewski, D.; Grochowski, Z.; Wójcik, J.; et al. Ninety-day mortality of thoracoscopic vs open lobectomy: A large multicenter cohort study. *Ann. Thorac. Surg.* **2023**, *115*, 693–699. [CrossRef] [PubMed]
7. Coco, D.; Leanza, S. Current perspective on uniportal and multiportal video-assisted thoracic surgery during lobectomy for lung cancer. *Kardiochir. Torakochir. Pol.* **2022**, *19*, 146–151. [CrossRef] [PubMed]
8. Ma, J.; Li, X.; Zhao, S.; Wang, J.; Zhang, W.; Sun, G. Robot-assisted thoracic surgery versus video-assisted thoracic surgery for lung lobectomy or segmentectomy in patients with non-small cell lung cancer: A meta-analysis. *BMC Cancer* **2021**, *21*, 498. [CrossRef]
9. Servais, E.L.; Miller, D.L.; Thibault, D.; Hartwig, M.G.; Kosinski, A.S.; Stock, C.T.; Price, T.; Quadri, S.M.; D'Agostino, R.S.; Burfeind, W.R. Conversion to thoracotomy during thoracoscopic vs robotic lobectomy: Predictors and outcomes. *Ann. Thorac. Surg.* **2022**, *114*, 409–417. [CrossRef]
10. Novellis, P.; Bottoni, E.; Voulaz, E.; Cariboni, U.; Testori, A.; Bertolaccini, L.; Giordano, L.; Dieci, E.; Granato, L.; Vanni, E.; et al. Robotic surgery, video-assisted thoracic surgery, and open surgery for early stage lung cancer: Comparison of costs and outcomes at a single institute. *J. Thorac. Dis.* **2018**, *10*, 790–798. [CrossRef]

11. Ginsberg, R.J.; Rubinstein, L.V. Randomized trial of lobectomy versus limited resection for T1 N0 non-small cell lung cancer. Lung Cancer Study Group. *Ann. Thorac. Surg.* **1995**, *60*, 615–622. [CrossRef]
12. Saji, H.; Okada, M.; Tsuboi, M.; Nakajima, R.; Suzuki, K.; Aokage, K.; Aoki, T.; Okami, J.; Yoshino, I.; Ito, H.; et al. Seg-mentectomy versus lobectomy in small-sized peripheral non-small-cell lung cancer (JCOG0802/WJOG4607L): A multicentre, open-label, phase 3, randomised, controlled, non-inferiority trial. *Lancet* **2022**, *399*, 1607–1617. [CrossRef]
13. Altorki, N.; Wang, X.; Kozono, D.; Watt, C.; Landrenau, R.; Wigle, D.; Port, J.; Jones, D.R.; Conti, M.; Ashrafi, A.S.; et al. Lobar or sublobar resection for peripheral stage IA non–small-cell lung cancer. *N. Engl. J. Med.* **2023**, *388*, 489–498. [CrossRef] [PubMed]
14. Cardillo, G.; Petersen, R.H.; Ricciardi, S.; Patel, A.; Lodhia, J.V.; Gooseman, M.R.; Brunelli, A.; Dunning, J.; Fang, W.; Gossot, D.; et al. European guidelines for the surgical management of pure ground-glass opacities and part-solid nodules: Task Force of the European Association of Cardio-Thoracic Surgery and the European Society of Thoracic Surgeons. *Eur. J. Cardiothorac. Surg.* **2023**, *64*, ezad222. [CrossRef] [PubMed]
15. Galanis, M.; Leivaditis, V.; Gioutsos, K.; Panagiotopoulos, I.; Kyratzopoulos, A.; Mulita, F.; Papaporfyriou, A.; Verras, G.I.; Tasios, K.; Antzoulas, A.; et al. Segmentectomy versus lobectomy. Which factors are decisive for an optimal oncological outcome? *Kardiochir. Torakochir. Pol.* **2023**, *20*, 179–186. [CrossRef] [PubMed]
16. Rami-Porta, R. The evolving concept of complete resection in lung cancer surgery. *Cancers* **2021**, *13*, 2583. [CrossRef] [PubMed]
17. Manfredini, B.; Zirafa, C.C.; Filosso, P.L.; Stefani, A.; Romano, G.; Davini, F.; Melfi, F. The Role of Lymphadenectomy in Early-Stage NSCLC. *Cancers* **2023**, *15*, 3735. [CrossRef] [PubMed]
18. Liang, R.-B.; Yang, J.; Zeng, T.-S.; Long, H.; Fu, J.-H.; Zhang, L.-J.; Lin, P.; Wang, X.; Rong, T.-H.; Hou, X.; et al. Incidence and distribution of lobe-specific mediastinal lymph node metastasis in non-small cell lung cancer: Data from 4511 resected cases. *Ann. Surg. Oncol.* **2018**, *25*, 3300–3307. [CrossRef] [PubMed]
19. Deng, H.Y.; Zhou, J.; Wang, R.L.; Jiang, R.; Zhu, D.X.; Tang, X.J.; Zhou, Q. Lobe-specific lymph node dissection for clinical early-stage (cIa) peripheral non-small cell lung cancer patients: What and how? *Ann. Surg. Oncol.* **2020**, *27*, 472–480. [CrossRef]
20. Shapiro, M.; Kadakia, S.; Lim, J.; Breglio, A.; Wisnivesky, J.P.; Kaufman, A.; Lee, D.S.; Flores, R.M. Lobe-specific mediastinal nodal dissection is sufficient during lobectomy by video-assisted thoracic surgery or thoracotomy for early-stage lung cancer. *Chest* **2013**, *144*, 1615–1621. [CrossRef]
21. Woo, W.; Shin, J.I.; Kipkorir, V.; Yang, Y.H.; Lee, S.; Lee, C.Y. Clinical benefits of lobe-specific lymph node dissection in surgery for non-small cell lung cancer: A systematic review and meta-analysis. *JTO Clin. Res. Rep.* **2023**, *4*, 100516. [CrossRef]
22. Wang, Z.; Qi, Z.; Cheng, D.; Hao, X.; Pu, Q.; Liu, L. Lobe-specific node dissection can be a suitable alternative to systematic lymph node dissection in highly selective early-stage non-small-cell lung cancer patients: A meta-analysis. *Ann. Thorac. Cardiovasc. Surg.* **2021**, *27*, 143–150. [CrossRef]
23. Kakuturu, J.; Abbas, G.; Toker, A. Evaluating the quality of lymphadenectomy in lung cancer resections: A narrative review. *AME Surg. J.* **2022**, *2*, 1–8. [CrossRef]
24. Ray, M.A.; Smeltzer, M.P.; Faris, N.R.; Osarogiagbon, R.U. Survival after mediastinal node dissection, systematic sampling, or neither for early stage NSCLC. *J. Thorac. Oncol.* **2020**, *15*, 1670–1681. [CrossRef] [PubMed]
25. Gabryel, P.; Skrzypczak, P.; Campisi, A.; Kasprzyk, M.; Roszak, M.; Piwkowski, C. Predictors of long-term survival of thoracoscopic lobectomy for stage ia non-small cell lung cancer: A large retrospective cohort study. *Cancers* **2023**, *15*, 3877. [CrossRef] [PubMed]
26. Osarogiagbon, R.U.; Yu, X. Nonexamination of lymph nodes and survival after resection of non-small cell lung cancer. *Ann Thorac Surg.* **2013**, *96*, 1178–1189. [CrossRef] [PubMed]
27. Butnor, K.J.; Asamura, H.; Travis, W.D. Node doubt: Rigorous surgical nodal procurement combined with thorough pathologic evaluation improves non-small cell lung carcinoma staging accuracy. *Ann. Thorac. Surg.* **2016**, *102*, 353–356. [CrossRef] [PubMed]
28. Gabryel, P.; Roszak, M.; Skrzypczak, P.; Gabryel, A.; Zielińska, D.; Sielewicz, M.; Campisi, A.; Kasprzyk, M.; Piwkowski, C. Identification of factors related to the quality of lymphadenectomy for lung cancer: Secondary analysis of prospective randomized trial data. *J. Clin. Med.* **2023**, *12*, 3780. [CrossRef] [PubMed]
29. Wojciechowska, U.; Barańska, K.; Michałek, I.; Olasek, P.; Miklewska, M.; Didkowska, J.A. Cancer in Poland in 2020. Narodowy Instytut Onkologii. 2020. Available online: https://onkologia.org.pl/en/publications (accessed on 23 July 2023).
30. National Comprehensive Cancer Network. NCCN Clinical Practice Guidelines in Oncology. In *Non-Small Cell Lung Cancer. Version 3.2022*; 2022. Available online: https://pubmed.ncbi.nlm.nih.gov/35545176/ (accessed on 4 November 2023).
31. Rami-Porta, R.; Call, S.; Dooms, C.; Obiols, C.; Sánchez, M.; Travis, W.D.; Vollmer, I. Lung cancer staging: A concise update. *Eur. Resp. J.* **2018**, *51*, 1800190. [CrossRef]
32. Al-Ibraheem, A.; Hirmas, N.; Fanti, S.; Paez, D.; Abuhijla, F.; Al-Rimawi, D.; Al-Rasheed, U.; Abdeljalil, R.; Hawari, F.; Alrabi, K.; et al. Impact of (18)F-FDG PET/CT, CT and EBUS/TBNA on preoperative mediastinal nodal staging of NSCLC. *BMC Med. Imaging.* **2021**, *21*, 49. [CrossRef]
33. Edwards, T.; Balata, H.; Elshafi, M.; Foden, P.; Bishop, P.; Fontaine, E.; Jones, M.; Krysiak, P.; Rammohan, K.; Shah, R.; et al. Adequacy of intraoperative nodal staging during surgical resection of NSCLC: Influencing factors and its relationship to survival. *J. Thorac. Oncol.* **2017**, *12*, 1845–1850. [CrossRef]
34. Pawelczyk, K.; Blasiak, P.; Szromek, M.; Nowinska, K.; Marciniak, M. Assessment of adequacy of intraoperative nodal staging and factors influencing the lack of its compliance with recommendations in the surgical treatment of non-small cell lung cancer (NSCLC). *J. Thorac. Dis.* **2018**, *10*, 4902–4911. [CrossRef]

35. Bott, M.J.; Patel, A.P.; Crabtree, T.D.; Colditz, G.A.; Kreisel, D.; Krupnick, A.S.; Patterson, G.A.; Broderick, S.; Meyers, B.F.; Puri, V. Pathologic upstaging in patients undergoing resection for stage I non-small cell lung cancer: Are there modifiable predictors? *Ann. Thorac. Surg.* **2015**, *100*, 2048–2053. [CrossRef] [PubMed]
36. Tsai, T.M.; Liu, C.Y.; Lin, M.W.; Hsu, H.H.; Chen, J.S. Factors associated with nodal upstaging in clinical T1a-bN0M0 non-small cell lung cancers. *Cancers* **2022**, *14*, 1277. [CrossRef]
37. Chmielewska, I.; Stencel, K.; Kalinka, E.; Ramlau, R.; Krawczyk, P. Neoadjuvant and adjuvant immunotherapy in non-small cell lung cancer—Clinical trials experience. *Cancers* **2021**, *13*, 5048. [CrossRef]
38. McKenna, R.J. Complications and learning curves for video-assisted thoracic surgery lobectomy. *Thorac. Surg. Clin.* **2008**, *18*, 275–280. [CrossRef] [PubMed]
39. Paladini, P.; Meniconi, F.; Ghisalberti, M.; Luzzi, L.; Ligabue, T.; de Leonibus, L.; Corzani, R. Review of the learning curve of video-assisted thoracic surgery & robotic-assisted thoracic surgery lobectomies—Similarities and differences. *Curr. Chall. Thorac. Surg.* **2021**, *3*, 16.
40. Amore, D.; Curcio, C. Steps in the development of a VATS lobectomy program. *J. Vis. Surg.* **2017**, *3*, 104. [CrossRef]
41. Petersen, R.H.; Hansen, H.J. Learning curve associated with VATS lobectomy. *Ann. Cardiothorac. Surg.* **2012**, *1*, 47–50. [CrossRef]
42. Gonfiotti, A.; Bongiolatti, S.; Borgianni, S.; Borrelli, R.; Jaus, M.O.; Politi, L.; Tancredi, G.; Viggiano, D.; Voltolini, L. Development of a video-assisted thoracoscopic lobectomy program in a single institution: Results before and after completion of the learning curve. *J. Cardiothorac. Surg.* **2016**, *11*, 130. [CrossRef]
43. Mazzella, A.; Olland, A.; Falcoz, P.E.; Renaud, S.; Santelmo, N.; Massard, G. Video-assisted thoracoscopic lobectomy: Which is the learning curve of an experienced consultant? *J. Thorac. Dis.* **2016**, *8*, 2444–2453. [CrossRef]
44. Osarogiagbon, R.U.; Ogbata, O.; Yu, X. Number of lymph nodes associated with maximal reduction of long-term mortality risk in pathologic node-negative non-small cell lung cancer. *Ann. Thorac. Surg.* **2014**, *97*, 385–393. [CrossRef]
45. Krantz, S.B.; Lutfi, W.; Kuchta, K.; Wang, C.H.; Kim, K.W.; Howington, J.A. Improved Lymph Node Staging in Early-Stage Lung Cancer in the National Cancer Database. *Ann. Thorac. Surg.* **2017**, *104*, 1805–1814. [CrossRef]
46. Mroczkowski, P.; Dziki, Ł.; Vosikova, T.; Otto, R.; Mercz-Sadowska, A.; Zajdel, R.; Zajdel, K.; Lippert, H.; Jannasch, O. Rectal cancer: Are 12 lymph nodes the limit? *Cancers* **2023**, *15*, 3447. [CrossRef]
47. Shapiro, M.; Mhango, G.; Kates, M.; Weiser, T.S.; Chin, C.; Swanson, S.J.; Wisnivesky, J.P. Extent of lymph node resection does not increase perioperative morbidity and mortality after surgery for stage I lung cancer in the elderly. *Eur. J. Surg. Oncol.* **2012**, *38*, 516–522. [CrossRef] [PubMed]
48. Darling, G.E.; Allen, M.S.; Decker, P.A.; Ballman, K.; Malthaner, R.A.; Inculet, R.I.; Jones, D.R.; McKenna, R.J.; Landreneau, R.J.; Rusch, V.W.; et al. Randomized trial of mediastinal lymph node sampling versus complete lymphadenectomy during pulmonary resection in the patient with N0 or N1 (less than hilar) non-small cell carcinoma: Results of the American College of Surgery Oncology Group Z0030 Trial. *J. Thorac. Cardiovasc. Surg.* **2011**, *141*, 662–670. [CrossRef] [PubMed]
49. Huang, X.; Wang, J.; Chen, Q.; Jiang, J. Mediastinal lymph node dissection versus mediastinal lymph node sampling for early stage non-small cell lung cancer: A systematic review and meta-analysis. *PLoS ONE* **2014**, *9*, e109979. [CrossRef] [PubMed]
50. Taleb, N.N. Black swans and the domains of statistics. *Am. Stat.* **2007**, *61*, 198–200. [CrossRef]
51. Safdie, F.M.; Sanchez, M.V.; Sarkaria, I.S. Prevention and management of intraoperative crisis in VATS and open chest surgery: How to avoid emergency conversion. *J. Vis. Surg.* **2017**, *3*, 87. [CrossRef]
52. Goldstraw, P.; Chansky, K.; Crowley, J.; Rami-Porta, R.; Asamura, H.; Eberhardt, W.E.; Nicholson, A.G.; Groome, P.; Mitchell, A.; Bolejack, V. The IASLC lung cancer staging project: Proposals for revision of the TNM stage groupings in the forthcoming (eighth) edition of the TNM classification for lung cancer. *J. Thorac. Oncol.* **2016**, *11*, 39–51. [CrossRef]
53. Ray, M.A.; Fehnel, C.; Akinbobola, O.; Faris, N.R.; Taylor, M.; Pacheco, A.; Smeltzer, M.P.; Osarogiagbon, R.U. Comparative effectiveness of a lymph node collection kit versus heightened awareness on lung cancer surgery quality and outcomes. *J. Thorac. Oncol.* **2021**, *16*, 774–783. [CrossRef]
54. Osarogiagbon, R.U.; Smeltzer, M.P.; Faris, N.R.; Ray, M.A.; Fehnel, C.; Ojeabulu, P.; Akinbobola, O.; Meadows-Taylor, M.; McHugh, L.M.; Halal, A.M.; et al. Outcomes after use of a lymph node collection kit for lung cancer surgery: A pragmatic, population-based, multi-institutional, staggered implementation study. *J. Thorac. Oncol.* **2021**, *16*, 630–642. [CrossRef]
55. Smeltzer, M.P.; Faris, N.R.; Fehnel, C.; Akinbobola, O.; Saulsberry, A.; Meadows-Taylor, M.; Pacheco, A.; Ray, M.; Osarogiagbon, R.U. Impact of a Lymph Node Specimen Collection Kit on the Distribution and Survival Implications of the Proposed Revised Lung Cancer Residual Disease Classification: A Propensity-Matched Analysis. *JTO Clin. Res. Rep.* **2021**, *2*, 100161. [CrossRef] [PubMed]
56. Gabryel, P.; Kasprzyk, M.; Roszak, M.; Campisi, A.; Smoliński, S.; Zieliński, P.; Piwkowski, C. Comparison of the LigaSure™ bipolar vessel sealer to monopolar electrocoagulation for thoracoscopic lobectomy and lymphadenectomy: A prospective randomized controlled trial. *Surg. Endosc.* **2023**, *37*, 4449–4457. [CrossRef] [PubMed]
57. Nakazawa, S.; Yajima, T.; Ohtaki, Y.; Ito, T.; Kosaka, T.; Shirabe, K. Tips on lymph node dissection using energy devices: A narrative review. *AME Surg. J.* **2022**, *2*, 1–7. [CrossRef]
58. ESTS Quality Certification Program. Available online: https://www.ests.org/professional_development/accreditation.aspx (accessed on 4 November 2023).
59. ESTS Silverbook, Database Annual Report 2023. Available online: https://www.ests.org/ests_database/database_reports/database_reports_silver_books.aspx (accessed on 4 November 2023).

60. Osarogiagbon, R.U.; Sareen, S.; Eke, R.; Yu, X.; McHugh, L.M.; Kernstine, K.H.; Putnam, J.B.; Robbins, E.T. Audit of lymphadenectomy in lung cancer resections using a specimen collection kit and checklist. *Ann. Thorac. Surg.* **2015**, *99*, 421–427. [CrossRef]
61. Riquet, M.; Legras, A.; Mordant, P.; Rivera, C.; Arame, A.; Gibault, L.; Foucault, C.; Dujon, A.; Le Pimpec Barthes, F. Number of mediastinal lymph nodes in non-small cell lung cancer: A Gaussian curve, not a prognostic factor. *Ann. Thorac. Surg.* **2014**, *98*, 224–231. [CrossRef]
62. Van de Graaf, F.W.; Eryigit, Ö.; Lange, J.F. Current perspectives on video and audio recording inside the surgical operating room: Results of a cross-disciplinary survey. *Updates Surg.* **2021**, *73*, 2001–2007. [CrossRef]
63. Eckhoff, J.A.; Rosman, G.; Altieri, M.S.; Speidel, S.; Stoyanov, D.; Anvari, M.; Meier-Hein, L.; März, K.; Jannin, P.; Pugh, C.; et al. SAGES consensus recommendations on surgical video data use, structure, and exploration (for research in artificial intelligence, clinical quality improvement, and surgical education). *Surg. Endosc.* **2023**, *37*, 8690–8707. [CrossRef]

cancers

MDPI

Article

Association between the Preoperative Standard Uptake Value (SUV) and Survival Outcomes after Robotic-Assisted Segmentectomy for Resectable Non-Small Cell Lung Cancer (NSCLC)

Aihab Aboukheir Aboukheir [1,2], Emilio Q. Villanueva III [3,4], Joseph R. Garrett [2], Carla C. Moodie [2], Jenna R. Tew [2], Eric M. Toloza [2], Jacques P. Fontaine [2] and Jobelle J. A. R. Baldonado [2,*]

1 Department of General Surgery, Saint Luke Episcopal Medical Center, General Surgery Residency, Ponce Health Sciences University, Ponce, PR 00716, USA; aihab.aboukheiraboukheir@moffitt.org
2 Department of Thoracic Oncology, Moffitt Cancer Center, Tampa, FL 33612, USA; joe.garrett@moffitt.org (J.R.G.); carla.moodie@moffitt.org (C.C.M.); jenna.tew@moffitt.org (J.R.T.); eric.toloza@moffitt.org (E.M.T.); jacques.fontaine@moffitt.org (J.P.F.)
3 Department of Pathology, University of the Philippines College of Medicine, Manila City 1000, Philippines; eqvillanueva@up.edu.ph
4 Expanded Hospital Research Office, UP–Philippine General Hospital, Manila City 1000, Philippines
* Correspondence: jobelle.baldonado@moffitt.org

Simple Summary: Early-stage lung cancers are best treated with lung resections such as segmentectomy. Despite curative lung resections, however, lung cancers can recur. In our study we present our outcomes for robotic segmentectomy performed for lung cancer and how outcomes could be related to standard uptake value (SUV) as reported in the patients' PET CT scan. We show here that robotic segmentectomy is safe and feasible for early-stage lung cancer, however recurrence was 28.4%. A higher preoperative SUV was associated with worse pathology outcomes and higher recurrence. A higher preoperative SUV was also associated with better long-term survival outcomes.

Abstract: Background: Lung-sparing procedures, specifically segmentectomies and wedge resections, have increased over the years to treat early-stage non-small cell lung cancer (NSCLC). We investigate here the perioperative and long-term outcomes of patients who underwent robotic-assisted segmentectomy (RAS) at an NCI-designated cancer center and aim to show associations between the preoperative standard update value (SUV) to tumor stage, recurrence patterns, and overall survival. Methods: A retrospective analysis was performed on 166 consecutive patients who underwent RAS at a single institution from 2010 to 2021. Of this number, 121 robotic-assisted segmentectomies were performed for primary NSCLC, and a total of 101 patients were evaluated with a PET-CT scan. The SUV from the primary tumor was determined from the PET-CT. The clinical, surgical, and pathologic profiles and perioperative outcomes were summarized via descriptive statistics. Numerical variables were described as the median and interquartile range because all numerical variables were not normally distributed as assessed by the Shapiro–Wilk test of normality. Categorical variables were described as the count and proportion. Chi-square or Fisher's exact test was used for association. The main outcomes were overall survival (OS) and recurrence-free survival (RFS). Kaplan–Meier (KM) curves were constructed to visualize the OS and RFS, which were also stratified according to tumor histology, the pathologic stage, and standard uptake value. A log-rank test for the equality of survival curves was performed to determine significant differences between groups. Results: The most common postoperative complications were atrial fibrillation (8.8%, 9/102), persistent air leak (7.84%, 8/102), and pneumonia (4.9%, 5/102). The median operative duration was 168.5 min (IQR 59), while the median estimated blood loss was 50 mL (IQR 125). The conversion rate to thoracotomy in this cohort was 3.9% (4/102). Intraoperative complications occurred in 2.9% (3/102). The median hospital length of stay was 3 days (IQR 3). The median chest tube duration was 3 days (IQR 2), but 4.9% (5/102) of patients were sent home with a chest tube. The recurrence for this cohort was 28.4% (29/102). The time to recurrence was 353 days (IQR 504), while the time to mortality was

505 days (IQR 761). The NSCLC patients were divided into the following two groups: low SUV (<5, n = 55) and high SUV (≥5, n = 47). Statistically significant associations were noted between SUV and the tumor histology (p = 0.019), tumor grade (p = 0.002), lymph-vascular invasion (p = 0.029), viscera-pleural invasion (p = 0.008), recurrence (p < 0.001) and the site of recurrence (p = 0.047). KM survival analysis showed significant differences in the curves for OS (log-rank p-value 0.0204) and RFS (log-rank p-value 0.0034) between the SUV groups. Conclusion: Robotic-assisted segmentectomy for NSCLC has reasonable perioperative and oncologic outcomes. Furthermore, we demonstrate here the prognostic implication of preoperative SUV to pathologic outcomes, recurrence-free survival, and overall survival.

Keywords: non-small cell lung cancer (NSCLC); segmentectomy; standard update value (SUV); lobectomy; overall survival (OS); recurrence-free survival (RFS)

1. Introduction

Non-small cell lung cancer (NSCLC) is the leading cause of cancer mortality worldwide. There are many risk factors for developing NSCLC, the most notable of which include smoking history, environmental exposure, and family history. Once diagnosed and staged as early, surgical resection is the standard of care for treatment.

Anatomic pulmonary segmentectomy is gaining popularity among thoracic surgeons with an improvement in diagnostic imaging and surgical techniques using minimally invasive surgery. Historically, segmentectomy has not always been accepted by surgeons from the beginning due to the technical complexity and high risk of prolonged air leaks and the supposed increase in local recurrence in comparison with lobectomy [1].

There are two types of sublobar resection NSCLC: wedge resection and segmentectomy. The distinction between the two is that segmentectomy requires the oncologic standard of lobectomies, such as the anatomy of the separation of pulmonary segmental veins, arteries, bronchi, and the removal of lung parenchymal tissue [2]. The European Respiratory Society (ERS) and the European Society of Thoracic Surgery (ESTS) established clinical guidelines for sublobar resections, including wedge and segmental resections. They recommend that anatomical segmentectomy could be performed in the following scenario: stage 1A (tumor size 2–3 cm) with margins of resection > 1 cm, a stage I patient with poor lung functions and lung resections after prior lobectomy all of them with a level of evidence 2 grade of recommendation D [3].

Some argue that the long-term reduction (>12 months) in lung function induced by segmentectomy is very small in comparison with lobectomy but that small differences could benefit lung cancer patients who need subsequent lung resections [4]. Segmentectomy could also be offered to high-risk patients who otherwise could not tolerate a major pulmonary resection and are expected to become ventilator-dependent postoperatively [5,6]. Data regarding differences comparing sublobar resection vs. lobectomy have been abundant. Some studies establish that sublobar resections are associated with an increased incidence of local recurrence when compared with lobectomy [7]. Regarding postoperative complications, segmentectomy patients experienced a prolonged air leak, more blood loss, and increased operative duration [8], but no statistical significance was found in terms of perioperative mortality and morbidity between lobar and sublobar resections [9].

A more recent multicenter study found that with sublobar resection, there were better perioperative outcomes without compromising the short-term survival of elderly patients with clinical stage I NSCLC, but lobectomy was still selected if accurate lymph node staging was needed [10]. With the newer published non-inferiority trial, the JCOG0802/WJOG4607L for small lung tumors (diameter ≤ 2 cm, consolidation-to-tumor ratio > 0.5) demonstrated segmentectomy to be non-inferior to lobectomy with regard to overall survival and a reduction in forced expiratory volume in 1 sec (FEV1), despite a higher proportion of patients with local relapse in the segmentectomy group. This landmark trial suggested that segmentectomy should be the standard surgical procedure for stage 1 small-sized, peripheral NSCLC [11,12].

Robotic surgery (RS) has advanced and become popular in many fields; robotic lobectomy was first reported in the field of thoracic surgery and has become a common surgical procedure with acceptable outcomes in terms of operative time and blood loss [13]. Advancements in RS include high-definition three-dimensional videos, improved ergonomics, a less steep learning curve, tremor suppression, and better maneuverability of instruments, which can promote complex movements in a closed space and influence perioperative outcomes [14,15]. Although advancements in RS have helped in the field of lung surgery, segmentectomy is associated with technical challenges because it requires a deep hilar dissection to identify the segmental branches that need to be divided or preserved and the division of multiple intersegmental planes [16,17].

In the preoperative workup, a 2-deoxy-2-[^{18}F] Fluro-D-glucose positron-emission tomography (^{18}F-FDG PET/CT) is widely used in lung cancer for staging, operative planning, restaging, and the evaluation of the treatment response. The PET/CT scan provides clinicians with additional prognostic indications regarding survival and the estimated risk of relapse utilizing the assessment of the standardized uptake value (SUV) [18,19], which has also been demonstrated to be a parameter for locally advanced disease and poor survival in esophageal cancer [20]. It was found that diagnosis using PET/CT resulted in a substantial detection rate of postoperative lymph node metastasis pathologically, leading to poor prognosis despite the successful complete resection in clinical stage I lung cancer [21].

We report here the perioperative outcomes, including clinical and pathologic, as well as recurrence-free survival and overall survival outcomes in patients who had a robotic-assisted segmentectomy at an NCI-designated comprehensive cancer center. We also aim to show associations between the preoperative SUV and tumor stage, grade, and long-term outcomes.

2. Patient and Methods

We retrospectively analyzed patients who underwent a robotic-assisted segmentectomy (RAS) at a single institution from 2010 to 2021. The Moffitt Cancer Center (MCC) robotic surgery database was used for this analysis. This is a database that has been retrospectively collected and prospectively maintained under an IRB-approved protocol in the Thoracic Oncology Program. This study was conducted in accordance with the Declaration of Helsinki (as revised in 2013). Ethical approval to report this study was obtained from our institution's Scientific Review Committee (MCC #16728, #18761, and #19304) and by our university's Institutional Review Boards (USF IRB #Pro00022263 and Chesapeake IRB #Pro00017745 and #00000790). Individual consent for this retrospective analysis was waived.

Multiple variables, including clinical, surgical, and pathologic profiles, as well as perioperative outcomes of patients with primary lung malignancy who underwent RAS, were collected, and data were summarized using descriptive statistics. Only patients with primary NSCLC staged with a [^{18}F]-fluorodeoxyglucose positron emission tomography/computed tomography (PET/CT) scan were included in the analysis. The preoperative SUVmax was determined from the primary tumor.

Numerical variables were described as a median and interquartile range (IQR) because all numerical variables were not normally distributed, as assessed by the Shapiro–Wilk test of normality. Categorical variables were described as the count and proportion. Chi-square or Fisher's exact test was used for association. The primary endpoints were overall survival (OS) and recurrence-free survival (RFS). Days-to-mortality and days-to-mortality/recurrence were right-censored to the date of their last known follow-up among those who did not die or did not have documented recurrence. Kaplan–Meier (KM) curves were used to demonstrate the OS and RFS of these patients, which were stratified according to tumor histology, pathologic stage, and preoperative SUV. In order to determine significant differences between groups, the log-rank test for equality of survival curves was performed.

3. Results

Between 2010 and 2021, 166 patients underwent RAS at MCC. Among these, 121 RASs were performed for primary early-stage NSCLC. The patients who had secondary malignancies, a history of prior primary NSCLC, and benign conditions were excluded. Of the 121 patients, 101 were evaluated with a PET-CT scan. Patient clinical characteristics are shown in Table 1. The median age was 72 years (IQR 12), and 60 patients (59.4%) were females. Most of our patients identified themselves as white (93/101, 92.1%) and were hypertensive (63/101, 62.4%). A left-sided segmentectomy was more common (66/101, 65.3%) than a right-sided one. The mean preoperative tumor size was 1.75 cm (IQR 1.2). A preoperative SUV $\geq$ 5 was identified in 46/101 patients (45.5%).

Table 1. Clinical profile of primary lung cancer patients who underwent RAS.

Clinical Profile	Summary Statistics	
	$\tilde{x}/n$	*IQR/%*
Age	72	12
Sex		
Male	41	40.6%
Female	60	59.4%
BMI	27.1	7.1
Race		
White	93	92.1%
Hispanic	2	2.0%
Black	5	4.9%
Others	1	1.0%
Pre-operative FEV1	2	0.745
Pre-operative FEV1%	80.5	31.5
Co-morbidities		
Hypertension	63	62.4%
Diabetes mellitus	16	15.8%
COPD	42	41.6%
Congestive heart failure	4	4.0%
ESRD	0	-
Ever-smoker	58	57.4%
Chronic steroid use	1	1.0%
Laterality		
Left	66	65.3%
Right	35	34.7%
Tumor size, clinical imaging	1.75	1.2
Standard uptake value		
SUV < 5	55	54.5%
SUV $\geq$ 5	46	45.5%

Table 2 shows the pathologic profile of our patients. Adenocarcinoma was the most common (65/101, 64.4%), and squamous cell carcinoma was second (24/101, 23.8%). Only 12 (11.8%) patients had other pathologies. In terms of tumor grade, 50/100 (50.00%) were moderately differentiated, and the mean pathologic tumor size was 1.8 cm (IQR 1.1), 12/101 (11.9%) patients had lympho-vascular invasion, 23/101 (22.8%) had viscero-pleural invasion and the majority had stage I disease 82/101 (81.2%).

Table 2. Pathologic profile of primary lung cancer patients who underwent RAS (n = 101).

Pathologic Profile	Summary Statistics	
	$\tilde{x}/n$	*IQR/%*
Tumor histology		
Adenocarcinoma	65	64.4%
Squamous	24	23.8%
Carcinoid/Neuroendocrine	11	10.9%
Other Lung Cancers	1	0.9%
Tumor grade *		
Well differentiated	25	25.0%
Moderately differentiated	50	50.0%
Poorly differentiated	25	25.0%
Tumor size, pathologic examination	1.8	1.1
Lymph-vascular space invasion **	12	11.9%
Viscero-pleural invasion **	23	22.8%
Positive margins of resection	1	1.0%
Total number of lymph nodes assessed	10	7
Number of mediastinal lymph nodes assessed	5	4
Positive lymph nodes	10	9.90%
Pathologic stage		
IA1	26	25.7%
IA2	30	29.7%
IA3	5	5.0%
IB	21	20.8%
IIA	4	4.0%
IIB	9	8.9%
IIIA	6	5.9%
IIIB	0	-
IIIC	0	-
IV	0	-

Note: * 2 cases were not graded, ** 1 case was not assessed for LVI and VPI.

In Table 3, we demonstrate the surgical outcomes. The median estimated blood loss was 50 mL (IQR 125), while the median operative duration was 168.5 min (IQR 59). The conversion rate to thoracotomy in this cohort was 4.0% (4/101). Intraoperative complications occurred in 3.0% (3/101).

Table 3. Surgical profile of primary lung cancer patients who underwent RAS.

Surgical Profile	Summary Statistics	
	$\tilde{x}/n$	*IQR/%*
Neoadjuvant therapy		
None	97	96.0%
Chemo/immunotherapy only	4	4.0%
Radiotherapy only	0	-
Combination chemoradiotherapy	0	-
Operative time	168.5	59
Estimated blood loss	50	125
Intraoperative complication	3	3.0%
Conversion to thoracotomy	4	4.0%

In Table 4, we further demonstrate our perioperative outcomes, including postoperative complications. The most common postoperative complications were atrial fibrillation (9.0%, 9/101), prolonged air leaks (8.0%, 8/101), pneumonia (5.0%, 5/101), and hypoxia (5.0%, 5/101). The thirty-day mortality rate was 0.0%. The median hospital length of stay was 3 days (IQR 3). The median chest tube duration was 3 days (IQR 2), but 5.0% (5/101) of patients were sent home with a chest tube. Recurrence for this cohort was at 27.8% (28/101). Time to recurrence was 353 days (IQR 504), while time to mortality was 505 days (IQR 761).

Table 4. Outcomes of primary lung cancer patients who underwent RAS.

Outcomes	Summary Statistics	
	$\bar{x}$/n	IQR/%
Postoperative complications *	33	32.7%
Atrial fibrillation	9	9.0%
Prolonged air leak	8	8.0%
Pneumonia	5	5.0%
Pneumothorax	5	5.0%
Hypoxia	5	5.0%
Empyema	4	4.0%
Shock	3	3.0%
Aspiration	3	3.0%
Mucus plug	2	2.0%
Respiratory failure	2	2.0%
Other arrhythmia	2	2.0%
Chyle leak	2	2.0%
Myocardial infarction	1	1.0%
Cardiopulmonary arrest	1	1.0%
Hemothorax	0	-
Cerebrovascular accident	0	-
Pulmonary embolism	0	-
Length of hospital stay	3	3
Days with chest tube	3	2
Sent home with chest tube	5	4.90%
Days at home with chest tube	24	20
30-day mortality	0	-
Mortality	25	24.8%
Time-to-mortality	505.5	761
Recurrence	28	28.43%
Time-to-recurrence	353	504
Site of recurrence		
Nodal	4	13.79% ^
Pleural	2	6.90%
Local	10	34.48%
Distant	13	44.83%

Note: * Several patients had more than one postoperative complication.

Table 5 demonstrates the association of SUV with pathologic factors. The 101 patients were divided into the following 2 groups: low SUV (<5, $n = 55$) and high SUV (≥5, $n = 46$). There were statistically significant associations between SUV and tumor histology ($p = 0.016$), tumor grade ($p = 0.002$), tumor size ($p = 0.001$), lympho-vascular invasion ($p = 0.029$), visceral-pleural invasion ($p = 0.008$), recurrence ($p < 0.001$) and the site of recurrence ($p = 0.047$). Interestingly, the pathologic stage and nodal metastasis were not associated with preoperative SUV in this cohort of patients.

Kaplan–Meier survival plots (Figures 1 and 2) showed significant differences in the curves for OS (log-rank *p*-value 0.0204) and RFS (log-rank *p*-value 0.0034) when stratifying for SUV uptake. The patients with a higher SUV uptake had a lower OS and RFS.

Table 5. Association of SUV with the following pathologic factors among primary lung cancer patients who underwent robotic surgery.

Factor	SUV < 5	SUV ≥ 5	*p*-Value
	n = 55 *n* (%)	*n* = 46 *n* (%)	
Tumor histology			0.016
Adenocarcinoma	42 (64.6%)	23 (35.4%)	
Squamous cell	9 (37.5%)	15 (62.5%)	
Neuroendocrine	4 (36.3%)	8 (66.7%)	
Tumor grade			0.002

Table 5. *Cont.*

Factor	SUV < 5	SUV ≥ 5	*p*-Value
Well differentiated	19 (76.00%)	6 (24.00%)	
Moderately differentiated	29 (58.00%)	21 (42.00%)	
Poorly differentiated	7 (28.00%)	18 (72.00%)	
Pathologic stage			0.244
Early (stages I–II)	53 (55.79%)	42 (44.21%)	
Late (stages III–IV)	2 (33.3%)	4 (66.7%)	
Tumor size			0.001
T1	45 (67.16%)	22 (32.84%)	
T2	9 (33.33%)	18 (66.67%)	
T3	1 (14.29%)	6 (85.71%0	
Lymph node metastasis			0.506
N0	51 (56.04%)	40 (43.96%)	
N1 + N2	4 (40.00%)	6 (60.00)	
Lymph-vascular space invasion			0.029
With	3 (25.00%)	9 (75.00%)	
Without	52 (58.43%)	37 (41.57%)	
Viscero-pleural invasion			0.008
With	7 (30.43%)	16 (69.57%)	
Without	48 (61.54%)	30 (38.46%)	
Recurrence			<0.001
With	7 (25.0%)	21 (75.0%)	
Without	48 (65.8%)	25 (34.2%)	
Site of recurrence			0.047
Nodal	0	4 (100.0%)	
Pleural	1 (50.0%)	1 (50.0%)	
Local	5 (55.6%)	4 (44.4%)	
Distant	1 (7.7%)	12 (92.3%)	

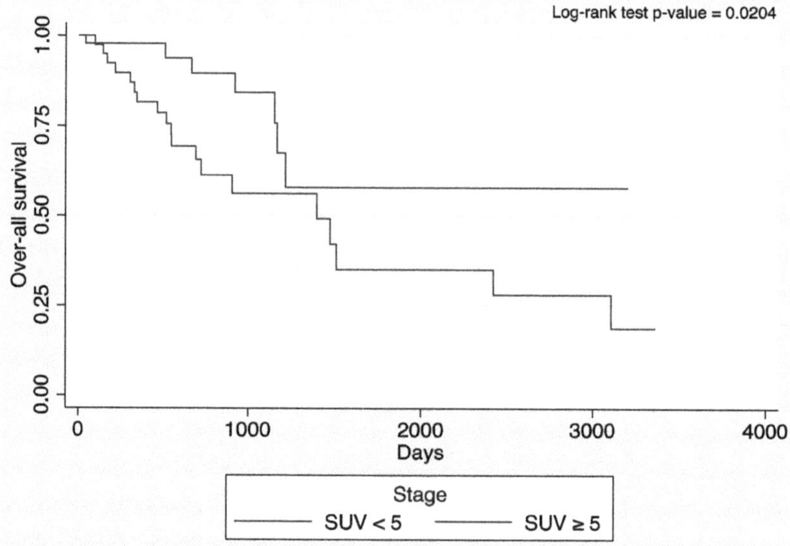

Figure 1. Kaplan–Meier curve of overall survival of primary lung cancer patients who underwent robotic surgery stratified to the standard uptake value.

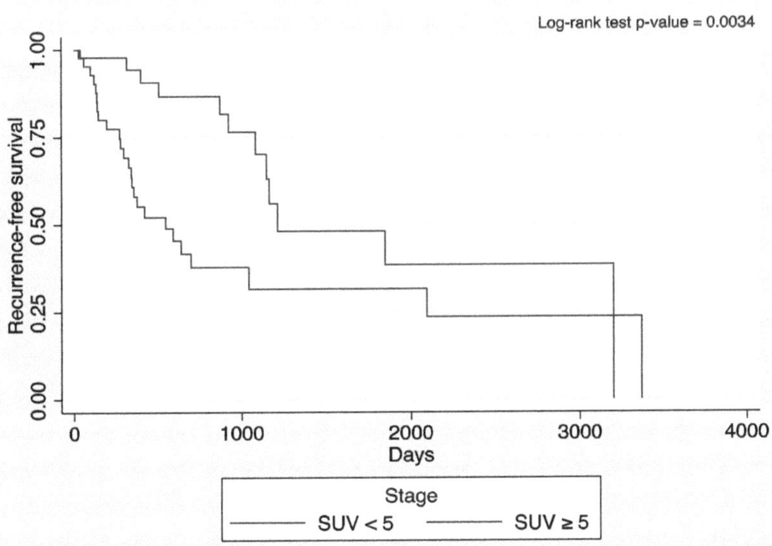

Figure 2. Kaplan–Meier curve of recurrence-free survival of primary lung cancer patients who underwent robotic surgery stratified to the standard uptake value.

4. Discussion

This study presents the experience of a single institution with robotic-assisted segmentectomy to treat NSCLC and the value of preoperative SUV. Segmentectomy has historically not been utilized due to the suggested increase in perioperative complications like prolonged air leaks, increased estimated blood loss (EBL), and the increased duration of chest tube days. These findings have been consistently demonstrated to be of no statistical significance when compared to lobectomy [22]. At our institution, perioperative events are comparable to single-institution robotic lobectomies with a similar population, where EBL, chest tube duration, and operative time are similar [23]. Our LOS comes from the standardized management of all our patients with enhanced recovery pathways, which are comparable to the early discharge described by Chevrollier et al. [24]. Our experience with RAS demonstrates an acceptable operative time and blood loss with only ~3% intraoperative complications. Most postoperative complications were atrial fibrillation and pneumonia, which are comparable to the literature [13,25–27].

Unfortunately, despite a curative resection for early-stage NSCLC, there continues to be a high rate of recurrence, which currently ranges from 30 to 60% [28]. The recurrence rate in our cohort is consistent with this at 28.4%. We hypothesized in our study that higher preoperative SUV could be a poor risk factor for pathologic outcomes as well as long-term survival outcomes, including recurrence and OS. In addition to its role in diagnosis and metastatic workups for NSCLC, a meta-analysis confirmed that the increased SUV of the primary tumor is a poor prognostic factor in patients with NSCLC, with a combined hazard ratio of 2.27 [29]. A retrospective review performed for NSCLC tumors $\geq$ 1 cm found that increasing tumor size was an independent predictor of a higher SUV_{max} and that a high SUV_{max} to tumor size ratio is a stronger predictor of survival than a high SUV_{max} alone [30]. Another study that looked at preoperative SUV in patients who underwent a lobectomy demonstrated that high SUVmax was associated with larger tumor size, poor differentiation, lymphovascular invasion, and shorter freedom from recurrence [31]. All these studies support the prognostic value that preoperative SUV_{max} affords.

We demonstrate here the value of preoperative SUV in relation to postoperative pathologic factors, showing that with a higher SUV, there is worse overall survival and worse recurrence-free survival. The standard uptake value has been an important determinant in lung cancer, with studies placing it as a risk factor for recurrence in small-sized early-stage NSCLC [32]. Both SUVmax and SUVmean values were also noted in one retrospective study to be significantly higher in those with lymph node metastasis compared to those without [33]. Kamigaichi et al. studied the predictive criteria of unexpected N2 disease findings in patients with preoperative SUV ≥ 3 and regarded it as an independent risk factor [34]. Likewise, higher SUVs were associated with worse survival for patients undergoing surgery and a marginal risk factor for OS [18].

Patients with preoperative SUV ≥ 5 in our cohort presented statistically significant associations in terms of tumor histology, tumor grade, lymph vascular invasion, visceral-pleural invasion, recurrence, and the site of recurrence. Sun et al. studied 200 patients who had lobectomies and identified preoperative SUV < 2.5 to be one of the prognostic variables for lower lymph node metastasis and cancers that could be treated with a segmentectomy [35]. This study showed that the probability of isolated lymph node metastasis in patients with a baseline SUVmax > 2.5 was 9 times that of patients whose SUVmax did not exceed 2.5, and concluded that the lower the SUVmax, the lower the chance of metastasis. All these data, including ours, suggest that a higher preoperative SUV portends a poorer prognosis. It could be a useful tool to predict lymph node metastases, recurrence patterns, and survival. More importantly, this prediction of tumor response and outcomes may offer clinical significance when optimizing treatment strategies.

A meta-analysis of previous studies on stage I lung cancer also demonstrated that patients with tumors with a higher metabolic activity have shorter survival than patients with tumors with lower metabolic activity via evaluating lympho-vascular invasion, SUV, and disease-free survival [36]. Kaplan–Meier survival analysis in our study showed significant differences in the curves for OS and RFS between the SUV groups, with a higher SUV portending poorer OS and RFS. With the publication of the JCOG 0802 and CALGB 140503 results, we now have strong data to support segmentectomy as a non-inferior alternative to lobectomy in treating early-stage, $\leq$2 cm NSCLC. We expect that based on these results, there could be an increase in the number of patients with early-stage, resectable NSCLC who are treated with segmentectomy. These two trials did not investigate and stratify patients based on preoperative SUV; however, and what we now know based on our study findings and the literature, future studies could dwell on how preoperative SUV can play a role in further influencing treatment decisions, including induction and adjuvant therapies.

5. Study Limitations

There are several limitations to this study. First, this is a retrospective analysis of prospectively collected data in a single-institution study only. In addition, there are no clear criteria as to the performance of robotic-assisted segmentectomy versus lobectomy for the population of patients in this study. In addition, SUV is affected by many factors, such as differences in body part composition, time-dependent factors, and PET scanner calibration. It is only a single-pixel value. There is no standardized cut-off value to establish a relationship between OS and RFS.

6. Conclusions

Robotic-assisted segmentectomy for NSCLC appears to have reasonable perioperative and oncologic outcomes. Furthermore, we demonstrate here the prognostic implication of how a higher preoperative SUV leads to higher recurrence, more lymph-vascular invasion, viscera-pleural invasion, worse overall survival, and recurrence-free survival. This study opens the discussion for taking SUV into consideration for the further treatment of stage 1 NSCLC postoperatively.

Author Contributions: Conceptualization, A.A.A., J.J.A.R.B., J.P.F. and E.M.T.; methodology, A.A.A., J.J.A.R.B., J.P.F. and E.M.T.; formal analysis, A.A.A., E.Q.V.III, J.J.A.R.B., J.P.F. and E.M.T.; investigation, A.A.A., J.J.A.R.B., J.P.F., E.M.T., J.R.G., C.C.M. and J.R.T.; resources, A.A.A., J.J.A.R.B., J.P.F., E.M.T., J.R.G., C.C.M. and J.R.T.; data curation, A.A.A., J.J.A.R.B., J.P.F., E.M.T., J.R.G., C.C.M. and J.R.T.; writing—original draft preparation, A.A.A., E.Q.V.III and J.J.A.R.B.; writing—review and editing, E.Q.V.III, J.J.A.R.B., J.P.F. and E.M.T.; visualization, A.A.A., E.Q.V.III and J.J.A.R.B.; supervision, J.J.A.R.B., J.P.F. and E.M.T.; project administration, J.J.A.R.B., J.P.F. and E.M.T.; All authors have read and agreed to the published version of the manuscript.

Funding: This research received no external funding.

Institutional Review Board Statement: The study was conducted in accordance with the Declaration of Helsinki (as revised in 2013). Ethical approval to report this study was obtained from Moffitt Cancer Center's Scientific Review Committee (MCC #16728, #18761, and #19304) and by our University of South Florida's Institutional Review Boards (USF IRB #Pro00022263 and Chesapeake IRB #Pro00017745 and #00000790).

Informed Consent Statement: Individual consent for this retrospective analysis was waived.

Data Availability Statement: The authors confirm that the data supporting the findings of this study are available within the article. Raw data that support the findings of the study are available from the corresponding author upon reasonable request.

Conflicts of Interest: E.M.T. and J.P.F. have had financial relationships with Intuitive Surgical, Inc., in the form of an honoraria received as robotic thoracic surgery observation sites and proctors. None of the other authors have any conflict of interest to disclose.

Abbreviations

CALGB: Cancer and Leukemia Group B; FEV1: forced expiratory volume in 1 sec; JCOG: Japanese Clinical Oncology Group; NSCLC: non-small cell lung cancer; OS: overall survival; RAS: robotic-assisted segmentectomy; RFS: recurrence-free survival; RS: robotic surgery; SUV: standardized uptake value; WJOG: West Japan Oncology Group.

References

1. Perroni, G.; Veronesi, G. Robotic segmentectomy: Indication and technique. *J. Thorac. Dis.* **2020**, *12*, 3404–3410. [CrossRef] [PubMed]
2. Wang, C.; Wu, S.; Zhang, R.; Jin, K.; Qian, Y.; Mao, N.; Liu, Y.; Zhang, M.; Zhang, K.; Wang, R.; et al. Identifying lung cancer patients suitable for Segmentectomy: A brief review. *Front. Surg.* **2021**, *8*, 637441. [CrossRef] [PubMed]
3. Brunelli, A. Commentary: The ERS/ESTS clinical guidelines for evaluating fitness for radical treatment for lung cancer. *Breathe* **2009**, *6*, 141–145. [CrossRef]
4. Charloux, A.; Quoix, E. Lung segmentectomy: Does it offer a real functional benefit over lobectomy? *Eur. Respir. Rev.* **2017**, *26*, 170079. [CrossRef] [PubMed]
5. Helminen, O.; Söderström, J.; Andersen, H.; Sihvo, E. How often segmentectomy is feasible in lung cancer surgery: A population-based evaluation. *Eur. J. Cardio-Thoracic Surg.* **2021**, *60*, 1286–1294. [CrossRef] [PubMed]
6. Roy, P. Preoperative pulmonary evaluation for lung resection. *J. Anaesthesiol. Clin. Pharmacol.* **2018**, *34*, 296–300. [CrossRef] [PubMed]
7. El-Sherif, A.; Gooding, W.E.; Santos, R.; Pettiford, B.; Ferson, P.F.; Fernando, H.C.; Urda, S.J.; Luketich, J.D.; Landreneau, R.J. Outcomes of Sublobar resection versus lobectomy for stage I non–small cell lung cancer: A 13-year analysis. *Ann. Thorac. Surg.* **2006**, *82*, 408–416. [CrossRef]
8. Ohtsuka, T.; Kamiyama, I.; Asakura, K.; Kohno, M. Thirty-day outcomes after lobectomy or segmentectomy for lung cancer surgery. *Asian Cardiovasc. Thorac. Ann.* **2015**, *23*, 828–831. [CrossRef]
9. Altorki, N.K.; Wang, X.; Wigle, D.; Gu, L.; Darling, G.; Ashrafi, A.S.; Landrenau, R.; Miller, D.; Liberman, M.; Jones, D.R.; et al. Perioperative mortality and morbidity after sublobar versus lobar resection for early-stage non-small-cell lung cancer: Post-hoc analysis of an international, randomised, phase 3 trial (CALGB/Alliance 140503). *Lancet Respir. Med.* **2018**, *6*, 915–924. [CrossRef]
10. Zhang, Z.; Feng, H.; Zhao, H.; Hu, J.; Liu, L.; Liu, Y.; Li, X.; Xu, L.; Li, Y.; Lu, X.; et al. Sublobar resection is associated with better perioperative outcomes in elderly patients with clinical stage I non-small cell lung cancer: A multicenter retrospective cohort study. *J. Thorac. Dis.* **2019**, *11*, 1838–1848. [CrossRef]

11. Nakamura, K.; Saji, H.; Nakajima, R.; Okada, M.; Asamura, H.; Shibata, T.; Nakamura, S.; Tada, H.; Tsuboi, M. A phase III randomized trial of lobectomy versus limited resection for small-sized peripheral non-small cell lung cancer (JCOG0802/WJOG4607L). *Ultrasound Med. Biol.* **2009**, *40*, 271–274. [CrossRef] [PubMed]
12. Saji, H.; Okada, M.; Tsuboi, M.; Nakajima, R.; Suzuki, K.; Aokage, K.; Aoki, T.; Okami, J.; Yoshino, I.; Ito, H.; et al. Segmentectomy versus lobectomy in small-sized peripheral non-small-cell lung cancer (JCOG0802/WJOG4607L): A multicentre, open-label, phase 3, randomised, controlled, non-inferiority trial. *Lancet* **2022**, *399*, 1607–1617. [CrossRef] [PubMed]
13. Kagimoto, A.; Tsutani, Y.; Izaki, Y.; Handa, Y.; Mimae, T.; Miyata, Y.; Okada, M. Initial experience of robotic anatomical segmentectomy for non-small cell lung cancer. *Ultrasound Med. Biol.* **2020**, *50*, 440–445. [CrossRef] [PubMed]
14. Ma, J.; Li, X.; Zhao, S.; Wang, J.; Zhang, W.; Sun, G. Robot-assisted thoracic surgery versus video-assisted thoracic surgery for lung lobectomy or Segmentectomy in patients with non-small cell lung cancer: A meta-analysis. *BMC Cancer* **2021**, *21*, 498. [CrossRef]
15. Li, C.; Han, Y.; Han, D.; Chen, X.; Chen, K.; Cerfolio, R.J.; Li, H. Robotic approach to combined anatomic pulmonary Subsegmentectomy: Technical aspects and early results. *Ann. Thorac. Surg.* **2018**, *107*, 1480–1486. [CrossRef]
16. Eguchi, T.; Miura, K.; Hamanaka, K.; Shimizu, K. Adoption of robotic core technology in minimally invasive lung Segmentectomy: Review. *J. Pers. Med.* **2022**, *12*, 1417. [CrossRef]
17. Eguchi, T.; Sato, T.; Shimizu, K. Technical advances in segmentectomy for lung cancer: A minimally invasive strategy for deep, small, and impalpable tumors. *Cancers* **2021**, *13*, 3137. [CrossRef]
18. Cistaro, A.; Quartuccio, N.; Mojtahedi, A.; Fania, P.; Filosso, P.L.; Campenni, A.; Ficola, U.; Baldari, S. Prediction of 2 years-survival in patients with stage I and II non-small cell lung cancer utilizing 18F-FDG PET/CT SUV quantifica. *Radiol. Oncol.* **2013**, *47*, 219–223. [CrossRef]
19. Paesmans, M.; Berghmans, T.; Dusart, M.; Garcia, C.; Hossein-Foucher, C.; Lafitte, J.-J.; Mascaux, C.; Meert, A.-P.; Roelandts, M.; Scherpereel, A.; et al. Primary tumor standardized uptake value measured on fluorodeoxyglucose positron emission tomography is of prognostic value for survival in non-small cell lung cancer: Update of a systematic review and meta-analysis by the European lung cancer working party for the international association for the study of lung cancer staging project. *J. Thorac. Oncol.* **2010**, *5*, 612–619. [CrossRef]
20. Mantziari, S.; Pomoni, A.; Prior, J.O.; Winiker, M.; Allemann, P.; Demartines, N.; Schäfer, M. 18f-Fdg pet/CT-derived parameters predict clinical stage and prognosis of esophageal cancer. *BMC Med. Imaging* **2020**, *20*, 7. [CrossRef]
21. Hino, H.; Utsumi, T.; Maru, N.; Matsui, H.; Taniguchi, Y.; Saito, T.; Murakawa, T. Clinical impact and utility of positron emission tomography on occult lymph node metastasis and survival: Radical surgery for stage I lung cancer. *Gen. Thorac. Cardiovasc. Surg.* **2021**, *69*, 1196–1203. [CrossRef] [PubMed]
22. Suzuki, K.; Saji, H.; Aokage, K.; Watanabe, S.-I.; Okada, M.; Mizusawa, J.; Nakajima, R.; Tsuboi, M.; Nakamura, S.; Nakamura, K.; et al. Comparison of pulmonary segmentectomy and lobectomy: Safety results of a randomized trial. *J. Thorac. Cardiovasc. Surg.* **2019**, *158*, 895–907. [CrossRef] [PubMed]
23. Herrera, L.J.; Wherley, E.M.; Agyabeng-Dadzie, K.; Ramsuchit, B.; Johnston, M.A.; Escalon, J.C. 500 Consecutive robotic lobectomies for non-small cell lung cancer: Perioperative and Oncologic outcomes. *Innov. Technol. Tech. Cardiothorac. Vasc. Surg.* **2021**, *16*, 441–447. [CrossRef] [PubMed]
24. Chevrollier, G.S.; Nemecz, A.K.; Devin, C.; Go, K.V.; Yi, M.; Keith, S.W.; Cowan, S.W.; Evans, N.R. Early discharge does not increase readmission rates after minimally invasive anatomic lung resection. *Innov. Technol. Tech. Cardiothorac. Vasc. Surg.* **2019**, *14*, 218–226. [CrossRef] [PubMed]
25. Nguyen, D.; Gharagozloo, F.; Tempesta, B.; Meyer, M.; Gruessner, A. Long-term results of robotic anatomical segmentectomy for early-stage non-small-cell lung cancer. *Eur. J. Cardio-Thoracic. Surg.* **2018**, *55*, 427–433. [CrossRef] [PubMed]
26. Toker, A.; Özyurtkan, M.O.; Kaba, E.; Ayalp, K.; Demirhan, Ö.; Uyumaz, E. Robotic anatomic lung resections: The initial experience and description of learning in 102 cases. *Surg. Endosc.* **2015**, *30*, 676–683. [CrossRef] [PubMed]
27. Terra, R.M.; Lauricella, L.L.; Haddad, R.; De-Campos, J.R.M.; Nabuco-De-Araujo, P.H.X.; Lima, C.E.T.; dos Santos, F.C.B.; Pego-Fernandes, P.M. Segmentectomia pulmonar anatômica robótica: Aspectos técnicos e desfechos. *Rev. Do Colégio Bras. De Cir.* **2019**, *46*. [CrossRef]
28. Winton, T.; Livingston, R.; Johnson, D.; Rigas, J.; Johnston, M.; Butts, C.; Cormier, Y.; Goss, G.; Inculet, R.; Vallieres, E.; et al. Vinorelbine plus cisplatin vs. observation in resected non–small-cell lung cancer. *N. Engl. J. Med.* **2005**, *352*, 2589–2597. [CrossRef]
29. Berghmans, T.; Dusart, M.; Paesmans, M.; Hossein-Foucher, C.; Buvat, I.; Castaigne, C.; Scherpereel, A.; Mascaux, C.; Moreau, M.; Roelandts, M.; et al. Primary tumor standardized uptake value (SUVmax) measured on fluorodeoxyglucose positron emission tomography (FDG-PET) is of prognostic value for survival in non-small cell lung cancer (NSCLC): A systematic review and meta-analysis (MA) by the European Lung Cancer Working Party for the IASLC Lung Cancer Staging Project. *J. Thorac. Oncol.* **2008**, *3*, 6–12.
30. Stiles, B.M.; Nasar, A.; Mirza, F.; Paul, S.; Lee, P.C.; Port, J.L.; McGraw, T.E.; Altorki, N.K. Ratio of Positron Emission Tomography Uptake to Tumor Size in Surgically Resected Non–Small Cell Lung Cancer. *Ann. Thorac. Surg.* **2013**, *95*, 397–404. [CrossRef]
31. Blumenthaler, A.N.; Hofstetter, W.L.; Mehran, R.J.; Rajaram, R.; Rice, D.C.; Roth, J.A.; Sepesi, B.; Swisher, S.G.; Vaporciyan, A.A.; Walsh, G.L.; et al. Preoperative Maximum Standardized Uptake Value Associated with Recurrence Risk in Early Lung Cancer. *Ann. Thorac. Surg.* **2021**, *113*, 1835–1844. [CrossRef] [PubMed]
32. Motono, N.; Mizoguchi, T.; Ishikawa, M.; Iwai, S.; Iijima, Y.; Uramoto, H. Adaptation criterion for segmentectomy in small-sized early stage non-small cell lung cancer. *Thorac. Cancer* **2022**, *13*, 2985–2991. [CrossRef] [PubMed]

33. Kandemir, O.; Demir, F. An Investigation of the Relationship Between ^{18}F-FDG PET/CT Parameters of Primary Tumors and Lymph Node Metastasis in Resectable Non-small Cell Lung Cancer. *Curr. Radiopharm.* **2023**. Epub ahead of print. [CrossRef] [PubMed]
34. Kamigaichi, A.; Tsutani, Y.; Mimae, T.; Miyata, Y.; Shimada, Y.; Ito, H.; Nakayama, H.; Ikeda, N.; Okada, M. Prediction of unexpected N2 disease associated with clinical T1-2N0-1M0 non–small-cell lung cancer. *Clin. Lung Cancer* **2020**, *22*, 120–126.e3. [CrossRef]
35. Sun, G.; Sun, Y.; Zou, Z.; Xu, S. Analysis of segmental lymph node metastasis and clinical features in cT1N0M0 lung adenocarcinoma. *BioMed Res. Int.* **2020**, *2020*, 2842604. [CrossRef] [PubMed]
36. Shiono, S.; Abiko, M.; Sato, T. Positron emission tomography/computed tomography and Lymphovascular invasion predict recurrence in stage I lung cancers. *J. Thorac. Oncol.* **2011**, *6*, 43–47. [CrossRef] [PubMed]

cancers

MDPI

Review

Integrating Artificial Intelligence in Bronchoscopy and Endobronchial Ultrasound (EBUS) for Lung Cancer Diagnosis and Staging: A Comprehensive Review

Sebastian Winiarski [1,*], Marcin Radziszewski [1,2], Maciej Wiśniewski [3], Jakub Cisek [4], Dariusz Wąsowski [1], Dariusz Plewczyński [3], Katarzyna Górska [5] and Piotr Korczyński [5]

1 Department of Thoracic Surgery, National Medical Institute of the Ministry of the Interior and Administration, 02-507 Warsaw, Poland; marcin.radziszewski@pimmswia.gov.pl (M.R.); dariusz.wasowski@pimmswia.gov.pl (D.W.)
2 Department of Histology and Embryology, Medical University of Warsaw, 02-004 Warsaw, Poland
3 Faculty of Mathematics and Information Science, Warsaw University of Technology, 00-662 Warsaw, Poland; m.wisniewski@datascience.edu.pl (M.W.); d.plewczynski@cent.uw.edu.pl (D.P.)
4 Faculty of Computer Science, Polish-Japanese Academy of Information Technology, 02-008 Warsaw, Poland; cisekjakub@wp.pl
5 Department of Pulmonary Diseases, Thoracic Oncology and Transplantology, National Medical Institute of the Ministry of the Interior and Administration, 02-507 Warsaw, Poland; katarzyna.gorska2@pimmswia.gov.pl (K.G.); piotr.korczynski@pimmswia.gov.pl (P.K.)
* Correspondence: sebastian.winiarski@pimmswia.gov.pl

Simple Summary: Interobserver variability remains a significant challenge in the accurate diagnosis and staging of lung cancer. This review analyzes existing artificial intelligence (AI) models for bronchoscopy and endobronchial ultrasound (EBUS) visual analysis, bridging engineering innovations with clinical needs to enhance diagnostic precision, standardize evaluations, and optimize procedural guidance. By providing a structured overview of current approaches, it lays the foundation for future system development and highlights the translational potential of these technologies to advance routine practice in thoracic oncology.

Abstract

Artificial intelligence (AI) is increasingly investigated as a potential adjunct in the diagnosis and staging of lung cancer, particularly through integration with bronchoscopy and endobronchial ultrasound (EBUS). Deep learning models have been applied to modalities such as white-light imaging, autofluorescence bronchoscopy, and spectroscopy, with the aim of assisting lesion detection, standardizing interpretation, and reducing interobserver variability. AI has also been explored in EBUS for lymph node assessment and guidance of transbronchial needle aspiration (EBUS-TBNA), with preliminary studies suggesting possible improvements in diagnostic yield. However, current evidence remains largely confined to small, retrospective, single-center datasets, often reporting performance under idealized conditions. External validation is rare, reproducibility is undermined by a lack of data and code availability, and workflow integration into real-world bronchoscopy practice has not been demonstrated. As such, most systems should still be regarded as experimental. Translating AI into routine thoracic oncology will require large-scale, prospective, multicenter validation studies, greater data transparency, and careful evaluation of cost-effectiveness, regulatory approval, and clinical utility.

Keywords: artificial intelligence (AI); deep learning (DL); endobronchial ultrasound (EBUS); endobronchial ultrasound-guided transbronchial needle aspiration (EBUS-TBNA); bronchoscopy; lung cancer

1. Introduction

Bronchoscopy, including endobronchial ultrasound (EBUS) and emerging robotic-assisted techniques, plays a central role in the diagnosis, staging, and management of lung cancer and mediastinal lymphadenopathy [1]. These minimally invasive procedures offer real-time imaging, precise tissue sampling, and guided navigation, all of which are critical for early diagnosis and informed clinical decision-making. Their effectiveness in evaluating central airway lesions and mediastinal lymph nodes has made them indispensable tools in thoracic oncology [2]. However, challenges such as operator-dependent variability, procedural complexity, and diagnostic uncertainty due to image interpretation and navigation issues persist [3,4].

Recent advances in artificial intelligence (AI) and machine learning (ML) are ushering in new possibilities for medical imaging and interventional pulmonology [5]. Specifically, deep learning (DL) and convolutional neural networks (CNNs) have demonstrated considerable promise in tasks such as automated image analysis, lesion detection, and clinical decision support. These AI technologies hold significant potential to enhance procedural accuracy and reproducibility, thereby reducing inter-operator variability. In the context of bronchoscopy and EBUS, AI can assist with lesion localization, biopsy tool guidance, and real-time interpretation of ultrasound images [6].

The integration of AI into bronchoscopy workflows could help address longstanding challenges in the field. By enabling automated image recognition, trajectory optimization, and real-time feedback, AI-enhanced systems could improve biopsy yield, shorten procedural times, and increase diagnostic confidence [7]. Additionally, AI may aid in standardizing procedures across different institutions and operator experience levels, thereby enhancing training, improving procedural safety, and ensuring consistent care. Notably, AI also holds promise in the analysis of cytological and histological specimens, further supporting diagnostic accuracy and overall procedural efficiency [8].

Despite promising advances, the clinical adoption of AI in bronchoscopy and EBUS remains limited. The available evidence is heterogeneous, and large-scale validation studies are still relatively scarce. This review provides a comprehensive overview of AI applications in bronchoscopy and EBUS, with a particular emphasis on lung cancer diagnosis and staging. It summarizes recent technological innovations, evaluates the current body of clinical evidence, and highlights future research directions, underscoring the translational potential of integrating engineering advances into clinical practice. The review is informed by a systematic literature search conducted in accordance with PRISMA guidelines, in which 2116 articles were screened and 35 studies were ultimately included. All included studies were assessed for risk of bias using the QUADAS-2 tool. To enhance readability, the findings are presented in a narrative format, structured around the results of the systematic review, with full methodological details provided in the Supplementary Material.

2. Core Concepts of Artificial Intelligence

AI is a rapidly evolving field focused on developing systems capable of performing tasks that traditionally require human intelligence, such as reasoning, decision-making, pattern recognition, and learning [9]. Within AI, ML emphasizes algorithms that enable systems to learn from data and adapt performance without explicit task-specific programming [10]. Unlike conventional software, which relies on predefined rules, ML models dynamically adjust their behavior based on input data. Figure 1 illustrates the fundamental concepts in AI, highlighting the principal learning approaches.

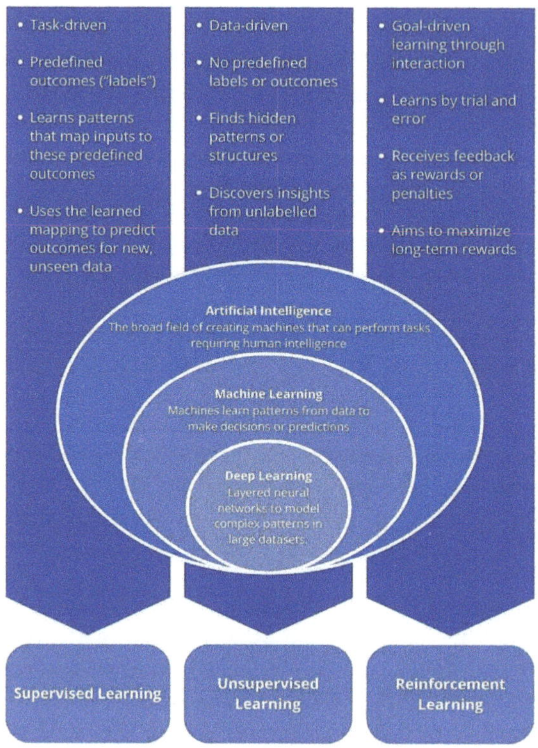

Figure 1. Hierarchical relationship between AI, ML, and DL, highlighting the three primary learning paradigms: supervised, unsupervised, and reinforcement learning. DL has gained particular prominence in medical imaging for its ability to improve accuracy, automate image analysis, and enhance diagnostic capabilities. Created with Canva.com.

ML approaches are commonly classified into three main categories: supervised learning, unsupervised learning, and reinforcement learning [11]. In supervised learning, models are trained on labeled datasets, where both inputs and corresponding outputs are known, allowing the algorithm to learn mappings between them [12]. This method is particularly useful for tasks such as image classification, outcome prediction, and diagnostics. In contrast, unsupervised learning analyzes unlabeled data to uncover hidden patterns, groupings, or anomalies, supporting applications such as identifying novel disease phenotypes, stratifying patient populations, and discovering subtypes [13]. Reinforcement learning, the third paradigm, involves models that learn through trial and error in dynamic environments, guided by rewards or penalties. This strategy is valuable for sequential decision-making, including optimizing treatment strategies over time and improving robotic performance in surgery [14].

DL, a specialized subset of ML, employs multilayered artificial neural networks (ANNs) to progressively extract higher-level features from raw data [15]. Unlike traditional ML, which often depends on manual feature engineering, DL models autonomously learn and refine features during training, making them particularly effective for unstructured data such as medical images, natural language, and audio signals [11]. Inspired by the human brain, DL architectures are composed of interconnected nodes arranged in input, hidden, and output layers [16]. Each layer transforms data into increasingly abstract representations: in medical imaging, for example, early layers detect edges, while deeper layers capture textures or lesion morphology. This hierarchical learning enables DL models to excel in disease classification, lesion detection, and image segmentation across radiological, pathological, and endoscopic domains [17].

Among DL methods, CNNs are especially powerful for visual data analysis [18]. Their convolutional layers scan images to detect spatial and hierarchical features, enabling direct interpretation of imaging modalities such as computed tomography (CT), ultrasound, and X-ray [19].

Critical Overview of Artificial Intelligence Applications in Medicine

While AI holds great promise in healthcare, its implementation requires critical evaluation. In medical imaging and diagnostics, algorithms show strong performance in disease detection and classification, yet challenges of data bias, transparency, and reproducibility limit clinical adoption [19]. In research and drug discovery, AI accelerates target identification and trial design but demands rigorous validation to ensure generalizability [20]. Invasive procedures and robotic platforms benefit from enhanced precision and reduced risk, though barriers such as cost, workflow integration, and surgeon training remain [21].

For patient care and rehabilitation, AI enables personalization and monitoring but raises ethical concerns regarding privacy, autonomy, and unequal access [22]. Administrative applications improve efficiency but introduce cybersecurity risks and potential workforce displacement [23]. Thus, despite its transformative potential, AI integration in healthcare must be accompanied by careful consideration of its limitations, risks, and ethical implications.

In this context, the application of AI in thoracic oncology, particularly in lung cancer diagnosis, treatment, and monitoring, exemplifies both the extraordinary potential and the complex challenges inherent in the adoption of AI-driven technologies in clinical practice [24]. Notably, the incorporation of AI into bronchoscopy and EBUS has shown potential to enhance lesion detection, navigation, and lymph node assessment; however, its clinical utility remains contingent upon rigorous validation, standardization of protocols, and careful integration into existing procedural workflows [25]. Figure 2 presents the broad applications of AI in healthcare, with specific areas marked by an asterisk (*) to highlight their relevance to bronchoscopy and EBUS.

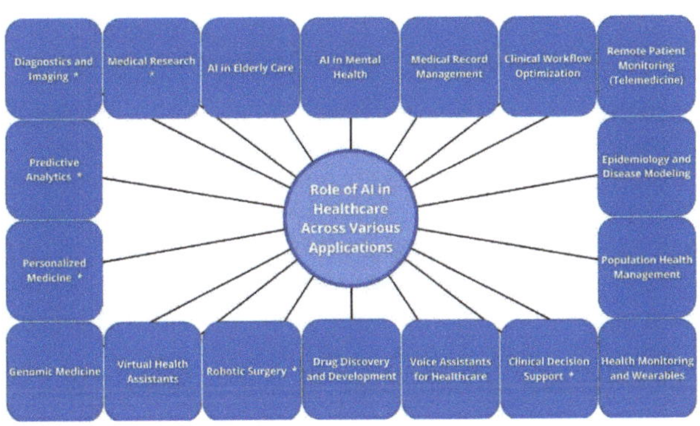

Figure 2. Diverse applications of AI in healthcare, with select domains marked by an asterisk (*) to indicate relevance to bronchoscopy and EBUS. Among these, diagnostics and imaging are most directly

applicable, where AI supports lesion detection, segmentation, and classification. While these tools show promise, their effectiveness depends on access to robust datasets and rigorous clinical validation. Clinical decision support can aid in biopsy target selection and malignancy risk assessment, though adoption is limited by workflow integration and clinician trust. In robotic surgery, AI enhances precision in bronchoscopic procedures but remains resource-intensive. Predictive analytics enables outcome forecasting, yet concerns about model generalizability persist. Other domains, such as medical research and personalized medicine, may benefit indirectly from bronchoscopy/EBUS data but require further translational development. Created with Canva.com.

3. Artificial Intelligence in Bronchoscopy for Lung Cancer Diagnosis

Bronchoscopy remains a cornerstone in the diagnosis of endobronchial lesions, providing direct visualization and vision-guided tissue sampling. Despite its established clinical utility, diagnostic yield is influenced by tumor location, accessibility, and operator expertise, and is subject to interobserver variability. Conventional approaches, including bronchial washing, brushing, and endobronchial biopsy, demonstrate variable yields ranging from 48% to 74%. When used in combination, these techniques can increase the overall diagnostic yield to approximately 88% [26]. Findings from the AEGIS trials further underscore these limitations: among 639 patients, 43% of bronchoscopic examinations were non-diagnostic for lung cancer, and 35% of patients with benign lesions underwent additional invasive procedures following bronchoscopy [27].

Recent advances in AI may help address some of these challenges by enhancing diagnostic precision, reducing interobserver variability, and promoting more standardized decision-making [28]. Table 1 summarizes key studies that have developed AI-based models for bronchoscopy image analysis across multiple modalities, including white light bronchoscopy (WLB), autofluorescence bronchoscopy (AFB), narrow-band imaging (NBI), and Raman spectroscopy (RS), with a focus on their application in the detection and diagnosis of lung cancer.

To date, the highest reported accuracy in lesion detection using WLB has been 97.8%, achieved with the multiscale attention residual network (MARN), a CNN-based model developed by Sun et al. [29]. This model was trained on 2900 frames from 615 patients, with the raw data made publicly available; however, no external validation was performed. Notably, its accuracy decreased by approximately 5% when the model was applied to distinguish malignant from benign lesions.

In another study, Deng et al. applied a ResNet101-based model to WLB images, achieving an accuracy of 95.1% for lesion detection and further demonstrating that DL can also support pathological subtype classification of lung cancer [30]. In a cohort comprising 312 squamous cell carcinoma (SCC), 178 adenocarcinoma (AC), and 129 small cell lung cancer (SCLC) cases, their model achieved an overall accuracy of 60% for three-class classification, which improved to 74.5% when restricted to SCC versus AC. Importantly, the system outperformed junior physicians and achieved diagnostic performance comparable to that of senior clinicians in distinguishing malignant lesions. In parallel, Tan et al. developed a DenseNet-based CNN with transfer learning through sequential fine-tuning (SFT), which successfully differentiated cancerous from tuberculous lesions in WLB [31].

Recent efforts have explored advanced knowledge distillation frameworks to enhance lesion detection in WLB. Yan et al. proposed the Prior Knowledge Distillation Network (PKDN), which integrates color and edge priors with spatial and channel attention mechanisms to better focus on lesion regions. Trained on more than 2000 bronchoscopic images from 200 patients, PKDN achieved an accuracy of 94.8% and an AUC of 98.2%, outperforming several state-of-the-art baselines [32]. Similarly, Liu et al. introduced the knowledge distillation–based memory feature unsupervised anomaly detection (KD-MFAD) model, which incorporates a downward deformable convolution (DDC) module and a convolutional block memory matrix (CB-Mem) to capture subtle airway abnormalities. On a self-built bronchoscopy dataset, KD-MFAD achieved an accuracy of 93.3% with an AUC of 97.6%, demonstrating robustness across both internal and external test sets [33]. Collectively, these studies indicate that knowledge distillation and anomaly detection strategies can achieve accuracies approaching 95% in bronchial lesion detection, while also improving model generalizability and interpretability.

A critical step in advancing AI-assisted bronchoscopy has been the introduction of publicly available datasets, which help overcome the limitations of restricted, institution-specific collections. The BI2K dataset, introduced alongside the MARN model, comprises 2900 bronchoscopic images from 615 patients and remains one of the largest open-access WLB resources to date, enabling reproducible benchmarking of lesion detection algorithms [29]. More recently, the BM-BronchoLC dataset has further enriched the field by providing meticulously annotated data from 208 patients (106 with lung cancer and 102 without), including detailed labels for both anatomical landmarks and airway lesions curated by senior bronchoscopists [34]. Together, these datasets provide diverse, high-quality material for training and validation, fostering transparency and comparability across studies. Their utility has already been demonstrated in the development of advanced detection models, such as BrYOLO-Mamba, which leverages optimized structured state-space modules to improve tracheal lesion detection, achieving significant performance gains while reducing computational cost [35].

In AFB, early studies confirmed the feasibility of computer-based lesion detection and classification. Chang et al. developed an automated video analysis pipeline using nearly 40,000 frames, achieving lesion detection accuracies exceeding 97%, although the dataset was limited to only four patients, thereby constraining generalizability [36]. Similarly, Haritou et al. proposed a texture- and color-based image analysis tool that achieved 95.4% accuracy in distinguishing malignant lesions from false positives caused by inflammation, though their evaluation was restricted to eleven patient cases [37]. Beyond detection, Feng et al. demonstrated that CAD systems applied to AFB images could also support pathological subtype classification, successfully differentiating AC from SCC with an accuracy of 83% (AUC of 81%) [38]. More recently, Chang et al. introduced ESFPNet, a transformer-based segmentation model trained on the first publicly available AFB dataset (20 patients), enabling real-time lesion detection and segmentation. ESFPNet achieved a Dice coefficient of 0.824 and an IoU of 0.707, outperforming established architectures such as UNet++ and CaraNet, while reducing computational cost [39].

Table 1. This table presents a curated summary of recent research studies leveraging AI for lung cancer diagnosis using bronchoscopy and related imaging modalities. Not all articles reported both the size of the patient cohort and the number of frames derived from the study population. It is important to note that a large dataset of frames generated from a small number of patients may lead to inflated accuracy estimates. Similarly, choosing only one frame per case may decrease the representativeness of the study. Owing to substantial heterogeneity in performance reporting, accuracy, sensitivity, and specificity were selected as the primary comparative metrics. For studies in which these parameters were not reported, precision was included as an alternative.

Input Data Type	Diagnostic Task	Model Type	Unit of Analysis	Dataset Size	Ground Truth	Performance Metrics	External Validation	Data Availability	Year	Authors [Ref.]
WLB	Lesion detection	CNN	Frames	2908	Expert consensus	Acc: 93.3%	Yes	Public	2025	Liu et al. [33]
WLB	Lesion detection	CNN	Patients/Frames	615/2900	Histopathology	Acc: 97.8%	No	Public	2024	Sun et al. [29]
WLB	Lesion detection	CNN	Frames	28,032	Expert consensus	Acc: 83.3%, Sen: 79.3%, Spe: 86.1%	No	On request	2024	Cao et al. [35]
WLB	Lesion classification	CNN	Patients/Frames	208/2921	Histopathology	Acc: 82–94%	No	Public	2023	Vu et al. [34]

Table 1. *Cont.*

Input Data Type	Diagnostic Task	Model Type	Unit of Analysis	Dataset Size	Ground Truth	Performance Metrics	External Validation	Data Availability	Year	Authors [Ref.]
WLB	Lesion detection	CNN	Patients/Frames	200/2029	Expert consensus	Acc: 94.8%	No	On request	2023	Yan et al. [32]
WLB	Lesion detection	CNN	Patients/Frames	818/2238	Histopathology	Acc: 95.1%, Sen: 97.8%, Spe: 83.3%	No	Not available	2022	Deng et al. [30]
WLB	Lesion classification	CNN	Patients	434	Histopathology	Acc: 82%	No	Not available	2018	Tan et al. [31]
AFB	Lesion detection	AE	Patients/Frames	20/685	Expert consensus	Prec: 86.2%	No	Public	2024	Chang et al. [39]
AFB	Lesion detection	SVM, ML	Patients/Frames	4/39,899	Expert consensus	Acc: ≥ 97%	No	Not available	2020	Chang et al. [36]
AFB	Lesion classification	ML	Patients	23	Histopathology	Acc: 83%, Sen: 73%, Spe: 92%	No	Not available	2018	Feng et al. [38]
AFB	Lesion classification	ML	Patients/Frames	11/715	Histopathology	Acc: 95.4%, Sen: 95.5%, Spe: 95.2%	No	Not available	2014	Haritou et al. [37]
NBI	Lesion detection	CNN	Patients/Frames	23/66,219	Expert consensus	Sen: 93%, Spe: 86%	No	Not available	2024	Daneshpajooh et al. [40]
RS	Lesion classification	ML	Patients/Spectra	70/78	Histopathology	Acc: 87.2%	No	On request	2024	Fousková et al. [41]

Abbreviations: convolutional neural network (CNN), autoEncoder (AE), support vector machine (SVM), machine learning (ML), white-light bronchoscopy (WLB), narrow-band imaging (NBI), autofluorescence bronchoscopy (AFB), Raman spectroscopy (RS), accuracy (Acc), sensitivity (Sen), specificity (Spe), precision (Prec).

AI models have also been extended to other bronchoscopic and optical modalities. In NBI bronchoscopy, Daneshpajooh et al. reported a two-stage DL-based system that achieved a sensitivity of 93% and specificity of 86% for lesion detection across 23 patient airway videos [40]. In parallel, RS has been investigated as a complementary diagnostic tool. A recent study demonstrated that an ML model applied to in vivo RS spectra attained a sensitivity of 89.7% and specificity of 84.6% for lung cancer diagnosis [41]. While NBI-based models primarily focus on localizing suspicious lesions, RS systems aim to characterize their molecular composition, highlighting their complementary potential in early lung cancer detection.

Overall, most AI models developed for bronchoscopy image analysis rely on DL, with a particular emphasis on CNN architectures. Both WLB- and AFB-based systems have shown strong potential for accurate lesion detection, including the recognition and classification of malignant lesions. Moreover, ML-based spectral classification of RS signals has demonstrated promise for malignancy detection without the need for biopsy. Nonetheless, the majority of models lack thorough clinical validation, which limits their integration into routine practice. Furthermore, although several publicly available datasets have recently been released, their number and diversity remain limited, continuing to restrict reproducibility and the standardized benchmarking of future models. In addition, the available studies carry considerable risk of bias, as they are most often single-center, retrospective, small-cohort investigations conducted under idealized conditions (Supplementary Figure S2). Prospective multicenter trials are essential to establish the validity and generalizability of these models before they can be implemented in clinical practice under regulatory approval.

3.1. The Role of Artificial Intelligence in Bronchonavigation

DL models are increasingly being explored as tools to enhance bronchoscopy, with potential applications in lesion detection, recognition, and navigation [42,43]. In principle, AI-assisted navigation in WLB could enable more precise lesion targeting and thereby improve the diagnostic yield of bronchoscopic biopsies. At present, however, these approaches remain largely experimental. For such systems to become clinically viable, AI models must first be trained to reliably identify a wide range of anatomical landmarks and bronchial branches throughout the airway tree [44,45].

A commonly proposed framework begins with the generation of a patient-specific three-dimensional (3D) model of the bronchial tree, derived from CT data [46]. Within this framework, AI may support automated airway segmentation and 3D reconstruction [47,48]. In addition, accurate localization of the target lesion would need to be extracted from CT imaging to define an optimal navigation path. During the procedure, real-time navigation would depend on adherence to this predefined route. Several proof-of-concept AI models are under development to assist in recognizing bronchial branches in WLB frames. By aligning the observed bronchial anatomy with the CT-derived map, these systems could, in the future, enable progression through the airways and guide the bronchoscope along the planned path to the lesion, thereby facilitating accurate localization and precise tissue acquisition (Figure 3).

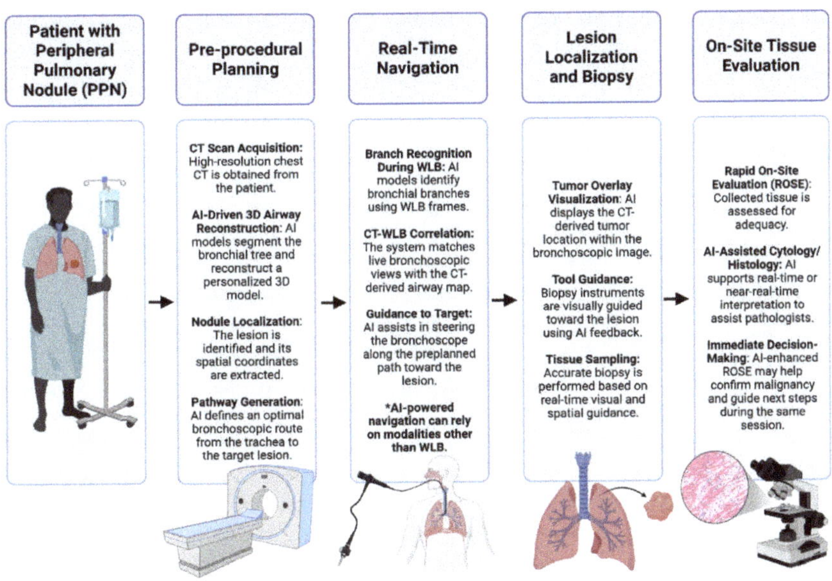

Figure 3. AI-enhanced workflow for WLB-based bronchonavigation in patients with peripheral pulmonary nodules (PPNs). The figure illustrates how AI can support each step of the procedure, from initial CT-based airway and lesion analysis to real-time guidance during bronchoscopy. AI models enable automated 3D reconstruction of the bronchial tree, accurate lesion localization, and path planning. During the procedure, WLB images are processed by AI to recognize anatomical landmarks, estimate bronchoscope position, and match the visual field to the preoperative CT map. This enables precise navigation to the target without reliance on expensive tracking systems or intraoperative radiation, underscoring the potential of AI to make advanced bronchoscopy more accurate, accessible, and efficient. Created with BioRender.com.

Even though this approach is still in its early phases, initial studies have yielded promising findings. Li et al. developed a CNN trained on 28,441 bronchial lumen images, achieving 91.8% accuracy in bronchial branch recognition under controlled conditions [49]. In clinical settings, however, performance declined to 82.7% for main and lobar bronchi and to 54.3% when segmental bronchi were included. Notably, clinical validation showed that three out of four physicians improved anatomical landmark recognition when assisted by the model. Similarly, Chen et al. designed a CNN that achieved 91% accuracy in identifying primary and secondary bronchial branches but encountered difficulty with segmental bronchi [50]. For comparison, physicians with more than six months of training achieved a mean accuracy of $84.33 \pm 7.52\%$. In another study, Yoo et al. demonstrated that a CNN model outperformed most clinicians in identifying primary bronchi, performing comparably only to the most experienced physicians [51]. These findings underscore the promise of AI in bronchial lumen recognition, though accurate identification of all airway branches leading to a target lesion remains essential, and current AI models still fall short of expert human performance.

To overcome these challenges, ongoing research is exploring various models designed to estimate bronchoscope pose using WLB images alone [52,53]. A particularly promising direction involves neural radiance fields (NeRF), a DL technique capable of reconstructing highly detailed 3D scenes by mapping spatial coordinates and viewing angles to color and density from 2D images [54]. The long-term objective is to achieve cost-effective navigation without expensive tracking systems or intraoperative radiation-based imaging [55].

Beyond WLB-based navigation, AI is also being applied to other modalities. Early clinical trials have reported encouraging results for AI-powered fluoroscopy-guided bronchonavigation [56,57]. In addition, shape-sensing technologies, such as fiber Bragg grating (FBG) catheters combined with AI software, provide a radiation-free alternative with promising accuracy and procedural support [58]. These technologies are especially impactful when integrated into robotic bronchoscopy systems, which are increasingly regarded as platforms for future autonomous interventions [59].

Robotic technologies are rapidly transforming bronchoscopy by offering enhanced precision, reach, and consistency compared with manual techniques [60]. Initial robotic platforms improved access to peripheral airways but remained dependent on operator expertise [61]. More recent innovations have produced semi-autonomous systems that integrate AI-driven navigation with user control, enabling novice clinicians to safely access distal bronchi via shared-control algorithms and shape-sensing feedback [62]. Specialized robotic bronchoscopes are also being developed to address the unique challenges of mechanically ventilated patients in critical care settings [63]. At the forefront of innovation, fully autonomous systems are being explored using vision transformers (ViT), surgical workflow recognition, and self-supervised learning to support real-time airway segmentation, tool tracking, and clinical decision-making [64–66].

In summary, AI holds substantial promise for improving bronchonavigation by enhancing lesion localization, airway recognition, and procedural accuracy. Among available modalities, WLB-based navigation is particularly appealing due to its cost-effectiveness and accessibility. However, WLB-only approaches remain in the early stages of development and currently lack the precision, robustness, and hardware integration required for standalone clinical use. By contrast, AI-guided navigation systems leveraging fluoroscopy or shape-sensing technologies are more advanced and clinically reliable. Looking ahead, the integration of AI with robotic bronchoscopy platforms represents a transformative direction, with the potential to increase biopsy yield, improve accessibility, and ultimately enable autonomous bronchoscopic procedures.

3.2. Artificial Intelligence in Competency-Based Endoscopy Training

There is a growing shift in endoscopy education from traditional volume-based training toward competency-based approaches, with increasing emphasis on the acquisition of practical skills in controlled simulation environments (Table 2) [67–69]. AI has significant potential to accelerate this transformation by providing immediate, objective feedback to trainees and reducing reliance on specialists, whose availability for direct supervision is often limited [70].

Table 2. Competency-based training focuses on learners mastering specific skills and progressing by demonstrating their abilities, while volume-based training emphasizes completing a set amount of time or sessions regardless of skill level.

Aspect	Competency-Based Training	Volume-Based Training
Focus	Skill mastery and application	Amount of training/time spent
Progression	Based on demonstration of skills	Based on time or sessions
Assessment	Performance-based	Time or attendance-based
Pace	Individualized	Fixed
Strength	Ensures readiness and proficiency	Easy to measure and manage

A randomized controlled trial by Agbontaen et al. demonstrated that AI-guided bronchoscopy training enabled intensive care unit (ICU) professionals to perform simulated procedures more quickly and efficiently compared with those trained under expert supervision alone [28]. Early trials further suggest that AI-based training systems can help novice endoscopists inspect more airway segments in a systematic manner and improve procedural speed [71,72]. For example, a randomized controlled trial by Cold et al. involving 24 novice bronchoscopists found that the group trained with an ML model completed the final assessment significantly faster than the control group trained without AI support [73].

AI-guided training can also be delivered using virtual, CT-derived bronchial tree models, making simulation-based education more accessible, particularly in resource-limited settings [74,75]. Preliminary evidence indicates that AI not only accelerates the learning curve but also serves as a valuable tool for performance assessment during bronchoscopy training [76]. Integration with standardized assessment instruments, such as the bronchoscopy-radiologic skills and task assessment tool (BRadSTAT), may further enhance evaluation by simultaneously measuring radiologic interpretation and navigational proficiency in reaching peripheral airways [77].

Despite these promising developments, evidence validating AI-guided training in real-world clinical practice remains scarce. Simulation environments cannot yet fully replicate the complexity and unpredictability of patient care, and current findings are largely confined to experimental or educational settings. At present, expert mentorship continues to represent the reference standard for bronchoscopy training and assessment, with AI best regarded as a complementary tool rather than a replacement [78].

4. Artificial Intelligence in Endobronchial Ultrasound (EBUS) for Lung Cancer Diagnosis and Staging

EBUS is an advanced bronchoscopic technique that integrates an ultrasound probe, enabling real-time imaging of structures beyond the airway wall. This allows for the visualization of lesions adjacent to the bronchial tree and facilitates transbronchial needle aspiration (EBUS-TBNA) for histopathological sampling [79]. EBUS is particularly valuable for assessing central thoracic lesions, including mediastinal and hilar lymph nodes, making it a critical tool for evaluating nodal metastases and staging lung cancer [80].

Reported diagnostic accuracy of EBUS-TBNA for lung cancer ranges from 81% to 98%, although considerable heterogeneity exists across published studies [81]. In addition to standard grayscale imaging, EBUS can assess vascularity using Doppler ultrasound and tissue stiffness via elastography, further enhancing its diagnostic capabilities [82,83]. For peripheral lesions, a specialized modality known as radial EBUS (rEBUS) enables the localization and sampling of peripheral pulmonary nodules (PPNs), thereby extending the clinical utility of EBUS in lung cancer diagnosis and management [84]. A recent meta-analysis of 41 studies involving 2988 lung nodules reported a pooled diagnostic accuracy of

72.4% (95% CI: 68.7–76.1) for rEBUS, underscoring both its clinical value and its limitations in the evaluation of peripheral lesions [85].

Several sonographic features observed across EBUS modalities are considered indicative of malignant lymph nodes. These include a short-axis diameter greater than 10 mm, absence of a central hilar structure, presence of necrosis, non-hilar vascular patterns, and elastography scores of 4 or 5 [86,87]. Beyond imaging features, blood-based biomarkers and clinical parameters can be integrated to develop predictive models for nodal metastasis [88]. Increasingly, AI models are demonstrating the ability to accurately identify malignant lesions based on ultrasound input alone or by incorporating multimodal diagnostic data [89,90]. Table 3 summarizes key studies that have developed AI models for EBUS image analysis across modalities, including B-mode grayscale, elastography, Doppler ultrasound, and rEBUS, with a specific focus on their application in detecting and diagnosing malignant lymph nodes and PPNs.

Accurate recognition of malignant lesions in EBUS imaging requires reliable detection and segmentation of lymph nodes or lesions. Ervik et al. introduced a U-Net–based framework for automated segmentation of mediastinal lymph nodes and blood vessels in grayscale images, reporting sensitivities of 0.71 ± 0.38 and 0.80 ± 0.25, with specificities of 0.98 ± 0.02 and 0.99 ± 0.01 [91]. Building on this, the group developed a DL model trained on 28,134 EBUS frames to classify lymph node stations, reaching an overall accuracy of $59.5 \pm 5.2\%$, with the best performance at station 4 L and the lowest at station 10 L [92]. These results highlight both the potential and current limitations of automated station recognition, particularly in anatomically complex regions.

In elastography-based EBUS, Zhou et al. proposed a dual-stream feature-fusion attention U-Net (DFA-UNet) integrating convolutional networks with lightweight ViT and hybrid attention mechanisms [93]. Their model outperformed nine state-of-the-art approaches in mediastinal lymph node segmentation, underscoring the value of combining local and global feature extraction to address indistinct boundaries and heterogeneous elasticity. Such developments illustrate rapid progress toward automated multimodal analysis in EBUS, though large-scale validation is still required before routine integration into bronchoscopic workflows.

Early AI applications in EBUS primarily employed ANNs. In 2008, Tagaya et al. trained layered ANNs on B-mode images to distinguish metastatic nodes from sarcoidosis, achieving accuracies of 75.8–91.2% and outperforming thoracic surgeons, whose accuracy was 78% [94]. Ozcelik et al. applied MATLAB-based (version 9.3.0.713579 [R2017b]) ANN modeling to 345 mediastinal nodes, yielding 82% accuracy (sensitivity 89%, specificity 72%, AUC 0.78) [95]. More recently, Koseoglu et al. trained an ML model on 992 nodes and reported 96% accuracy in distinguishing malignant from benign cases [96]. Comparative studies suggest that while ANNs provide strong baseline performance, advanced architectures such as SVMs and DL models can surpass them when trained on curated datasets [96,97].

These findings illustrate the progression from ANN-based classifiers to modern ML frameworks incorporating radiomics and advanced architectures. Although diagnostic accuracies exceeding 90% have been reported, heterogeneity in design, dataset size, and input features limits generalizability. Multi-institutional datasets with rigorous external validation are essential for reproducible performance and clinical translation.

CNN-based models are increasingly applied to grayscale EBUS for metastatic node diagnosis. Churchill et al. evaluated NeuralSeg, training it on 298 nodes and prospectively validating on 108, achieving 72.9% accuracy and 90.8% specificity, thereby demonstrating its utility in ruling out metastasis when biopsy results are inconclusive [98]. Ito et al. trained an Xception-based CNN on more than 5000 frames from 166 nodes, reporting accuracies up to 87.9% and specificities of 95% [99]. Ishiwata et al. used SqueezeNet with transfer learning, achieving 96.7% accuracy with Adam optimization and slightly lower but more stable results with stochastic gradient descent [100]. Yong et al. employed a modified VGG-16 with global average pooling and a custom loss, reaching 75.8% accuracy and an AUC of 0.80, while enabling real-time inference at 63 fps on a single GPU [101].

These approaches reflect a trajectory toward clinical use. Early models were proof-of-concept, while recent work emphasizes robustness through cross-validation, augmentation, and prospective testing. Lightweight architectures such as SqueezeNet demonstrate that high performance can be achieved without excessive computational cost, facilitating real-time deployment on standard GPUs. Despite reported accuracies ranging from 73% to 97%, evidence remains constrained by single-center datasets, modest sample sizes, and limited external validation. Large, multicenter trials with standardized protocols are needed to establish CNNs as reliable adjuncts in nodal staging. Notably, reliance on ultrasound input alone enhances their practicality [102].

Elastography provides a complementary modality by reflecting tissue stiffness, a correlate of malignancy. Zhi et al. developed an ML model for automatic frame selection in strain elastography videos using clustering and color histograms, achieving accuracies of 78–83.5%, comparable to experts and superior to trainees [103]. Xu et al. advanced this with a sparse graph attention mechanism to classify nodes from 727 videos, reaching 81.3% accuracy and an AUC of 0.875 [104]. Patel et al. validated NeuralSeg for lymph node segmentation and stiffness area ratio (SAR) calculation in a prospective trial of 187 nodes, reporting 70.6% accuracy, 90.7% specificity, and an AUC of 0.82, supporting its role in ruling out metastasis when combined with EBUS-TBNA [105].

These studies highlight the potential of AI-enhanced elastography to improve nodal staging through automated frame selection, standardized SAR assessment, and reduced operator dependence. High specificity results warrant further multicenter validation for real-time integration.

Multimodal frameworks further enhance diagnostic performance. Li et al. reported that EBUSNet, combining grayscale, Doppler, and elastography, achieved 88.6% accuracy and an AUC of 0.95, outperforming experts and unimodal models [106]. Lin et al. introduced TransEBUS, a CNN-Transformer hybrid fusing grayscale, Doppler, and elastography with temporal dynamics, achieving 82% accuracy and an AUC of 0.88 [107]. Although multimodal approaches improve predictive reliability, they require longer acquisition and higher computational resources, potentially limiting real-time use.

AI has also been applied to rEBUS for PPN assessment and biopsy guidance. Chen et al. showed that CNNs with transfer learning distinguished benign from malignant lesions with 85.4% accuracy, outperforming texture-based methods [108]. Hotta et al. trained a CNN on over 2.4 million rEBUS frames from 213 patients, reporting 83.4% accuracy and 95.3% sensitivity, surpassing four bronchoscopists whose accuracy was 68.4% [109]. Yu et al. validated a CNN across three centers, reporting an internal AUC of 0.88 and feasibility for malignancy classification and histological subtype prediction, though subtype performance remained modest (AUC 0.64–0.70) [110].

Beyond binary classification, ensemble strategies have shown promise. Khomkham and Lipikorn combined CNNs with radiomic and clinical data in a weighted ensemble with random forests, reaching 95% accuracy and 100% sensitivity in 200 rEBUS images [111]. Xing et al. proposed a fuzzy k-nearest neighbor (FKNN) classifier optimized with a manta ray foraging algorithm, trained on multimodal datasets from 156 patients, achieving 99.4% accuracy in distinguishing malignant from benign lesions [112].

Table 3. This table provides an overview of recent research studies that employ AI techniques for the diagnosis and staging of lung cancer, using various forms and modalities of EBUS. A large number of frames derived from only a few patients can artificially inflate reported accuracy, whereas restricting analyses to a single frame per case may reduce the representativeness of the findings. Notably, some models demonstrated higher specificity than sensitivity, while others showed the opposite trend. Diagnostic tools with high sensitivity are valuable for screening, as they minimize the risk of missing affected patients, although confirmatory testing remains necessary. Conversely, tests with high specificity are useful for ruling in disease, meaning that models with very high specificity have the potential to reduce the number of unnecessary biopsies.

Input Data Type	Diagnostic Task	Model Type	Unit of Analysis	Dataset Size	Ground Truth	Performance Metrics	External Validation	Data Availability	Year	Authors [Ref.]
EBUS	Malignant LN recognition	CNN	Patients/frames	773/2569	Histopathology	Acc: 80.6%, Sen: 43.2%, Spe: 96.9%	No	Not available	2024	Patel et al. [102]
EBUS	Malignant LN recognition	CNN	Videos/LNs	53/90	Histopathology	Acc: 96.7%	No	Not available	2024	Ishiwata et al. [100]
EBUS	Malignant LN recognition	SVM	Patients/Lesions	197/205	Histopathology	Acc: 74.2%, Sen: 70.3%, Spe: 74.1%	No	Not available	2024	Hu et al. [97]
EBUS	Malignant LN recognition	SVM/KNN	LNs	992	Histopathology	Acc: 95.9–96.4%	No	Not available	2023	Koseoglu et al. [96]
EBUS	Malignant LN recognition	AE	Patients/LNs	140/298	Histopathology	Acc: 72.9–73.8%	No	Not available	2022	Churchill et al. [98]
EBUS	Malignant LN recognition	CNN	Patients/LNs/frames	91/166/11,699	Histopathology/ follow-up	Acc: 87.9%, Sen: 76.9%, Spe: 95.0%	No	Not available	2022	Ito et al. [99]
EBUS	Malignant LN recognition	CNN	LNs/frames	2394/2396	Histopathology	Acc: 75.8%, Sen: 72.7%, Spe: 79.0%	No	On request	2022	Yong et al. [101]
EBUS	Malignant LN recognition	ANN	LNs/frames	345/345	Histopathology/ follow-up	Acc: 82%, Sen: 89%, Spe: 72%	No	Not available	2020	Ozcelik et al. [95]
EBUS	Malignant LN recognition	ANN	Patients/LNs	91/91	Histopathology	Acc: 75.8–91.2%, Sen: 84.9–98.5%, Spe: 48–84%	No	Not available	2008	Tagaya et al. [94]
EBUS	LN segmentation	CNN	Patients/frames	56/28,134	Expert consensus	Acc: 59.5%	No	On request	2025	Ervik et al. [92]
EBUS	LN segmentation	AE	Patients/frames	40/1161	Expert consensus	Sen: 71%, Spe: 98%	No	On request	2024	Ervik et al. [91]
EBUS (elastography)	Malignant LN recognition	CNN	Patients/LNs	124/187	Histopathology	Acc: 70.6%, Sen: 43.0%, Spe: 90.7%	No	Not available	2024	Patel et al. [105]
EBUS (elastography)	Malignant LN recognition	CNN	Videos	727	Histopathology/ follow-up	Acc: 81.3%	No	Not available	2023	Xu et al. [104]
EBUS (elastography)	Malignant LN recognition	ML	Patients/LNs	351/415	Histopathology/ follow-up	Acc: 82.4%	No	On request	2021	Zhi et al. [103]
EBUS (elastography)	LN segmentation	AE, ViT	Patients/frames	206/263	Expert consensus	Prec: 84.4%	No	On request	2024	Zhou et al. [93]
EBUS (gray scale, Doppler, elastography)	Malignant LN recognition	CNN, ViT	Patients/videos	150/330	Histopathology/ follow-up	Acc: 82%, Sen: 84.2%, Spe: 80.7%	No	Not available	2025	Lin et al. [107]
EBUS (gray scale, Doppler, elastography)	Malignant LN recognition	AE	Patients/LNs	267/294	Histopathology/ follow-up	Acc: 88.6%, Sen: 92.4%, Spe: 83.0%	No	Not available	2021	Li et al. [106]
rEBUS	Malignant PPN recognition	KNN	Patients	156	Histopathology/ follow-up	Acc: 99.4%, Sen: 100.0%, Spe: 98.9%	No	Not available	2024	Xing et al. [112]
rEBUS	Malignant PPN recognition	CNN	Patients/PPNs/frames	260/265/769	Histopathology/ follow-up	Sen: 58–80%, Spe: 75–92%	Yes	On request	2023	Yu et al. [110]
rEBUS	Malignant PPN recognition	CNN	PPNs	200	Histopathology	Acc: 95%, Sen: 100%, Spe: 86.7%	No	Not available	2022	Khomkham et al. [111]
rEBUS	Malignant PPN recognition	CNN	Patients/frames	213/2421,360	Histopathology/ follow-up	Acc: 83.4%, Sen: 95.3%, Spe: 53.6%	No	On request	2022	Hotta et al. [109]
rEBUS	Malignant PPN recognition	CNN	Patients/frames	164/164	Histopathology/ follow-up	Acc: 85.4%, Sen: 87.0%, Spe: 82.1%	No	Not available	2019	Chen et al. [108]

Abbreviations: endobronchial ultrasound (EBUS), radial endobronchial ultrasound (rEBUS), lymph nodes (LNs), peripheral pulmonary nodules (PPNs), convolutional neural network (CNN), support vector machine (SVM), autoEncoder (AE), vision transformer (ViT), k-nearest neighbors (KNN), machine learning (ML), artificial neural network (ANN), accuracy (Acc), sensitivity (Sen), specificity (Spe), precision (Prec).

These findings suggest CNN-based methods can surpass physicians in identifying malignant features, while advanced ensembles may further enhance diagnostic power through integration of radiomics and clinical data. Nonetheless, external validation and prospective trials remain essential to ensure robustness and generalizability.

Overall, CNN-based models dominate AI applications in both B-mode EBUS and rEBUS imaging. While elastography and Doppler integration can improve accuracy, their use may prolong procedures. Models combining radiomic and clinical data often yield superior performance, but progress remains limited by scarce public datasets, a lack of open-source code, and insufficient real-world validation. Addressing these challenges will be crucial for establishing AI as a reliable adjunct in EBUS-based nodal staging and lung cancer diagnosis. Similarly to models analyzed in the context of bronchoscopy, studies describing DL systems in EBUS are also subject to potential bias, as large multicenter cohorts remain rare and the literature is dominated by retrospective, single-center designs (Supplementary Figure S2). Prospective multicenter evaluations will be essential to achieve regulatory approval and enable clinical implementation.

5. Artificial Intelligence Assistance in Histopathological Examination and Rapid On-Site Evaluation (ROSE)

Although minimally invasive techniques such as bronchoscopy and EBUS offer several advantages over traditional approaches like mediastinoscopy for lung cancer diagnosis, the amount of biopsy material obtained is often limited [113,114]. This limitation poses challenges for pathologists in establishing a definitive diagnosis and may necessitate additional procedures. To address this issue, rapid on-site evaluation (ROSE) was introduced, allowing real-time assessment of sample adequacy during the procedure [115]. Current evidence also suggests that ROSE can reduce the overall cost of EBUS [116]. However, ROSE generally requires the physical presence of a pathologist, which may not always be feasible in clinical practice [117]. Recent studies indicate that AI can effectively analyze ROSE smears, thereby improving both efficiency and diagnostic accuracy in bronchoscopy and EBUS [118,119].

AI algorithms employing CNNs have demonstrated high accuracy in identifying cancerous cells in cytological specimens, with reported performance exceeding 98% [120]. Their efficiency can be further enhanced by integration with automated sample preparation systems, such as ASP Health's ROSE Prep™ [121]. Notably, diagnostic concordance between AI-driven ROSE systems and experienced cytopathologists in identifying major lung cancer subtypes, including SCC, AC, and SCLC, has shown near perfect agreement [122]. The highest accuracy to date was achieved using cytological images analyzed with a ResNet101-based system, which reported 98.8% accuracy, sensitivity, and specificity [123]. In addition, Wang et al. have proposed the use of whole slide EBUS images to further improve diagnostic performance and processing speed when applying AI models [124].

Despite these encouraging results, expectations should remain cautious. Many reported accuracies approaching 98–99% are derived from retrospective studies of highly curated datasets, which may not capture the variability of routine clinical workflows. Prospective workflow-integrated validations of AI-assisted ROSE remain scarce, and real-world performance across diverse patient populations is yet to be fully established. Consequently, while AI shows considerable potential as an adjunct to ROSE, its role should currently be regarded as supportive rather than definitive until more robust prospective evidence becomes available.

The performance of AI-based ROSE systems may be further optimized by incorporating serum biomarkers and leveraging advanced imaging modalities such as higher harmonic generation microscopy [125,126]. Another promising development is the emergence of cloud-based platforms for AI-powered ROSE assessment, which could improve both accessibility and scalability [127]. A schematic representation of AI applications in ROSE and histopathological analysis within airway endoscopy is provided in Figure 4.

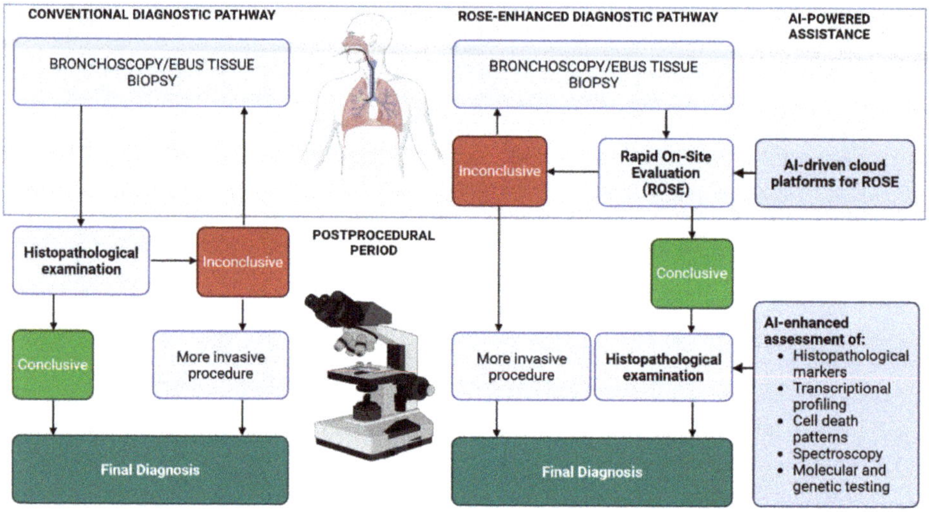

Figure 4. Comparison of the conventional diagnostic pathway relying solely on histopathological examination with the ROSE-enhanced pathway. The steps within the light blue box occur during the endoscopic procedure, whereas those outside the box take place in the postprocedural period. ROSE enables intraoperative tissue assessment, reducing the need for repeated procedures when samples are inconclusive, which is often required in the conventional pathway. The figure highlights key points at which AI-powered solutions can further improve the modern diagnostic workflow following bronchoscopy or EBUS-derived tissue analysis. Created with BioRender.com.

The primary role of ROSE is to confirm sample adequacy and minimize repeat procedures or diagnostic delays. However, definitive diagnosis ultimately depends on comprehensive histopathological assessment, including staining, immunohistochemistry, and molecular or genetic testing [128]. The application of AI in histopathological analysis is expanding across both research and early clinical settings, offering opportunities to support diagnostic accuracy and workflow efficiency [129,130].

Recent advances in ML have contributed to progress in tumor cellularity assessment in clinical practice [131]. Beyond conventional histopathological markers, ML approaches have been investigated for their potential to integrate multidimensional data sources, such as whole-transcriptome RNA sequencing and airway epithelial transcriptional profiling, with the aim of improving risk stratification and diagnostic yield, particularly in patients with indeterminate bronchoscopy results [132,133]. Predictive models based on programmed cell death signatures have also been proposed to generate prognostic indices in lung AC that could eventually inform therapeutic decision-making [134].

Complementary technologies such as RS suggest a role for AI-driven spectral analysis in the rapid detection of malignant lesions, although current evidence remains limited to early studies and controlled research environments [135]. Similarly, ML classifiers trained on histopathological and microenvironmental features from transbronchial lung biopsy specimens have shown promising performance in distinguishing malignant from benign conditions in previously non-diagnostic samples [136].

Taken together, these developments indicate that AI may support the integration of molecular, morphological, and spectroscopic data to advance diagnostic precision and clinical decision-making in thoracic oncology. Nonetheless, most approaches remain at a proof-of-concept stage, and large-scale, workflow-embedded prospective validations are still scarce.

Overall, AI holds promise for augmenting bronchoscopy and EBUS by supporting real-time sample assessment, intraprocedural tissue evaluation, and subsequent histopathological review. These tools could help reduce pathologists' workload while maintaining diagnostic reliability, though ultimate confirmation continues to rely on comprehensive histopathological evaluation. Beyond sample adequacy assessment, AI may also contribute to the integration of tissue-derived molecular and genomic data. Importantly, rigorous prospective validation remains essential, and the expertise of experienced pathologists continues to be indispensable for ensuring diagnostic accuracy and guiding effective lung cancer management.

6. Artificial Intelligence in Other Imaging Modalities and Lung Cancer Screening

The advent of AI has profoundly reshaped medical imaging and its interpretation. While the clinical expertise of radiologists remains indispensable, ML models increasingly complement image analysis across modalities such as CT and positron emission tomography (PET) [137]. These imaging techniques are integral to the diagnosis, staging, and management of lung cancer, providing critical information on tumor localization, morphology, and metabolic activity.

Although histopathological evaluation of tissue specimens remains the gold standard for definitive diagnosis and treatment planning, imaging features, such as lesion morphology and metabolic behavior, can often suggest malignancy or benignity with considerable reliability [137,138]. In recent years, a growing number of AI-based models have been developed to manage the vast imaging datasets generated in clinical practice. These models are capable of detecting subtle, clinically meaningful patterns that may elude human observers [139,140]. As illustrated in Figure 5, AI-driven approaches can extract diverse diagnostic information from advanced imaging modalities, thereby enhancing lung cancer detection and screening.

For lung cancer staging, PET/CT-based ML classifiers have demonstrated high sensitivity in identifying malignant lymph nodes, frequently achieving low misclassification rates [141,142]. The integration of clinical variables, such as patient demographics and primary tumor characteristics, further improves predictive performance [143,144]. Moreover, certain PET/CT-based AI models can distinguish between histological subtypes of lung cancer [145]. Despite these advances, overall diagnostic accuracy generally remains comparable to that of experienced clinicians. A major barrier to widespread clinical implementation is the lack of large-scale, externally validated studies across diverse patient populations. Emerging evidence also highlights the potential of combining CT-based radiomics with ML algorithms to predict molecular biomarker expression, including PD-L1, EGFR, and Ki-67, as well as functional outcomes such as spirometric indices; however, more research is needed [146–150].

AI applied to low-dose CT (LDCT) is further transforming early lung cancer screening by providing scalable, efficient, and cost-effective solutions [151,152]. Predictive accuracy can be enhanced by integrating additional parameters, including circulating tumor biomarkers and exhaled breath analyses [153,154]. By enabling comprehensive, patient-specific interpretation of large-scale datasets, AI offers the potential for earlier lung cancer detection. This capability may ultimately redefine the paradigm of lung cancer screening and diagnosis, supporting more timely and individualized interventions and improving patient outcomes [155,156].

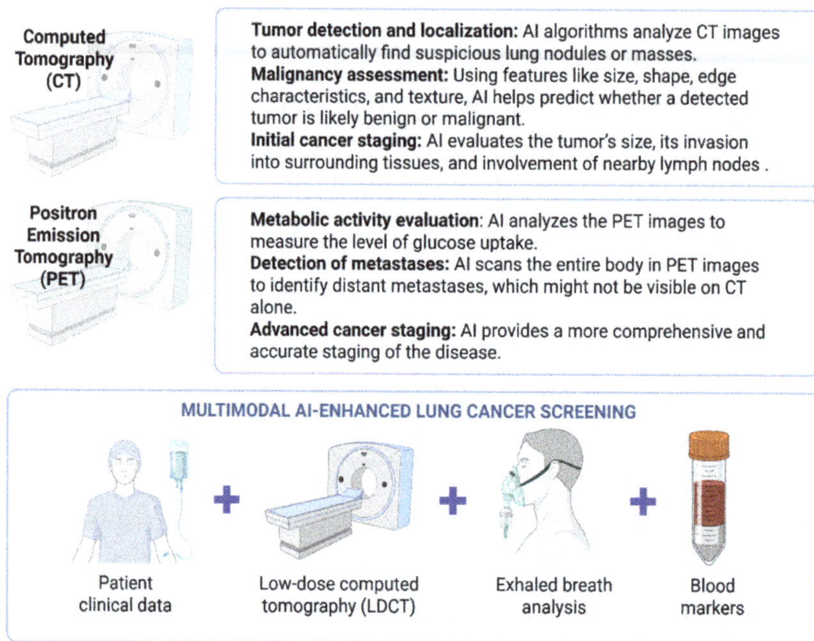

Figure 5. AI integration across various diagnostic tools offers a more comprehensive approach to lung cancer screening. The top panels illustrate AI's role in analyzing CT and PET images, while the bottom panel highlights a multimodal strategy combining patient clinical data, LDCT, exhaled breath analysis, and blood biomarkers. By merging AI-enhanced insights from both imaging and non-imaging sources, this approach aims to improve early detection, increase diagnostic accuracy, and refine lung cancer staging. Created with BioRender.com.

7. Conclusions

AI models applied to bronchoscopy and EBUS have demonstrated considerable potential in lesion recognition, with performance in specific tasks approaching or even exceeding that of experienced clinicians. DL techniques, particularly CNNs, have shown efficacy in processing visual input across multiple modalities, including WLB, AFB, ultrasound, and elastography. Integration with clinical data and radiomics further enhances diagnostic precision, offering the potential to improve biopsy accuracy and, by extension, diagnostic outcomes in lung cancer.

However, despite these advances, important limitations remain. Most models lack external validation, and source code or datasets are rarely made publicly available, restricting reproducibility and the development of more generalizable approaches. The majority of studies are retrospective, single-center, and rely on carefully curated image sets, with poor-quality or complex cases frequently excluded, conditions that do not reflect routine clinical practice. Consequently, while reported performances are often promising, they likely represent optimistic estimates that may not translate directly to real-world clinical settings. Moreover, limited integration with bronchoscopy hardware continues to pose a significant barrier to real-time, intra-procedural application.

Beyond diagnostic assistance, AI holds promise in bronchonavigation and endoscopic education. The concept of navigation based solely on white-light images is particularly intriguing, although current models lack sufficient accuracy for clinical deployment. Established navigation methods, such as fluoroscopy and electromagnetic guidance, remain more reliable. AI is also increasingly used for pre-procedural imaging analysis and intra-procedural histopathological assessment, where it may assist in evaluating sample adequacy and guiding real-time decisions. In the context of education, AI-based tools may support a shift from volume-based to competency-based training by enabling objective, standardized assessment of trainee performance. However, these systems have largely been evaluated in simulated environments, and experienced clinical educators continue to play a critical role in real-world training.

Overall, while AI offers substantial opportunities to enhance bronchoscopy and EBUS across diagnostic, procedural, and educational domains, widespread clinical implementation will depend on rigorous validation, greater data transparency, and closer integration with existing procedural technologies.

Supplementary Materials: The following supporting information can be downloaded at: https://www.mdpi.com/article/10.3390/cancers17172835/s1, Figure S1: Inclusion scheme for relevant publications; Figure S2. Articles from the systematic review were evaluated for bias using QUADAS-2. Most of these studies carry a considerable risk of bias, primarily due to their reliance on small, single-center datasets and retrospective designs. Images are often carefully curated, with poor-quality or complex cases excluded, which does not reflect routine clinical practice. Reference standards are frequently based on expert annotations rather than pathology, while external validation across centers or devices is uncommon, raising concerns about overfitting and limited generalizability. As a result, while reported performances are often promising, they likely represent optimistic estimates that may not translate directly to real-world clinical settings.

Author Contributions: Conceptualization, S.W. and M.R.; methodology, S.W., M.R., M.W. and J.C.; formal analysis, S.W., M.R., M.W., J.C., D.W., D.P., K.G. and P.K.; writing: original draft preparation, S.W. and M.R.; writing: review and editing, S.W., M.R., M.W., J.C., D.W., D.P., K.G. and P.K.; visualization, S.W. and M.R.; supervision, D.P., K.G. and P.K. All authors have read and agreed to the published version of the manuscript.

Funding: This research received no external funding.

Institutional Review Board Statement: Not applicable.

Informed Consent Statement: Not applicable.

Data Availability Statement: The datasets analyzed in this study are described in the Supplementary Material. Additional details are available from the corresponding author upon reasonable request.

Conflicts of Interest: The authors declare no conflicts of interest.

Abbreviations

The following abbreviations are used in this manuscript:

EBUS	endobronchial ultrasound
AI	artificial intelligence
EBUS-TBNA	endobronchial ultrasound-guided transbronchial needle aspiration
ML	machine learning
DL	deep learning
CNN	convolutional neural network
CT	computed tomography
WLB	white light bronchoscopy
AFB	autofluorescence bronchoscopy
NBI	narrow band imaging
RS	Raman spectroscopy

AE	autoEncoder
SVM	support vector machine
Acc	accuracy
AUC	area under the curve
Sen	sensitivity
Spe	specificity
Prec	precision
MARN	multiscale attention residual network
TL	transfer learning
SFT	sequential fine-tuning
PKDN	prior knowledge distillation network
KD MFAD	knowledge distillation-based memory feature unsupervised anomaly detection
DDC	downward deformable convolution
CB Mem	convolutional block focused memory matrix
PPN	peripheral pulmonary nodule
NeRF	neural radiance fields
FBG	fiber Bragg grating
ICU	intensive care unit
BRadSTAT	bronchoscopy–radiologic skills and task assessment tool
rEBUS	radial endobronchial ultrasound
LN	lymph node
ViT	vision transformer
KNN	K-nearest neighbors
ANN	artificial neural network
ROI	region of interest
GPU	graphics processing unit
ROSE	rapid on-site evaluation
PET	positron emission tomography
LDCT	low-dose computed tomography
SCC	squamous cell carcinoma
AC	adenocarcinoma
SCLS	small cell lung carcinoma

References

1. Prabhakar, B.; Shende, P.; Augustine, S. Current trends and emerging diagnostic techniques for lung cancer. *Biomed. Pharmacother.* **2018**, *106*, 1586–1599. [CrossRef]
2. Dollin, Y.; Munoz Pineda, J.A.; Sung, L.; Hasteh, F.; Fortich, M.; Lopez, A.; Van Nostrand, K.; Patel, N.M.; Miller, R.; Cheng, G. Diagnostic modalities in the mediastinum and the role of bronchoscopy in mediastinal assessment: A narrative review. *Mediastinum* **2024**, *8*, 51. [CrossRef]
3. Minami, H.; Ando, Y.; Nomura, F.; Sakai, S.; Shimokata, K. Interbronchoscopist variability in the diagnosis of lung cancer by flexible bronchoscopy. *Chest* **1994**, *105*, 1658–1662. [CrossRef]
4. Mwesigwa, N.W.; Tentzeris, V.; Gooseman, M.; Qadri, S.; Maxine, R.; Cowen, M. Electromagnetic Navigational Bronchoscopy Learning Curve Regarding Pneumothorax Rate and Diagnostic Yield. *Cureus* **2024**, *16*, e58289. [CrossRef]
5. Ishiwata, T.; Yasufuku, K. Artificial intelligence in interventional pulmonology. *Curr. Opin. Pulm. Med.* **2024**, *30*, 92–98. [CrossRef]
6. Bertolaccini, L.; Guarize, J.; Diotti, C.; Donghi, S.M.; Casiraghi, M.; Mazzella, A.; Spaggiari, L. Harnessing artificial intelligence for breakthroughs in lung cancer management: Are we ready for the future? *Front. Oncol.* **2024**, *14*, 1450568. [CrossRef] [PubMed]
7. Luo, X.; Mori, K.; Peters, T.M. Advanced Endoscopic Navigation: Surgical Big Data, Methodology, and Applications. *Annu. Rev. Biomed. Eng.* **2018**, *20*, 221–251. [CrossRef]
8. Shafi, S.; Parwani, A.V. Artificial intelligence in diagnostic pathology. *Diagn. Pathol.* **2023**, *18*, 109. [CrossRef]
9. Amisha Malik, P.; Pathania, M.; Rathaur, V.K. Overview of artificial intelligence in medicine. *J. Fam. Med. Prim. Care* **2019**, *8*, 2328–2331. [CrossRef] [PubMed]
10. Bellini, V.; Cascella, M.; Cutugno, F.; Russo, M.; Lanza, R.; Compagnone, C.; Bignami, E.G. Understanding basic principles of Artificial Intelligence: A practical guide for intensivists. *Acta Biomed.* **2022**, *93*, e2022297.

11. Choi, R.Y.; Coyner, A.S.; Kalpathy-Cramer, J.; Chiang, M.F.; Campbell, J.P. Introduction to Machine Learning, Neural Networks, and Deep Learning. *Transl. Vis. Sci. Technol.* **2020**, *9*, 14.
12. Jiang, T.; Gradus, J.L.; Rosellini, A.J. Supervised Machine Learning: A Brief Primer. *Behav. Ther.* **2020**, *51*, 675–687. [CrossRef] [PubMed]
13. Eckhardt, C.M.; Madjarova, S.J.; Williams, R.J.; Ollivier, M.; Karlsson, J.; Pareek, A.; Nwachukwu, B.U. Unsupervised machine learning methods and emerging applications in healthcare. *Knee Surg. Sports Traumatol. Arthrosc.* **2023**, *31*, 376–381. [CrossRef] [PubMed]
14. Al-Hamadani, M.N.A.; Fadhel, M.A.; Alzubaidi, L.; Balazs, H. Reinforcement Learning Algorithms and Applications in Healthcare and Robotics: A Comprehensive and Systematic Review. *Sensors* **2024**, *24*, 2461. [CrossRef]
15. Sarker, I.H. Deep Learning: A Comprehensive Overview on Techniques, Taxonomy, Applications and Research Directions. *SN Comput. Sci.* **2021**, *2*, 420. [CrossRef]
16. LeCun, Y.; Bengio, Y.; Hinton, G. Deep learning. *Nature* **2015**, *521*, 436–444. [CrossRef] [PubMed]
17. Kufel, J.; Bargieł-Łączek, K.; Kocot, S.; Koźlik, M.; Bartnikowska, W.; Janik, M.; Czogalik, Ł.; Dudek, P.; Magiera, M.; Lis, A.; et al. What Is Machine Learning, Artificial Neural Networks and Deep Learning?—Examples of Practical Applications in Medicine. *Diagnostics* **2023**, *13*, 2582. [CrossRef]
18. Ayachi, R.; Said, Y.; Atri, M. A Convolutional Neural Network to Perform Object Detection and Identification in Visual Large-Scale Data. *Big Data* **2021**, *9*, 41–52. [CrossRef]
19. Yamashita, R.; Nishio, M.; Do, R.K.G.; Togashi, K. Convolutional neural networks: An overview and application in radiology. *Insights Imaging* **2018**, *9*, 611–629. [CrossRef]
20. Paul, D.; Sanap, G.; Shenoy, S.; Kalyane, D.; Kalia, K.; Tekade, R.K. Artificial intelligence in drug discovery and development. *Drug Discov. Today* **2021**, *26*, 80–93. [CrossRef]
21. Chatterjee, S.; Das, S.; Ganguly, K.; Mandal, D. Advancements in robotic surgery: Innovations, challenges and future prospects. *J. Robot. Surg.* **2024**, *18*, 28. [CrossRef]
22. Lanotte, F.; O'Brien, M.K.; Jayaraman, A. AI in Rehabilitation Medicine: Opportunities and Challenges. *Ann. Rehabil. Med.* **2023**, *47*, 444–458. [CrossRef]
23. Olawade, D.B.; Wada, O.J.; David-Olawade, A.C.; Kunonga, E.; Abaire, O.; Ling, J. Using artificial intelligence to improve public health: A narrative review. *Front. Public. Health* **2023**, *11*, 1196397. [CrossRef]
24. Bellini, V.; Valente, M.; Del Rio, P.; Bignami, E. Artificial intelligence in thoracic surgery: A narrative review. *J. Thorac. Dis.* **2021**, *13*, 6963–6975. [CrossRef]
25. Mehta, V. Artificial intelligence augmentation raises questions about the future of bronchoscopy. *ERJ Open Res.* **2025**, *11*, 00931–02024. [CrossRef]
26. Lee, P.; Colt, H.G. Bronchoscopy in lung cancer: Appraisal of current technology and for the future. *J. Thorac. Oncol.* **2010**, *5*, 1290–1300. [CrossRef] [PubMed]
27. Silvestri, G.A.; Vachani, A.; Whitney, D.; Elashoff, M.; Porta Smith, K.; Ferguson, J.S.; Parsons, E.; Mitra, N.; Brody, J.; Lenburg, M.E.; et al. A Bronchial Genomic Classifier for the Diagnostic Evaluation of Lung Cancer. *N. Engl. J. Med.* **2015**, *373*, 243–251. [CrossRef] [PubMed]
28. Agbontaen, K.O.; Cold, K.M.; Woods, D.; Grover, V.; Aboumarie, H.S.; Kaul, S.; Konge, L.; Singh, S. Artificial Intelligence-Guided Bronchoscopy is Superior to Human Expert Instruction for the Performance of Critical-Care Physicians: A Randomized Controlled Trial. *Crit. Care Med.* **2025**, *53*, e1105. [CrossRef] [PubMed]
29. Sun, W.; Yan, P.; Li, M.; Li, X.; Jiang, Y.; Luo, H.; Zhao, Y. An accurate prediction for respiratory diseases using deep learning on bronchoscopy diagnosis images. *J. Adv. Res.* **2024**. [CrossRef] [PubMed]
30. Deng, Y.; Chen, Y.; Xie, L.; Wang, L.; Zhan, J. The investigation of construction and clinical application of image recognition technology assisted bronchoscopy diagnostic model of lung cancer. *Front. Oncol.* **2022**, *12*, 1001840. [CrossRef] [PubMed]
31. Tan, T.; Li, Z.; Liu, H.; Zanjani, F.G.; Ouyang, Q.; Tang, Y.; Hu, Z.; Li, Q. Optimize Transfer Learning for Lung Diseases in Bronchoscopy Using a New Concept: Sequential Fine-Tuning. *IEEE J. Transl. Eng. Health Med.* **2018**, *6*, 1800808. [CrossRef]
32. Yan, P.; Sun, W.; Li, X.; Li, M.; Jiang, Y.; Luo, H. PKDN: Prior Knowledge Distillation Network for bronchoscopy diagnosis. *Comput. Biol. Med.* **2023**, *166*, 107486. [CrossRef]
33. Liu, Q.; Zheng, H.; Jia, Z.; Shi, Z. Tumor detection on bronchoscopic images by unsupervised learning. *Sci. Rep.* **2025**, *15*, 245. [CrossRef]
34. Vu, V.G.; Hoang, A.D.; Phan, T.P.; Nguyen, N.D.; Nguyen, T.T.; Nguyen, D.N.; Dao, N.P.; Doan, T.P.L.; Nguyen, T.T.H.; Trinh, T.H.; et al. BM-BronchoLC—A rich bronchoscopy dataset for anatomical landmarks and lung cancer lesion recognition. *Sci. Data* **2024**, *11*, 321. [CrossRef] [PubMed]
35. Cao, Y.; Zhang, J.; Zhuo, R.; Zhao, J.; Dong, Y.; Liu, T.; Zhao, H. BrYOLO-Mamba: A Approach to Efficient Tracheal Lesion Detection in Bronchoscopy. *IEEE Access* **2024**, *12*, 174630–174639. [CrossRef]

36. Chang, Q.; Bascom, R.; Toth, J.; Ahmad, D.; Higgins, W.E. Autofluorescence Bronchoscopy Video Analysis for Lesion Frame Detection. *Annu. Int. Conf. IEEE Eng. Med. Biol. Soc.* **2020**, *2020*, 1556–1559.
37. Haritou, M.; Bountris, P.; Passalidou, E.; Koklonis, K.; Koutsouris, D. An image analysis tool for the classification of lesions suspicious for malignancy in autofluorescence bronchoscopy. *Biomed. Spectrosc. Imaging* **2014**, *3*, 167–183. [CrossRef]
38. Feng, P.H.; Chen, T.T.; Lin, Y.T.; Chiang, S.Y.; Lo, C.M. Classification of lung cancer subtypes based on autofluorescence bronchoscopic pattern recognition: A preliminary study. *Comput. Methods Programs Biomed.* **2018**, *163*, 33–38. [CrossRef]
39. Chang, Q.; Ahmad, D.; Toth, J.; Bascom, R.; Higgins, W.E. ESFPNet: Efficient Stage-Wise Feature Pyramid on Mix Transformer for Deep Learning-Based Cancer Analysis in Endoscopic Video. *J. Imaging* **2024**, *10*, 191. [CrossRef] [PubMed]
40. Daneshpajooh, V.; Ahmad, D.; Toth, J.; Bascom, R.; Higgins, W.E. Automatic lesion detection for narrow-band imaging bronchoscopy. *J. Med. Imaging* **2024**, *11*, 036002. [CrossRef] [PubMed]
41. Fousková, M.; Habartová, L.; Vališ, J.; Nahodilová, M.; Vaňková, A.; Synytsya, A.; Šestáková, Z.; Votruba, J.; Setnička, V. Raman spectroscopy in lung cancer diagnostics: Can an in vivo setup compete with ex vivo applications? *Spectrochim. Acta A Mol. Biomol. Spectrosc.* **2024**, *322*, 124770. [CrossRef]
42. Kiraly, A.P.; Odry, B.L.; Godoy, M.C.; Geiger, B.; Novak, C.L.; Naidich, D.P. Computer-aided diagnosis of the airways: Beyond nodule detection. *J. Thorac. Imaging* **2008**, *23*, 105–113. [CrossRef] [PubMed]
43. Ramírez, E.; Sánchez, C.; Gil, D. Localizing Pulmonary Lesions Using Fuzzy Deep Learning. In Proceedings of the 2019 21st International Symposium on Symbolic and Numeric Algorithms for Scientific Computing (SYNASC), Timisoara, Romania, 4–7 September 2019; pp. 290–294.
44. Zhang, M.; Gu, Y. Towards Connectivity-Aware Pulmonary Airway Segmentation. *IEEE J. Biomed. Health Inform.* **2023**, *28*, 321–332. [CrossRef] [PubMed]
45. Yang, H.W.; Wang, Y.; Zhu, H.; Zhang, J.; Deng, X.; Liu, W. A Cascaded Network for Airway Tree Segmentation Incorporating Multiple Attention Mechanisms. In Proceedings of the 2024 7th International Symposium on Autonomous Systems (ISAS), Chongqing, China, 7–9 May 2024; pp. 1–5.
46. Meng, Q.; Kitasaka, T.; Nimura, Y.; Oda, M.; Ueno, J.; Mori, K. Automatic segmentation of airway tree based on local intensity filter and machine learning technique in 3D chest CT volume. *Int. J. Comput. Assist. Radiol. Surg.* **2017**, *12*, 245–261. [CrossRef]
47. Mori, K.; Ota, S.; Deguchi, D.; Kitasaka, T.; Suenaga, Y.; Iwano, S.; Hasegawa, Y.; Takabatake, H.; Mori, M.; Natori, H. Automated anatomical labeling of bronchial branches extracted from CT datasets based on machine learning and combination optimization and its application to bronchoscope guidance. *Med. Image Comput. Comput. Assist. Interv.* **2009**, *12*, 707–714.
48. Zhou, Z.Q.; Guo, Z.Y.; Zhong, C.H.; Qiu, H.Q.; Chen, Y.; Rao, W.Y.; Chen, X.B.; Wu, H.K.; Tang, C.L.; Su, Z.Q.; et al. Deep Learning-Based Segmentation of Airway Morphology from Endobronchial Optical Coherence Tomography. *Respiration* **2023**, *102*, 227–236. [CrossRef]
49. Li, Y.; Zheng, X.; Xie, F.; Ye, L.; Bignami, E.; Tandon, Y.K.; Rodríguez, M.; Gu, Y.; Sun, J. Development and validation of the artificial intelligence (AI)-based diagnostic model for bronchial lumen identification. *Transl. Lung Cancer Res.* **2022**, *11*, 2261–2274. [CrossRef] [PubMed]
50. Chen, C.; Herth, F.J.; Zuo, Y.; Li, H.; Liang, X.; Chen, Y.; Ren, J.; Jian, W.; Zhong, C.; Li, S. Distinguishing bronchoscopically observed anatomical positions of airway under by convolutional neural network. *Ther. Adv. Chronic Dis.* **2023**, *14*, 20406223231181495. [CrossRef]
51. Yoo, J.Y.; Kang, S.Y.; Park, J.S.; Cho, Y.J.; Park, S.Y.; Yoon, H.I.; Park, S.J.; Jeong, H.G.; Kim, T. Deep learning for anatomical interpretation of video bronchoscopy images. *Sci. Rep.* **2021**, *11*, 23765. [CrossRef]
52. Borrego-Carazo, J.; Sanchez, C.; Castells-Rufas, D.; Carrabina, J.; Gil, D. BronchoPose: An analysis of data and model configuration for vision-based bronchoscopy pose estimation. *Comput. Methods Programs Biomed.* **2023**, *228*, 107241. [CrossRef]
53. Wang, C.; Oda, M.; Hayashi, Y.; Kitasaka, T.; Itoh, H.; Honma, H.; Takebatake, H.; Mori, M.; Natori, H.; Mori, K. Anatomy Aware-Based 2.5D Bronchoscope Tracking for Image-Guided Bronchoscopic Navigation. *Comput. Methods Biomech. Biomed. Eng. Imaging Vis.* **2022**, *11*, 1122–1129. [CrossRef]
54. Zhu, L.; Zheng, J.; Wang, C.; Jiang, J.; Song, A. A bronchoscopic navigation method based on neural radiation fields. *Int. J. Comput. Assist. Radiol. Surg.* **2024**, *19*, 2011–2021. [CrossRef]
55. Keuth, R.; Heinrich, M.; Eichenlaub, M.; Himstedt, M. Airway label prediction in video bronchoscopy: Capturing temporal dependencies utilizing anatomical knowledge. *Int. J. Comput. Assist. Radiol. Surg.* **2024**, *19*, 713–721. [CrossRef]
56. Cicenia, J.; Sethi, S. Navigation to peripheral lung nodules using an artificial intelligence-driven augmented image fusion platform (LungVision): A pilot study. *Chest* **2019**, *156*, A830. [CrossRef]
57. Whitten, P. Artificial intelligence driven diagnosis of lung cancer in patients with multiple pulmonary nodules. *Chest* **2019**, *156*, A534. [CrossRef]
58. Gruionu, L.G.; Udriștoiu, A.L.; Iacob, A.V.; Constantinescu, C.; Stan, R.; Gruionu, G. Feasibility of a lung airway navigation system using fiber-Bragg shape sensing and artificial intelligence for early diagnosis of lung cancer. *PLoS ONE* **2022**, *17*, e0277938. [CrossRef]

59. Fried, I.; Hoelscher, J.; Akulian, J.A.; Pizer, S.; Alterovitz, R. Landmark Based Bronchoscope Localization for Needle Insertion Under Respiratory Deformation. In Proceedings of the 2023 IEEE/RSJ International Conference on Intelligent Robots and Systems (IROS), Detroit, MI, USA, 1–5 October 2023; pp. 6593–6600.
60. Chahla, B.; Ozen, M. Fluoroscopy and Cone Beam CT Guidance in Robotic Interventions. *Tech. Vasc. Interv. Radiol.* **2024**, *27*, 101007. [CrossRef]
61. Boac, B.M.; Kanathanavanich, M.; Li, X.; Imai, T.; Fan, X.; Walts, A.E.; Marchevsky, A.M.; Bose, S. Accuracy and efficacy of Ion robotic-assisted bronchoscopic fine needle aspiration of lung lesions. *J. Am. Soc. Cytopathol.* **2024**, *13*, 420–430. [CrossRef] [PubMed]
62. Zhang, J.; Liu, L.; Xiang, P.; Fang, Q.; Nie, X.; Ma, H.; Hu, J.; Xiong, R.; Wang, Y.; Lu, H. AI co-pilot bronchoscope robot. *Nat. Commun.* **2024**, *15*, 241. [CrossRef] [PubMed]
63. Mitros, Z.; Thamo, B.; Bergeles, C.; da Cruz, L.; Dhaliwal, K.; Khadem, M. Design and Modelling of a Continuum Robot for Distal Lung Sampling in Mechanically Ventilated Patients in Critical Care. *Front. Robot. AI* **2021**, *8*, 611866. [CrossRef] [PubMed]
64. Xu, S.; Wang, X.; Qin, Y.; Wang, H.; Yu, N.; Han, J. Depth-Awareness Shared Self-Supervised Bronchial Orifice Segmentation for Center Detection in Vision-Based Robotic Bronchoscopy. In Proceedings of the 2024 IEEE 14th International Conference on CYBER Technology in Automation, Control, and Intelligent Systems (CYBER), Copenhagen, Denmark, 16–19 July 2024; pp. 345–351.
65. Zheng, M.; Ye, M.; Rafii-Tari, H. Automatic Biopsy Tool Presence and Episode Recognition in Robotic Bronchoscopy Using a Multi-Task Vision Transformer Network. In Proceedings of the 2022 International Conference on Robotics and Automation (ICRA), Philadelphia, PA, USA, 23–27 May 2022; pp. 7349–7355.
66. Zhao, J.; Chen, H.; Tian, Q.; Chen, J.; Yang, B.; Zhang, Z.; Liu, H. BronchoCopilot: Towards Autonomous Robotic Bronchoscopy via Multimodal Reinforcement Learning. In Proceedings of the 2024 IEEE/RSJ International Conference on Intelligent Robots and Systems (IROS), Abu Dhabi, United Arab Emirates, 14–18 October 2024; pp. 6923–6930.
67. Sachdeva, A.; Sethi, S. Motivation and Learning: Leveraging Artificial Intelligence to Improve Bronchoscopy Performance. *Chest* **2024**, *165*, 243–245. [CrossRef] [PubMed]
68. Hostetter, L.J.; Nelson, D.R. Competency-based medical education in interventional pulmonology: Current state and future opportunities. *Curr. Opin. Pulm. Med.* **2025**, *31*, 65–71. [CrossRef] [PubMed]
69. Healy, W.J.; Musani, A.; Fallaw, D.J.; Islam, S.U. Emerging Role of Artificial Intelligence in Academic Pulmonary Medicine. *South. Med. J.* **2024**, *117*, 369–370. [CrossRef]
70. Cold, K.M.; Vamadevan, A.; Nielsen, A.O.; Konge, L.; Clementsen, P.F. Systematic Bronchoscopy: The Four Landmarks Approach. *J. Vis. Exp.* **2023**, e65358. [CrossRef]
71. Cold, K.M.; Agbontaen, K.; Nielsen, A.O.; Andersen, C.S.; Singh, S.; Konge, L. Artificial intelligence improves bronchoscopy performance: A randomised crossover trial. *ERJ Open Res.* **2025**, *11*, 00395–02024. [CrossRef] [PubMed]
72. Cold, K.M.; Xie, S.; Nielsen, A.O.; Clementsen, P.F.; Konge, L. Artificial Intelligence Improves Novices' Bronchoscopy Performance: A Randomized Controlled Trial in a Simulated Setting. *Chest* **2024**, *165*, 405–413. [CrossRef]
73. Cold, K.M.; Wei, W.; Agbontaen, K.; Singh, S.; Konge, L. Mastery Learning Guided by Artificial Intelligence Is Superior to Directed Self-Regulated Learning in Flexible Bronchoscopy Training: An RCT. *Respiration* **2025**, *104*, 206–215. [CrossRef]
74. Xu, W.; Hou, G.; Deng, M. A novel artificial intelligence feedback system boosts novice bronchoscopy performance based on chest-CT simulated tracheal models: A randomized controlled trial. *Eur. Respir. J.* **2024**, *64*, RCT998. [CrossRef]
75. Mora, A.; Debiasi, E. Leveraging artificial intelligence for development of a cost-effective bronchoscopy simulator for resource-constrained settings. *Chest* **2023**, *164*, A3896. [CrossRef]
76. Cold, K.M.; Agbontaen, K.; Nielsen, A.O.; Andersen, C.S.; Singh, S.; Konge, L. Artificial intelligence for automatic and objective assessment of competencies in flexible bronchoscopy. *J. Thorac. Dis.* **2024**, *16*, 5718–5726. [CrossRef] [PubMed]
77. Yap, E.L.C.; Vandal, A.C.; Williamson, J.P.; Nguyen, P.; Colt, H. Development of a Bronchoscopy-Radiologic Skills and Task Assessment Tool (BRadSTAT): A Tool for Evaluating the Radiological Skills of Bronchoscopists with Different Experience. *Respiration* **2022**, *101*, 990–1005. [CrossRef]
78. Huang, J.; Lin, J.; Lin, Z.; Li, S.; Zhong, C. Artificial Intelligence Feedback for Bronchoscopy Training: Old Wine in a New Bottle or True Innovation? *Chest* **2024**, *165*, e60–e61. [CrossRef] [PubMed]
79. Jaliawala, H.A.; Farooqui, S.M.; Harris, K.; Abdo, T.; Keddissi, J.I.; Youness, H.A. Endobronchial Ultrasound-Guided Transbronchial Needle Aspiration (EBUS-TBNA): Technical Updates and Pathological Yield. *Diagnostics* **2021**, *11*, 2331. [CrossRef]
80. Fielding, D.I.; Kurimoto, N. EBUS-TBNA/staging of lung cancer. *Clin. Chest Med.* **2013**, *34*, 385–394. [CrossRef]
81. Torre, M.; Reda, M.; Musso, V.; Danuzzo, F.; Mohamed, S.; Conforti, S. Diagnostic accuracy of endobronchial ultrasound-transbronchial needle aspiration (EBUS-TBNA) for mediastinal lymph node staging of lung cancer. *Mediastinum* **2021**, *5*, 15. [CrossRef] [PubMed]
82. Zhou, X.; Li, Y. Diagnostic utility of endobronchial ultrasound elastography for detecting benign and malignant lymph nodes: A retrospective study. *J. Thorac. Dis.* **2025**, *17*, 614–622. [CrossRef]

83. Nosotti, M.; Palleschi, A.; Tosi, D.; Mendogni, P.; Righi, I.; Carrinola, R.; Rosso, L. Color-Doppler sonography patterns in endobronchial ultrasound-guided transbronchial needle aspiration of mediastinal lymph-nodes. *J. Thorac. Dis.* **2017**, *9*, S376–S380. [CrossRef]
84. Chen, A.; Chenna, P.; Loiselle, A.; Massoni, J.; Mayse, M.; Misselhorn, D. Radial probe endobronchial ultrasound for peripheral pulmonary lesions. A 5-year institutional experience. *Ann. Am. Thorac. Soc.* **2014**, *11*, 578–582. [CrossRef] [PubMed]
85. McGuire, A.L.; Myers, R.; Grant, K.; Lam, S.; Yee, J. The Diagnostic Accuracy and Sensitivity for Malignancy of Radial-Endobronchial Ultrasound and Electromagnetic Navigation Bronchoscopy for Sampling of Peripheral Pulmonary Lesions: Systematic Review and Meta-analysis. *J. Bronchol. Interv. Pulmonol.* **2020**, *27*, 106–121. [CrossRef]
86. Wang, B.; Guo, Q.; Wang, J.Y.; Yu, Y.; Yi, A.J.; Cui, X.W.; Dietrich, C.F. Ultrasound Elastography for the Evaluation of Lymph Nodes. *Front. Oncol.* **2021**, *11*, 714660. [CrossRef]
87. Huang, Z.; Wang, L.; Chen, J.; Zhi, X.; Sun, J. A risk-scoring model based on endobronchial ultrasound multimodal imaging for predicting metastatic lymph nodes in lung cancer patients. *Endosc. Ultrasound* **2024**, *13*, 107–114. [CrossRef] [PubMed]
88. Choi, J.; Zo, S.; Kim, J.H.; Oh, Y.J.; Ahn, J.H.; Kim, M.; Lee, K.; Lee, H.Y. Nondiagnostic, radial-probe endobronchial ultrasound-guided biopsy for peripheral lung lesions: The added value of radiomics from ultrasound imaging for predicting malignancy. *Thorac. Cancer* **2023**, *14*, 177–185. [CrossRef] [PubMed]
89. Wu, J.; Wu, C.; Zhou, C.; Zheng, W.; Li, P. Recent advances in convex probe endobronchial ultrasound: A narrative review. *Ann. Transl. Med.* **2021**, *9*, 419. [CrossRef]
90. Achim, C.; Rusu-Both, R.; Chira, R.I. Computerised application for lung cancer diagnosis based on transthoracic ultrasonography. In Proceedings of the 2018 IEEE-EMBS Conference on Biomedical Engineering and Sciences (IECBES), Sarawak, Malaysia, 3–6 December 2018; pp. 211–216.
91. Ervik, Ø.; Tveten, I.; Hofstad, E.F.; Langø, T.; Leira, H.O.; Amundsen, T.; Sorger, H. Automatic Segmentation of Mediastinal Lymph Nodes and Blood Vessels in Endobronchial Ultrasound (EBUS) Images Using Deep Learning. *J. Imaging* **2024**, *10*, 190. [CrossRef] [PubMed]
92. Ervik, Ø.; Rødde, M.; Hofstad, E.F.; Tveten, I.; Langø, T.; Leira, H.O.; Amundsen, T.; Sorger, H. A New Deep Learning-Based Method for Automated Identification of Thoracic Lymph Node Stations in Endobronchial Ultrasound (EBUS): A Proof-of-Concept Study. *J. Imaging* **2025**, *11*, 10. [CrossRef]
93. Zhou, Q.; Zhou, Y.; Hou, N.; Zhang, Y.; Zhu, G.; Li, L. DFA-UNet: Dual-stream feature-fusion attention U-Net for lymph node segmentation in lung cancer diagnosis. *Front. Neurosci.* **2024**, *18*, 1448294. [CrossRef]
94. Tagaya, R.; Kurimoto, N.; Osada, H.; Kobayashi, A. Automatic objective diagnosis of lymph nodal disease by B-mode images from convex-type echobronchoscopy. *Chest* **2008**, *133*, 137–142. [CrossRef]
95. Ozcelik, N.; Ozcelik, A.E.; Bulbul, Y.; Oztuna, F.; Ozlu, T. Can artificial intelligence distinguish between malignant and benign mediastinal lymph nodes using sonographic features on EBUS images? *Curr. Med. Res. Opin.* **2020**, *36*, 2019–2024. [CrossRef]
96. Koseoglu, F.D.; Alıcı, I.O.; Er, O. Machine learning approaches in the interpretation of endobronchial ultrasound images: A comparative analysis. *Surg. Endosc.* **2023**, *37*, 9339–9346. [CrossRef]
97. Hu, W.; Wen, F.; Zhao, M.; Li, X.; Luo, P.; Jiang, G.; Yang, H.; Herth, F.J.F.; Zhang, X.; Zhang, Q. Endobronchial Ultrasound-Based Support Vector Machine Model for Differentiating between Benign and Malignant Mediastinal and Hilar Lymph Nodes. *Respiration* **2024**, *103*, 675–685. [CrossRef]
98. Churchill, I.F.; Gatti, A.A.; Hylton, D.A.; Sullivan, K.A.; Patel, Y.S.; Leontiadis, G.I.; Farrokhyar, F.; Hanna, W.C. An Artificial Intelligence Algorithm to Predict Nodal Metastasis in Lung Cancer. *Ann. Thorac. Surg.* **2022**, *114*, 248–256. [CrossRef] [PubMed]
99. Ito, Y.; Nakajima, T.; Inage, T.; Otsuka, T.; Sata, Y.; Tanaka, K.; Sakairi, Y.; Suzuki, H.; Yoshino, I. Prediction of Nodal Metastasis in Lung Cancer Using Deep Learning of Endobronchial Ultrasound Images. *Cancers* **2022**, *14*, 3334. [CrossRef]
100. Ishiwata, T.; Inage, T.; Aragaki, M.; Gregor, A.; Chen, Z.; Bernards, N.; Kafi, K.; Yasufuku, K. Deep learning-based prediction of nodal metastasis in lung cancer using endobronchial ultrasound. *JTCVS Tech.* **2024**, *28*, 151–161. [CrossRef]
101. Yong, S.H.; Lee, S.H.; Oh, S.I.; Keum, J.S.; Kim, K.N.; Park, M.S.; Chang, Y.S.; Kim, E.Y. Malignant thoracic lymph node classification with deep convolutional neural networks on real-time endobronchial ultrasound (EBUS) images. *Transl. Lung Cancer Res.* **2022**, *11*, 14–23. [CrossRef]
102. Patel, Y.S.; Gatti, A.A.; Farrokhyar, F.; Xie, F.; Hanna, W.C. Artificial Intelligence Algorithm Can Predict Lymph Node Malignancy from Endobronchial Ultrasound Transbronchial Needle Aspiration Images for Non-Small Cell Lung Cancer. *Respiration* **2024**, *103*, 741–751. [CrossRef]
103. Zhi, X.; Li, J.; Chen, J.; Wang, L.; Xie, F.; Dai, W.; Sun, J.; Xiong, H. Automatic Image Selection Model Based on Machine Learning for Endobronchial Ultrasound Strain Elastography Videos. *Front. Oncol.* **2021**, *11*, 673775. [CrossRef]
104. Xu, M.; Chen, J.; Li, J.; Zhi, X.; Dai, W.; Sun, J.; Xiong, H. Automatic Representative Frame Selection and Intrathoracic Lymph Node Diagnosis With Endobronchial Ultrasound Elastography Videos. *IEEE J. Biomed. Health Inform.* **2023**, *27*, 29–40. [CrossRef]
105. Patel, Y.S.; Gatti, A.A.; Farrokhyar, F.; Xie, F.; Hanna, W.C. Clinical utility of artificial intelligence-augmented endobronchial ultrasound elastography in lymph node staging for lung cancer. *JTCVS Tech.* **2024**, *27*, 158–166. [CrossRef]

106. Li, J.; Zhi, X.; Chen, J.; Wang, L.; Xu, M.; Dai, W.; Sun, J.; Xiong, H. Deep learning with convex probe endobronchial ultrasound multimodal imaging: A validated tool for automated intrathoracic lymph nodes diagnosis. *Endosc. Ultrasound* **2021**, *10*, 361–371. [CrossRef] [PubMed]
107. Lin, C.K.; Wu, S.H.; Chua, Y.W.; Fan, H.J.; Cheng, Y.C. TransEBUS: The interpretation of endobronchial ultrasound image using hybrid transformer for differentiating malignant and benign mediastinal lesions. *J. Formos. Med. Assoc.* **2025**, *124*, 28–37. [CrossRef] [PubMed]
108. Chen, C.H.; Lee, Y.W.; Huang, Y.S.; Lan, W.R.; Chang, R.F.; Tu, C.Y.; Chen, C.Y.; Liao, W.C. Computer-aided diagnosis of endobronchial ultrasound images using convolutional neural network. *Comput. Methods Programs Biomed.* **2019**, *177*, 175–182. [CrossRef] [PubMed]
109. Hotta, T.; Kurimoto, N.; Shiratsuki, Y.; Amano, Y.; Hamaguchi, M.; Tanino, A.; Tsubata, Y.; Isobe, T. Deep learning-based diagnosis from endobronchial ultrasonography images of pulmonary lesions. *Sci. Rep.* **2022**, *12*, 13710. [CrossRef]
110. Yu, K.L.; Tseng, Y.S.; Yang, H.C.; Liu, C.J.; Kuo, P.C.; Lee, M.R.; Huang, C.T.; Kuo, L.C.; Wang, J.Y.; Ho, C.C.; et al. Deep learning with test-time augmentation for radial endobronchial ultrasound image differentiation: A multicentre verification study. *BMJ Open Respir. Res.* **2023**, *10*, e001602. [CrossRef]
111. Khomkham, B.; Lipikorn, R. Pulmonary Lesion Classification Framework Using the Weighted Ensemble Classification with Random Forest and CNN Models for EBUS Images. *Diagnostics* **2022**, *12*, 1552. [CrossRef]
112. Xing, J.; Li, C.; Wu, P.; Cai, X.; Ouyang, J. Optimized fuzzy K-nearest neighbor approach for accurate lung cancer prediction based on radial endobronchial ultrasonography. *Comput. Biol. Med.* **2024**, *171*, 108038. [CrossRef]
113. Um, S.W.; Kim, H.K.; Jung, S.H.; Han, J.; Lee, K.J.; Park, H.Y.; Choi, Y.S.; Shim, Y.M.; Ahn, M.J.; Park, K.; et al. Endobronchial ultrasound versus mediastinoscopy for mediastinal nodal staging of non-small-cell lung cancer. *J. Thorac. Oncol.* **2015**, *10*, 331–337. [CrossRef]
114. Czarnecka-Kujawa, K.; Yasufuku, K. The role of endobronchial ultrasound versus mediastinoscopy for non-small cell lung cancer. *J. Thorac. Dis.* **2017**, *9*, S83–S97. [CrossRef]
115. Jain, D.; Allen, T.C.; Aisner, D.L.; Beasley, M.B.; Cagle, P.T.; Capelozzi, V.L.; Hariri, L.P.; Lantuejoul, S.; Miller, R.; Mino-Kenudson, M.; et al. Rapid On-Site Evaluation of Endobronchial Ultrasound-Guided Transbronchial Needle Aspirations for the Diagnosis of Lung Cancer: A Perspective From Members of the Pulmonary Pathology Society. *Arch. Pathol. Lab. Med.* **2018**, *142*, 253–262. [CrossRef]
116. Kalluri, M.; Puttagunta, L.; Ohinmaa, A.; Thanh, N.X.; Wong, E. Cost Analysis of Intra Procedural Rapid on Site Evaluation of Cytopathology with Endobronchial Ultrasound. *Int. J. Technol. Assess. Health Care* **2015**, *31*, 273–280. [CrossRef] [PubMed]
117. Witt, B.L. Rapid On Site Evaluation (ROSE): A Pathologists' Perspective. *Tech. Vasc. Interv. Radiol.* **2021**, *24*, 100767. [CrossRef] [PubMed]
118. Asfahan, S.; Elhence, P.; Dutt, N.; Niwas Jalandra, R.; Chauhan, N.K. Digital-Rapid On-site Examination in Endobronchial Ultrasound-Guided Transbronchial Needle Aspiration (DEBUT): A proof of concept study for the application of artificial intelligence in the bronchoscopy suite. *Eur. Respir. J.* **2021**, *58*, 2100915. [CrossRef]
119. Koratala, A.; Chandra, N.C.; Pulipaka, S.P.; Colleti, S.; Lee-Mateus, A.Y.; Barrios-Ruiz, A.; Neshat, S.; Diaz-Churion, F.; Johnson, M.M.; Abia Trujillo, D.; et al. Artificial Intelligence in Rapid On-Site Evaluation of Bronchoscopy Samples. *Am. J. Respir. Crit. Care Med.* **2023**, *207*, A4467.
120. Lan, H.; Chen, P.; Wang, C.; Chen, C.; Yao, C.; Jin, F.; Wan, T.; Lv, X.; Wang, J. A Multiscale Connected UNet for the Segmentation of Lung Cancer Cells in Pathology Sections Stained Using Rapid On-Site Cytopathological Evaluation. *Am. J. Pathol.* **2024**, *194*, 1712–1723. [CrossRef]
121. Subramanian, H.; Oleari, N.; Bluestone, A.; Danczuk, J.; Randolph, M.; Costaldi, M. Improving the Efficiency of Rapid Onsite Evaluation Utilizing Artificial Intelligence. *J. Am. Soc. Cytopathol.* **2024**, *13*, S6–S7. [CrossRef]
122. Yan, S.; Li, Y.; Pan, L.; Jiang, H.; Gong, L.; Jin, F. The application of artificial intelligence for Rapid On-Site Evaluation during flexible bronchoscopy. *Front. Oncol.* **2024**, *14*, 1360831. [CrossRef]
123. Lin, C.K.; Chang, J.; Huang, C.C.; Wen, Y.F.; Ho, C.C.; Cheng, Y.C. Effectiveness of convolutional neural networks in the interpretation of pulmonary cytologic images in endobronchial ultrasound procedures. *Cancer Med.* **2021**, *10*, 9047–9057. [CrossRef]
124. Wang, C.W.; Khalil, M.A.; Lin, Y.J.; Lee, Y.C.; Huang, T.W.; Chao, T.K. Deep Learning Using Endobronchial-Ultrasound-Guided Transbronchial Needle Aspiration Image to Improve the Overall Diagnostic Yield of Sampling Mediastinal Lymphadenopathy. *Diagnostics* **2022**, *12*, 2234. [CrossRef] [PubMed]
125. Chen, J.; Zhang, C.; Xie, J.; Zheng, X.; Gu, P.; Liu, S.; Zhou, Y.; Wu, J.; Chen, Y.; Wang, Y.; et al. Automatic lung cancer subtyping using rapid on-site evaluation slides and serum biological markers. *Respir. Res.* **2024**, *25*, 391. [CrossRef]
126. van Huizen, L.M.G.; Blokker, M.; Daniels, J.M.A.; Radonic, T.; von der Thüsen, J.H.; Veta, M.; Annema, J.T.; Groot, M.L. Rapid On-Site Histology of Lung and Pleural Biopsies Using Higher Harmonic Generation Microscopy and Artificial Intelligence Analysis. *Mod. Pathol.* **2025**, *38*, 100633. [CrossRef] [PubMed]

127. Zhang, S.; Raff, R.; Rossi, J.; Zukovsky, E.; Thosani, N. Rapid Onsite Evaluation (ROSE) Anywhere and Anytime: Developing a Cloud Based Artificial Intelligence (AI) Platform Service. *J. Am. Soc. Cytopathol.* **2023**, *12*, S76. [CrossRef]
128. Travis, W.D. Lung Cancer Pathology: Current Concepts. *Clin. Chest Med.* **2020**, *41*, 67–85. [CrossRef] [PubMed]
129. Hays, P. Artificial intelligence in cytopathological applications for cancer: A review of accuracy and analytic validity. *Eur. J. Med. Res.* **2024**, *29*, 553. [CrossRef] [PubMed]
130. Vaickus, L.J.; Kerr, D.A.; Velez Torres, J.M.; Levy, J. Artificial Intelligence Applications in Cytopathology: Current State of the Art. *Surg. Pathol. Clin.* **2024**, *17*, 521–531. [CrossRef]
131. Kiyuna, T.; Cosatto, E.; Hatanaka, K.C.; Yokose, T.; Tsuta, K.; Motoi, N.; Makita, K.; Shimizu, A.; Shinohara, T.; Suzuki, A.; et al. Evaluating Cellularity Estimation Methods: Comparing AI Counting with Pathologists' Visual Estimates. *Diagnostics* **2024**, *14*, 1115. [CrossRef]
132. Tomlinson, G.S.; Thomas, N.; Chain, B.M.; Best, K.; Simpson, N.; Hardavella, G.; Brown, J.; Bhowmik, A.; Navani, N.; Janes, S.M.; et al. Transcriptional Profiling of Endobronchial Ultrasound-Guided Lymph Node Samples Aids Diagnosis of Mediastinal Lymphadenopathy. *Chest* **2016**, *149*, 535–544. [CrossRef]
133. Choi, Y.; Qu, J.; Wu, S.; Hao, Y.; Zhang, J.; Ning, J.; Yang, X.; Lofaro, L.; Pankratz, D.G.; Babiarz, J.; et al. Improving lung cancer risk stratification leveraging whole transcriptome RNA sequencing and machine learning across multiple cohorts. *BMC Med. Genomics.* **2020**, *13*, 151. [CrossRef]
134. Wang, S.; Wang, R.; Hu, D.; Zhang, C.; Cao, P.; Huang, J. Machine learning reveals diverse cell death patterns in lung adenocarcinoma prognosis and therapy. *NPJ Precis. Oncol.* **2024**, *8*, 49. [CrossRef]
135. Leblond, F.; Dallaire, F.; Tran, T.; Yadav, R.; Aubertin, K.; Goudie, E.; Romeo, P.; Kent, C.; Leduc, C.; Liberman, M. Subsecond lung cancer detection within a heterogeneous background of normal and benign tissue using single-point Raman spectroscopy. *J. Biomed. Opt.* **2023**, *28*, 090501. [CrossRef]
136. Sano, H.; Okoshi, E.N.; Tachibana, Y.; Tanaka, T.; Lami, K.; Uegami, W.; Ohta, Y.; Brcic, L.; Bychkov, A.; Fukuoka, J. Machine-Learning-Based Classification Model to Address Diagnostic Challenges in Transbronchial Lung Biopsy. *Cancers* **2024**, *16*, 731. [CrossRef]
137. Guglielmo, P.; Marturano, F.; Bettinelli, A.; Sepulcri, M.; Pasello, G.; Gregianin, M.; Paiusco, M.; Evangelista, L. Additional Value of PET and CT Image-Based Features in the Detection of Occult Lymph Node Metastases in Lung Cancer: A Systematic Review of the Literature. *Diagnostics* **2023**, *13*, 2153. [CrossRef] [PubMed]
138. Flechsig, P.; Frank, P.; Kratochwil, C.; Antoch, G.; Rath, D.; Moltz, J.; Rieser, M.; Warth, A.; Kauczor, H.U.; Schwartz, L.H.; et al. Radiomic Analysis using Density Threshold for FDG-PET/CT-Based N-Staging in Lung Cancer Patients. *Mol. Imaging Biol.* **2017**, *19*, 315–322. [CrossRef]
139. Kawaguchi, Y.; Matsuura, Y.; Kondo, Y.; Ichinose, J.; Nakao, M.; Okumura, S.; Mun, M. The predictive power of artificial intelligence on mediastinal lymphnode metastasis. *Gen. Thorac. Cardiovasc. Surg.* **2021**, *69*, 1545–1552. [CrossRef] [PubMed]
140. Teramoto, A.; Tsujimoto, M.; Inoue, T.; Tsukamoto, T.; Imaizumi, K.; Toyama, H.; Saito, K.; Fujita, H. Automated Classification of Pulmonary Nodules through a Retrospective Analysis of Conventional CT and Two-phase PET Images in Patients Undergoing Biopsy. *Asia Ocean. J. Nucl. Med. Biol.* **2019**, *7*, 29–37. [PubMed]
141. Guberina, M.; Herrmann, K.; Pöttgen, C.; Guberina, N.; Hautzel, H.; Gauler, T.; Ploenes, T.; Umutlu, L.; Wetter, A.; Theegarten, D.; et al. Prediction of malignant lymph nodes in NSCLC by machine-learning classifiers using EBUS-TBNA and PET/CT. *Sci. Rep.* **2022**, *12*, 17511. [CrossRef] [PubMed]
142. Rogasch, J.M.M.; Michaels, L.; Baumgärtner, G.L.; Frost, N.; Rückert, J.C.; Neudecker, J.; Ochsenreither, S.; Gerhold, M.; Schmidt, B.; Schneider, P.; et al. A machine learning tool to improve prediction of mediastinal lymph node metastases in non-small cell lung cancer using routinely obtainable [18F]FDG-PET/CT parameters. *Eur. J. Nucl. Med. Mol. Imaging* **2023**, *50*, 2140–2151. [CrossRef] [PubMed]
143. Laros, S.S.A.; Dieckens, D.; Blazis, S.P.; van der Heide, J.A. Machine learning classification of mediastinal lymph node metastasis in NSCLC: A multicentre study in a Western European patient population. *EJNMMI Phys.* **2022**, *9*, 66. [CrossRef]
144. Ouyang, M.L.; Wang, Y.R.; Deng, Q.S.; Zhu, Y.F.; Zhao, Z.H.; Wang, L.; Wang, L.X.; Tang, K. Development and Validation of a 18F-FDG PET-Based Radiomic Model for Evaluating Hypermetabolic Mediastinal-Hilar Lymph Nodes in Non-Small-Cell Lung Cancer. *Front. Oncol.* **2021**, *11*, 710909. [CrossRef]
145. Zhou, Y.; Ma, X.L.; Zhang, T.; Wang, J.; Zhang, T.; Tian, R. Use of radiomics based on 18F-FDG PET/CT and machine learning methods to aid clinical decision-making in the classification of solitary pulmonary lesions: An innovative approach. *Eur. J. Nucl. Med. Mol. Imaging* **2021**, *48*, 2904–2913. [CrossRef] [PubMed]
146. Hashimoto, K.; Murakami, Y.; Omura, K.; Takahashi, H.; Suzuki, R.; Yoshioka, Y.; Oguchi, M.; Ichinose, J.; Matsuura, Y.; Nakao, M.; et al. Prediction of Tumor PD-L1 Expression in Resectable Non-Small Cell Lung Cancer by Machine Learning Models Based on Clinical and Radiological Features: Performance Comparison With Preoperative Biopsy. *Clin. Lung Cancer* **2024**, *25*, e26–e34.e6. [CrossRef]

147. Digumarthy, S.R.; Padole, A.M.; Gullo, R.L.; Sequist, L.V.; Kalra, M.K. Can CT radiomic analysis in NSCLC predict histology and EGFR mutation status? *Medicine* **2019**, *98*, e13963. [CrossRef]
148. Yamazaki, M.; Yagi, T.; Tominaga, M.; Minato, K.; Ishikawa, H. Role of intratumoral and peritumoral CT radiomics for the prediction of EGFR gene mutation in primary lung cancer. *Br. J. Radiol.* **2022**, *95*, 20220374. [CrossRef]
149. Sun, H.; Zhou, P.; Chen, G.; Dai, Z.; Song, P.; Yao, J. Radiomics nomogram for the prediction of Ki-67 index in advanced non-small cell lung cancer based on dual-phase enhanced computed tomography. *J. Cancer Res. Clin. Oncol.* **2023**, *149*, 9301–9315. [CrossRef]
150. Boulogne, L.H.; Charbonnier, J.P.; Jacobs, C.; van der Heijden, E.H.F.M.; van Ginneken, B. Estimating lung function from computed tomography at the patient and lobe level using machine learning. *Med. Phys.* **2024**, *51*, 2834–2845. [CrossRef]
151. Ziegelmayer, S.; Graf, M.; Makowski, M.; Gawlitza, J.; Gassert, F. Cost-Effectiveness of Artificial Intelligence Support in Computed Tomography-Based Lung Cancer Screening. *Cancers* **2022**, *14*, 1729. [CrossRef] [PubMed]
152. Trujillo, J.C.; Soriano, J.B.; Marzo, M.; Higuera, O.; Gorospe, L.; Pajares, V.; Olmedo, M.E.; Arrabal, N.; Flores, A.; García, J.F.; et al. Cost-effectiveness of a machine learning risk prediction model (LungFlag) in the selection of high-risk individuals for non-small cell lung cancer screening in Spain. *J. Med. Econ.* **2025**, *28*, 147–156. [CrossRef]
153. Ye, M.; Tong, L.; Zheng, X.; Wang, H.; Zhou, H.; Zhu, X.; Zhou, C.; Zhao, P.; Wang, Y.; Wang, Q.; et al. A Classifier for Improving Early Lung Cancer Diagnosis Incorporating Artificial Intelligence and Liquid Biopsy. *Front. Oncol.* **2022**, *12*, 853801. [CrossRef]
154. Mohamed, E.I.; Mohamed, M.A.; Abdel-Mageed, S.M.; Abdel-Mohdy, T.S.; Badawi, M.I.; Darwish, S.H. Volatile organic compounds of biofluids for detecting lung cancer by an electronic nose based on artificial neural network. *J. Appl. Biomed.* **2019**, *17*, 67. [CrossRef] [PubMed]
155. Hesso, I.; Kayyali, R.; Zacharias, L.; Charalambous, A.; Lavdaniti, M.; Stalika, E.; Ajami, T.; Acampa, W.; Boban, J.; Gebara, S.N. Cancer care pathways across seven countries in Europe: What are the current obstacles? And how can artificial intelligence help? *J. Cancer Policy* **2024**, *39*, 100457. [CrossRef] [PubMed]
156. Purohit, L.; Kiamos, A.; Ali, S.; Alvarez-Pinzon, A.M.; Raez, L. Incidental Pulmonary Nodule (IPN) Programs Working Together with Lung Cancer Screening and Artificial Intelligence to Increase Lung Cancer Detection. *Cancers* **2025**, *17*, 1143. [CrossRef]

cancers

MDPI

Review

Equity and Opportunities in Lung Cancer Care—Addressing Disparities, Challenges, and Pathways Forward

Dena G. Shehata [1], Jennifer Megan Pan [2], Zhuxuan Pan [3], Janani Vigneswaran [4], Nicolas Contreras [4], Emily Rodriguez [5], Sara Sakowitz [6], Jessica Magarinos [4], Sara Pereira [4], Fatima G. Wilder [7] and Ammara A. Watkins [1,*]

1 Division of Thoracic and Cardiovascular Surgery, Lahey Hospital and Medical Center, Burlington, MA 01805, USA; dena.shehata@lahey.org
2 Department of General Surgery, Beth Israel Deaconess Medical Center, Boston, MA 02115, USA; jmpan@bidmc.harvard.edu
3 UMass Chan Medical School, Worcester, MA 01655, USA; zhuxuan.pan@umassmed.edu
4 Department of Thoracic Surgery, University of Utah, Salt Lake City, UT 84132, USA; janani.vigneswaran@gmail.com (J.V.); jessicamagarinos@gmail.com (J.M.)
5 School of Medicine, The Johns Hopkins University, Baltimore, MD 21218, USA; erodri47@jhmi.edu
6 David Geffen School of Medicine, University of California, Los Angeles, CA 90024, USA; ssakowitz@mednet.ucla.edu
7 Division of Thoracic Surgery, Department of Surgery, Brigham and Women's Hospital, Boston, MA 02115, USA
* Correspondence: ammara.watkins@lahey.org

Simple Summary: Lung cancer is the leading cause of cancer-related mortality in the United States, with racial and ethnic minorities experiencing worse outcomes due to disparities in screening, diagnosis, and treatment. This review aims to identify the underlying causes of these disparities and explore strategies to improve lung cancer care for underserved populations. The findings highlight gaps in screening and treatment, suggest policy changes, and discuss targeted interventions to improve access to care and reduce health disparities in lung cancer outcomes.

Abstract: Background: Lung cancer is the leading cause of cancer-related mortality in the United States, which disproportionately affect racial and ethnic minorities. Disparities in lung cancer screening, diagnosis, treatment, and survival outcomes are due to a complex interplay of socioeconomic factors, structural racism, and limited access to high-quality care. This review aims to examine the underlying causes of these disparities and explore potential mitigation strategies to improve lung cancer care equity. Methods: A review of the literature was conducted, evaluating racial and ethnic disparities in lung cancer care. Disparities in lung cancer screening, genomic testing, surgical and systemic treatment, and survival were explored. Additionally, interventional strategies such as risk-based screening, patient navigation programs, and policy reforms were examined. Results: Racial and ethnic minority patients are diagnosed at younger ages with fewer pack-years yet are less likely to qualify for screening under current guidelines. They receive lower rates of guideline-concordant treatment, including surgery, radiation, chemotherapy, and biomarker testing, and have reduced access to specialty care. Socioeconomic barriers, medical mistrust, and geographic disparities further contribute to these inequities. Targeted interventions, including mobile screening programs, financial assistance initiatives, and culturally competent care, have shown promise in improving lung cancer outcomes. Conclusion: A multi-level approach, incorporating healthcare policy changes, improved screening criteria, and an enhanced community engagement strategy, is essential for achieving equitable lung cancer care, ultimately improving outcomes for racial minority populations.

Keywords: lung cancer disparities; social determinants of health; lung cancer screening; race; ethnicity; survival; surgical treatment

1. Introduction

Lung cancer is the leading cause of cancer-related deaths in the United States, with a disproportionate impact on racial and ethnic minorities [1]. After a lung cancer diagnosis, the estimated 5-year survival rate is 26.7% [2,3] across all stages. The reasons for poor survival are multifaceted and are related to tobacco use, late-stage diagnosis, and under-utilization of effective treatments [4]. County-level spatial analyses have highlighted that social determinants, including income inequality, education level, and rurality, are tightly linked to geographic disparities in cancer mortality [5].

It is evident in the literature that race and gender impact lung cancer diagnosis and treatment. The incidence of lung cancer is 40.7 per 100,000 in White individuals and 43.5 per 100,000 in Black individuals [3,4]. Studies have found that Black patients develop lung cancer earlier than White patients, with a median age of 67 compared to 70 [4]. Of the patients with lung cancer outside of the screening age range (50–80 years old), Black patients were almost twice as likely as White patients to be diagnosed (14.2 vs. 8.2%, $p < 0.05$) [1,6]. Furthermore, the rates of lung cancer death are disproportionate. Death rates are estimated at 35.1% for non-Hispanic Whites, 33.4% for non-Hispanic Blacks, 18.5% for Asian/Pacific Islanders, 26.3% for American Indian/Alaska Natives, and 14.2% for Latinos. Gender also has an impact on mortality rates. From 2016 to 2020, mortality rates were highest among Black males (51.0 per 100,000), followed by White males (44.7 per 100,000; 14% lower) and American Indian/Alaska Native males (39.9 per 100,000; 28% lower) [7]. Among women, White women had the highest death rates (32.8 per 100,000), followed by American Indian/Alaska Native women (29.9 per 100,000; 10% lower) and Black women (27.8 per 100,000; 18% lower) [7].

Elements of social determinants of health (SDOH) play an important role in these disparities. Socioeconomic status (SES) significantly impacts lung cancer disparities and influences incidence, treatment, and outcomes (Figure 1). Lower SES is associated with higher lung cancer rates, late diagnoses, and worse survival, with this discrepancy being most evident in Black patients [8]. The etiology of these disparities is multifactorial and often includes downstream effects of systemic racism such as education access, decreased access to healthcare, higher smoking prevalence, and limited economic opportunities [8,9]. In a comprehensive review of how lung cancer risk and structural racism are linked, Bonner et al. summarize seven main domains in the literature. They highlight that poor housing conditions disproportionately affect Black and Hispanic patients. Additionally, Black patients experienced higher occupational exposures to factors known to increase lung cancer risk. The impact of structural racism in policies contributes to increased poverty, decreased access to high-quality health insurance, as well as implicit medical biases [9]. Health literacy, often lower among individuals with low SES, further exacerbates challenges in accessing and understanding healthcare, affecting clinical decision-making and outcomes [9,10]. Ultimately, these social determinants perpetuate the disparities observed in lung cancer incidence and survival rates among disadvantaged populations. Addressing disparities in lung cancer screening, treatment, and survival could significantly reduce the morbidity and mortality burden of this disease.

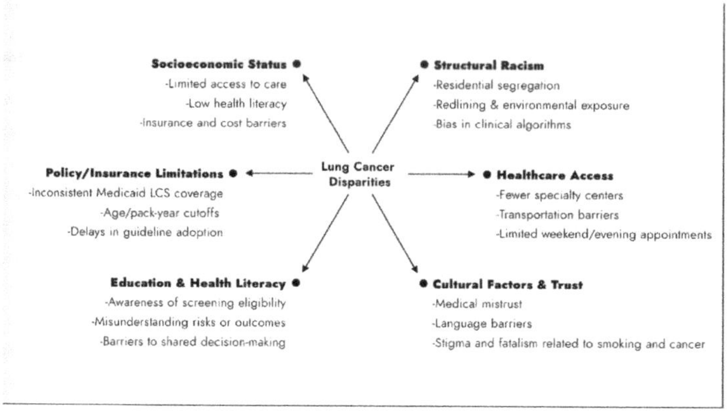

Figure 1. Social determinants of health contributing to lung cancer disparities. LCS, lung cancer screening.

2. Methods

This is a narrative review based on targeted literature searches conducted in PubMed and Google Scholar. We searched for studies published between 2000 and 2024 using combinations of terms such as lung cancer disparities, screening, treatment, genomics, and survival. Studies were selected for inclusion based on relevance, recency, and impact within each thematic section.

3. Lung Cancer Screening and Surveillance

Screening with an annual low-dose computed tomography (CT) scan can reduce lung cancer mortality by 16% to 24% among high-risk individuals by identifying asymptomatic cancers suitable for curative treatment [11]. However, overall screening rates remain low, with only about 6% of the 14.2 million eligible Americans screened annually [7]. Similar low screening rates are observed internationally [12]. Early detection through screening is crucial for improving lung cancer survival rates, yet significant disparities in screening eligibility and access persist [1,11–13].

New guidelines from the American Cancer Society recommend annual lung cancer screening (LCS) for healthy individuals aged 50 to 80 years with a smoking history of 20 pack-years or more, regardless of when they quit. This has expanded eligibility to an additional 5 million people and increased the potential to prevent lung cancer deaths [13]. However, these guidelines fail to address racial and ethnic differences. Data indicate that Black individuals develop lung cancer with fewer pack-years of smoking [13–16]. Black individuals are less likely to qualify for lung cancer screening due to lower tobacco exposure and younger age at diagnosis. Non-Black patients were 90% more likely to meet USPSTF (United States Preventive Services Task Force) criteria for lung cancer screening compared to Black patients. However, this disparity may be reduced with the use of more detailed risk-based screening criteria ($PLCO_{m2012}$) [4,17,18]. Further existing data demonstrate that Black patients who are eligible for screening based on USPSTF criteria are less likely to be screened compared to White patients. Poulson et al. examined redlined areas in the Boston area. They found that Black patients had 61% lower odds of completing lung cancer screening than White patients in those areas despite meeting the USPSTF eligibility criteria at that time [19]. In another screening program in Philadelphia, Black patients had significantly lower odds of undergoing lung cancer screening compared to White patients after a referral. Among patients with a negative baseline screening CT, Black patients experienced longer intervals before subsequent screening compared to White patients and had higher rates of loss to follow-up [20].

The National Lung Screening Trial (NLST) found that White patients had statistically higher rates of follow-up care after screening tests compared to Black patients (89.6% vs. 82.8%; $p < 0.05$) [10]. A study on LCS barriers among veterans found racial disparities, with Black veterans having lower odds of completing initial LCS compared to White veterans (30.5% vs. 41.3%). Key barriers included a higher proportion of current smokers among Black veterans (71.6% vs. 61.6%), a lower pack-year smoking history, and a higher prevalence of mental health or substance use diagnoses (65.6% vs. 54.6%). Despite living closer to VA screening centers, Black veterans faced lower screening completion rates [21]. In a larger study of the VA cohort, Black veterans had higher odds of delayed or no follow-up compared to White veterans [22].

Inequity in lung cancer screening is prevalent in other races and ethnicities as well. A study examining racial and ethnic differences in LCS completion and follow-up rates in Hawaii revealed significant disparities. Asian individuals had the highest completion rate at 86%, with Korean (94%) and Japanese (88%) subgroups having the highest screening rates. In contrast, lower rates were observed among Native Hawaiians (80%), non-Hispanic Whites (80%), Pacific Islanders (79%), and other racial and ethnic groups (77%), highlighting a 14% to 15% gap in LCS completion rates among the groups studied [23].

Disparities in LCS rates are often attributed to various factors [18–30] including insurance coverage. The Affordable Care Act mandates that most insurance plans cover LCS; however, Medicaid coverage varies. While 46 states' Medicaid programs cover LCS, three do not. The Centers for Medicare and Medicaid Services provide LCS coverage for high-risk individuals aged 55–77. While Medicaid expansion has improved 2-year survival rates for non-older adult men with non-small-cell lung cancer (NSCLC) in expansion states, it has not had the same effect for women [24]. Income also plays a role, as studies reported that higher annual income is associated with higher completion rates or intent to undergo screening [25].

Geographic disparities also exist, with southern and western states having lower LCS completion rates [26]. One study highlighted that geographic disparities, including limited access to low-dose computed tomography facilities in rural and underserved areas, were more prevalent in these regions [26]. Another study conducted in rural settings found that 47% of participants cited financial constraints as a barrier to LCS. Thirty-five percent mentioned limited access to healthcare facilities, while 28% highlighted transportation issues. Additionally, 22% reported stigma and fear of false positives as deterrents [27]. Factors such as environmental or occupational exposures beyond tobacco use, access to care, transportation challenges, stigma and beliefs, difficulties in patient-practitioner communication, and shared decision-making all contribute to disparities in LCS [21–30].

Studies have reported differences in beliefs and attitudes among smokers. Black smokers were more likely than White smokers to believe they were at lower risk (28% vs. 15%) and that early detection would not improve survival (33% vs. 19%) [28]. Hispanic smokers expressed greater concern about screening costs (64% vs. 48% for Whites) and felt screening could cause unnecessary worry (47% vs. 34%) [29]. A qualitative study found that smoking-related stigma, characterized by shame and self-blame, was a major barrier to LCS. In a small group of majority White smokers, one cohort had been screened and the other had never been screened. They identified three major barriers to screening: inconvenience, smoking-related stigma, and distrust of the medical system [29].

4. Lung Cancer Preoperative Workup and Diagnosis

Accurate staging is pivotal in managing NSCLC, as it dictates both prognosis and treatment decisions [31–34]. Staging methods for NSCLC encompass both non-invasive and invasive techniques. Non-invasive methods, such as imaging modalities like CT and positron emission tomography (PET) scans, are widely employed for diagnosis and staging, but their utilization can vary considerably [32,33]. Guidelines from the American College of Chest Physicians and the National Comprehensive Cancer Network (NCCN) emphasize the role of PET scans in staging NSCLC patients eligible for curative treatments [31–33].

In a multi-site, prospective, observational study analyzing data from the Cancer Care Outcomes Research and Surveillance (CanCORS) Consortium between 2003 and 2005, PET scans were used 13% less often among non-White and Hispanic patients [32]. This disparity remained consistent across subgroups and could not be explained by variations in income, education, or insurance status. Although these data were published more than a decade ago, these findings persist. A more recent study using the national Surveillance, Epidemiology, and End Results (SEER)–Medicare linked database found similar results [34]. After accounting for demographic, community, and facility characteristics, Black individuals were still significantly less likely to undergo PET or CT imaging at the time of diagnosis compared to non-Hispanic Whites. Similarly, Hispanic individuals had a lower likelihood of receiving PET imaging [34].

5. Lung Cancer Genetic Testing

Genetic testing, fundamental to precision medicine, plays an essential role in diagnosing NSCLC and pinpointing mutations that guide the selection of targeted treatments [4,35]. Next-generation sequencing has identified numerous genetic anomalies in lung cancer, highlighting a panel of twenty genes with the highest mutation frequencies [4,35]. Based on a large Medicare study, molecular testing rates for NSCLC have risen in recent years but still fall short of recommended levels [36]. Despite increased molecular testing tools, disparities are pervasive in the use of this implement. In an analysis of the SEER database, 28,511 patients were identified with any stage of NSCLC [37]. Of these patients, 40.4% of White patients received molecular genetic testing compared to only 27.9% of Black patients ($p < 0.001$). There was not a sufficient number of patients of other races and ethnicities to perform additional comparison [37].

Despite a 19.7% increase in epidermal growth factor receptor (EGFR) testing from 2011 to 2013, Lynch et al. identified socioeconomic and geographic disparities in testing. Patients living in the northeastern regions had the highest likelihood of undergoing testing, and Asian/Pacific Islanders were the most likely racial group to undergo testing [38]. In contrast, Medicaid recipients, Hispanics, and Blacks were less likely to receive testing. Similarly, Illei et al. studied the trends and patterns of anaplastic lymphoma kinase (ALK) testing and found that patients with Medicare and Medicaid were less likely to undergo ALK testing [39]. However, unlike Lynch et al., they found that those residing in non-western states were also less likely to receive this testing. Using the SEER database, Kehl et al. reported molecular testing rates of 32.8% for Asian/other descents, 26.2% for Whites, and 14.1% for Blacks, with median survival times of 8.2 months for those tested and 6.1 months for those not tested [40]. Using data from the Kentucky Cancer Registry, Larson et al. found that factors like male sex, enrollment in Medicaid or Medicare, older age, geographic region, and smoking were linked to a lack of EGFR testing, and those tested had higher overall survival rates [41]. Interestingly, Cheng et al. discovered that among patients with EGFR-mutated NSCLC, Black patients had shorter survival rates compared to non-Black patients, with 2-year survival rates of 33% vs. 61%, respectively [42]. Begnaud et al. found no significant difference in mutation testing between American Indians and non-American Indians in Minnesota, suggesting that other factors contribute to higher mortality rates in this group [43].

Although broad-based genomic sequencing (BGS) has improved access to the genomic profile of advanced NSCLC tumors, as recommended by NCCN guidelines, disparities in testing still persist [35–46]. Riaz et al. observed significant age-related and racial disparities in the use of BGS among NSCLC patients treated in community settings. Black patients were less likely to receive BGS compared to White patients, and patients aged 76–85 were less likely to receive BGS compared to those under 45 years of age [44]. Likewise, Wu et al., in their analysis of real-world biomarker testing trends and overall survival among US patients with advanced NSCLC, reported that PD-L1 testing before first-line treatment was less frequently performed in older patients, those treated in a community setting, and those with squamous NSCLC, recurrent disease, or no distant metastasis. Testing was also less common, albeit to a lesser degree, among Black patients and those with Medicare insurance [45]. A recent systematic review of studies spanning 2007 to 2022 highlighted persistent racial and ethnic disparities in genomic testing for lung cancer patients, with Black patients consistently having lower testing rates compared to Asian and White patients [46].

A number of studies have examined the impact of race on lung cancer genetics but have reported conflicting results. In a prospective study of multiple Baltimore hospitals with an overrepresentation of Black patients, authors identified distinctly different elements in the NSCLC transcriptome when comparing African Americans to European Americans [47]. MicroRNA expression also varied between the two groups [47]. Another study analyzed over 509 lung cancers for the frequencies of genomic changes between Black and White patients, identifying 504 genes but finding no significant differences in genetic alterations between the groups [48]. With further advancements in genetic testing, it is crucial to improve genetic testing to identify any transcriptomic nuances present in patients.

Minority representation has been consistently lower in clinical trials and studies, despite minorities express a similar willingness to participate in medical research [49]. In an analysis of lung cancer clinical trials, Kanuparthy et al. found that although racial and gender minority enrollment has increased, it still has not reached parity across different races, ethnicities, and gender [50]. Similarly, Kwak et al. analyzed NSCLC patients from the National Cancer Database and found that Black and Hispanic patients were significantly less likely to be enrolled in lung cancer trials [51]. This underrepresentation was further confirmed in a more recent analysis of clinical trials enrolled on ClinicalTrials.gov (accessed on 10 April 2025) [52].

6. Lung Cancer Treatment

Disparities in lung cancer treatment have been well documented [53–63], with significant concerns regarding adherence to guideline-concordant treatment for minoritized groups. Notably, Black patients with resectable NSCLC are less likely to receive surgery and more likely to be treated with radiation therapy (RT) and/or chemotherapy—treatments not standard for this stage—even after adjusting for confounders such as comorbidities and age [53–58].

A SEER study found that Black patients underwent lung resection less frequently than White patients (69% vs. 83%, a 14% difference, 99% CI 11–18%), despite both groups being recommended to undergo surgical therapy [53]. Additionally, a notable delay from diagnosis to treatment for minorities has been reported [55]. Black patients were found to experience a longer time from diagnosis to treatment compared to White patients, with an approximate delay of eight days following multivariable analysis [55].

Contributing factors include socioeconomic vulnerabilities, limited access to experienced surgeons, misconceptions about surgery, and inadequate insurance coverage or reliance on public insurance. Distrust of healthcare providers is also a significant issue in this population [53–59]. Disparities in patient–surgeon interactions reveal that Black patients are less frequently offered surgery and have higher refusal rates when it is recommended [53,54]. This refusal is often linked to beliefs about accelerated tumor spread, potential for cure without surgery, and general distrust of healthcare providers [53]. Annesi and colleagues found that structural racism through residential segregation contributes to worse lung cancer outcomes for Black patients, including advanced disease at diagnosis, lower rates of early-stage surgery, and higher cancer-specific mortality, particularly in highly segregated areas [56].

A statewide quality collaborative involving high-volume centers in Michigan identified disparities in surgical quality for resectable NSCLC. Black patients received fewer lymph node resections and sampling than White patients. Unadjusted analysis found that Black patients were more likely to undergo wedge resection (limited resection); however, this difference was not observed in adjusted analyses. Further examination of the covariates found that Black patients were more likely to have lower predicted DLCO (diffusing capacity of the lung for carbon monoxide), higher rates of hypertension and diabetes, and a greater likelihood of requiring dialysis [58].

These disparities align with broader trends observed in national databases. Analysis from the SEER and New York Statewide Planning and Research Cooperative Database found that limited resection, increasingly used among patients with comorbidities (from 68% in the 1990s to 83% by 2007–2012), may lead to fewer in-hospital complications and shorter lengths of stay compared to lobectomy [59]. However, lobectomy with lymph node dissection is still regarded as the standard of care for the majority of operative lung cancer cases. Taioli and Flores further demonstrated that Black patients were significantly less likely to undergo surgery, and when they did, they were more likely to undergo a limited resection rather than a lobectomy compared to White patients [60]. Furthermore, Black patients had significantly less lymph nodes resected compared to White patients and had overall worse survival [60]. Similarly, SEER data show significant variability in resection rates for Black patients compared to White patients [61].

Specialty care is vital in thoracic oncology, with thoracic surgeons playing a pivotal role in evaluating and managing lung cancer patients. Cardiothoracic surgeons specializing in thoracic surgery perform the majority of minimally invasive (MIS) lobectomies compared to general surgeons or cardiac-track surgeons [61,62]. Notably, an analysis of the Premier database found that Black patients were less likely to undergo minimally invasive operations because they were less likely to be treated by thoracic surgeons [62]. A cohort analysis of the STS GTSD (Society of Thoracic Surgeons General Thoracic Surgery Database) also found that Black and Hispanic patients were less likely to undergo MIS surgery [63]. Additionally, Black patients, those with Medicaid insurance, and patients in smaller hospitals, the western region, and rural areas are less likely to have a thoracic surgeon perform their lobectomy, resulting in lower rates of MIS lobectomies for these groups [61,62].

7. Lung Cancer Survival

Lung cancer survival rates exhibit notable disparities across racial and ethnic groups despite advances in cancer awareness, screening, and treatment [4,64]. As shown by Wolf et al., Black patients with Stage I NSCLC were less likely to be treated with surgery and more likely to receive radiation or chemotherapy compared to their White counterparts. However, when analyzed according to treatment type, there were no differences in rate of survival [54]. Therefore, when provided comparable treatment, Black patients with Stage I NSCLC had similar rates of survival to White patients [54,56]. As highlighted by Wolf et al., socioeconomic factors, such as a lack of access to experienced surgeons, inadequate insurance coverage, and misconceptions associated with surgery, contribute to disparities in treatment [4,54,56]. Further, as discussed by Annesi et al., structural factors, such as residential segregation, exacerbate these disparities [56]. Studies have shown that Black patients residing in highly segregated areas are more likely to be diagnosed at an advanced stage and less likely to undergo surgical resection, leading to higher cancer-specific mortality rates [56]. This pattern underscores the role of structural racism in healthcare outcomes, where the geographic, socioeconomic, and cultural context significantly affects access to timely and appropriate care [4,54,56,64].

These disparities extend beyond Black patients and are present in other minority groups as well. Hispanic and Asian patients have been shown to have similar disparities, especially regarding the frequency of surgical interventions offered and the stage at diagnosis. Using the STS database, Weksler et al. found that for NSCLC, Hispanic and Asian patients had fewer operations for early-stage NSCLC than White and Black patients [65]. Hispanic and Asian patients were shown to have fewer surgical interventions and were diagnosed at a later stage compared to White patients [4,64,65]. These differences were reflected in the disparities in survival. Structural challenges, such as the impacts of immigration status, language concordance between providers and patients, and lack of cultural sensitivity, compounded with other structural barriers noted above, contribute to inferior survival outcomes [4,64,65].

The attribution of genetics as a key component in the differences in health outcomes is controversial and finds historical roots in eugenics [4,46,64]. While there may be certain genetic differences in lung cancers among races and ethnicities [66], these are not the sole reason why minorities are more likely to be diagnosed at later stages and have worse outcomes [67]. Further understanding of genetic differences is important for precision medicine. Additionally, studies analyzing genetic factors have repeatedly found that social determinants hinder access to diagnosis and treatment, often leading to later-stage presentation and substandard care, both of which have a more profound impact on outcomes and long-term survival [54,55,64]. Therefore, targeted interventions that consider the concepts of SDOH can work towards reducing racial disparities in lung cancer survival.

Survival disparities in patients with lung cancer are primarily driven by unequal access to timely diagnosis and the acceptance of appropriate guideline-directed treatment. These disparities are both compounded and influenced by socioeconomic, structural, and cultural barriers within the healthcare system and built environment that disproportionately affect minority populations. To improve survival outcomes and achieve equity in lung cancer care, it is essential to address these systemic issues, ensuring that all patients receive the best possible care regardless of their racial or ethnic background. This involves not only policy reforms and increased access to healthcare but also targeted efforts to overcome cultural and language barriers to provide culturally competent care.

8. Challenges and Future Opportunities

Race is a social construct. Thus, race-adjusted equations may increase health disparities by normalizing the differences in pulmonary function, limiting early diagnosis and intervention with pulmonary disease. In March 2023, the American Thoracic Society made an official recommendation to replace race- and ethnicity-specific equations with race-neutral reference equations for pulmonary function test (PFT) interpretation [68]. With these changes in how PFTs are calculated, Black patients' FEV1 and DLCO measurements will appear lower (with a higher reference range in use). As a result, many patients previously calculated as having borderline function may end up being excluded from surgical intervention due to lower PFT calculations. It is unclear if these patients with borderline pulmonary function who previously underwent surgical intervention due to a perceived better function may have had better clinical outcomes with non-surgical intervention for their cancer. Providers need to be intentional about how these borderline patients are evaluated for surgical intervention and if PFTs are the best assessment for their surgical candidacy. There is an opportunity for continued research and education on how changes in PFT calculations alter surgical risk assessment.

The cultural factors that impact cancer outcomes can be challenging to address. For example, Black Americans have higher rates of medical distrust, potentially stemming from a history of medical experimentation and exploitation of Black Americans [29,53–59]. Among minority patients, there are higher rates of negative beliefs around standardized treatments compared to their White counterparts, even when patients are evaluated at high-volume centers and recommended for appropriate guideline-directed treatments [29,53–59]. Further investigations incorporating community-based research addressing barriers experienced by underserved groups need to be explored. Barriers such as low health literacy, medical mistrust, cancer fatalism, stigma, language barriers, time and transportation limitations, and cost constraints with insurance issues need to be studied and addressed [69]. It would be useful to evaluate local interventions in other diseases where providers have been successful in engaging the community. One suggested approach to bridging and mitigating some of these barriers is the utilization of Community Health Workers (CHWs) [70], by supporting the role of community partners who have pre-existing relationships with their communities [71].

A review of community engagement initiatives utilizing CHWs to promote cancer prevention and education in underserved communities in both high- and low–middle-income countries found that CHWs served as vital links between healthcare systems and the community they support. By providing culturally tailored education, outreach, and support, CHWs play crucial roles in breast cancer screening, including disseminating information, assisting with the screening process, and navigating patients through healthcare services. These initiatives led to significantly improved cancer screening rates and awareness which enhanced early detection and reduced barriers to care. Post-intervention evaluations demonstrated increased cancer awareness and screening rates, underscoring the effectiveness of employing CHWs in reducing cancer disparities [70]. A notable initiative in California, the "Fe en Acción" community intervention, significantly enhanced breast cancer screening rates among churchgoing Latinas [72]. The program, implemented in 8 of 16 randomly assigned churches, notably increased self-reported mammography (OR = 4.64) and breast exams (OR = 2.82), while also reducing barriers to breast cancer screening [72]. Efforts to implement CHWs in lung cancer screening have successfully increased awareness but face barriers to improving actual screening uptake. A pilot study in Alabama's Black Belt highlighted challenges such as limited access to primary care providers, reluctance among providers to recommend screening, and logistical issues such as transportation and facility availability [73]. While CHWs effectively address knowledge gaps, systemic barriers must be overcome to translate awareness into action [73].

The U.S. Department of Health and Human Services created a priority area, "Healthy People 2030", to mitigate the health disparities that exist by focusing on the domains of SODH [74]. As described earlier in this chapter, structural racism and residential segregation contributes to these disparities [56]. Distinguishing the individual roles of socioeconomic status, geography, and race as root causes of these disparities is difficult. The all-cause mortality of Black Americans with lung cancer is higher than that of their matched White counterparts. While some of this disparity is related to differences in cancer treatment, most excess mortality can be attributed to various SDOH beyond the scope of lung cancer diagnosis and treatment. These factors include occupational and environmental exposures, socioeconomic status, neighborhood characteristics, and health behaviors beyond smoking status [56].

One opportunity, albeit extraordinarily difficult to achieve, is improving access to high-quality medical care across racial and gender groups. Appropriate management and treatment of smoking-related chronic conditions and disease can help reduce the all-cause mortality of Black patients with lung cancer. One place to start is with individual groups, studying why there is unequal care presented to minority patients within a specific health system or community. For example, assessing the reason for loss of follow-up care for positive LCS imaging in minority patients within a specific healthcare system can help develop targeted interventions. Institutional assessments of inherent biases or factors that lead to lower guideline-concordant care or curative intent surgery in minority patients are critical. A major cause of disparity in Black and Hispanic patients is limited access to experienced surgeons and high-volume centers—disparities that lead to treatment delay and higher morality [62]. These disparities highlight underlying societal issues that need to be addressed and the importance of moving away from a one-size-fits-all approach. Instead, health policies should focus on investing in tailored strategies that assess and address the unique risk factors and needs of individual communities, acknowledging their distinct challenges and priorities.

9. Intervention Strategies

There are several proposed solutions for improving health disparities in the literature, many of which emphasize multilevel approaches that target change across the healthcare ecosystem (Figure 2). Black patients are diagnosed with lung cancer at younger ages with fewer pack-years of smoking than their white counterparts. As a result, the current USPSTF guidelines (ages 50–80 with 20 pack-year history) may fail to capture all high-risk individuals. Creating LCS eligibility criteria that accurately reflect the cancer risk across the different racial and ethnic groups is the key to reducing screening disparities [18]. A change in formal LCS recommendations to include a risk assessment algorithm that includes race, smoking duration and intensity, environmental factors, and socioeconomic status may better capture higher-risk individuals [75]. Potter et al. proposed changes to the USPSTF guidelines. In their analysis of the Southern Community Cohort, the authors found that significantly more White patients would have undergone lung cancer screening based on the current USPSTF guidelines (57.6% of Black patients vs. 74% of White patients, $p < 0.001$) [76]. The authors proposed using a 20-year smoking duration rather than a 20-pack-year smoking cutoff. With this change, the percentage of Black and White patients who qualified for screening were similar (85.3% vs. 82%). The authors found a similar trend when using their proposed guidelines in the Black Women's Health Study. Of the patients with lung cancer, 63.8% would have qualified for screening as opposed to the 42.5% ($p < 0.001$) with the USPSTF guidelines [76].

A system-based intervention can also serve as a potential solution. An example of this is the multi-institutional "ACCURE" study, which implemented a system-based intervention to address disparities in cancer treatment completion and outcomes. This intervention included a real-time warning system based on electronic health records, feedback to clinical teams on treatment disparities by race, and the support of a nurse navigator [76]. By comparing patients from 2013–2015 to historical controls from 2007–2011, the study found significant improvements in survival rates for both Black and White patients with breast cancer and White patients with lung cancer. The intervention reduced the racial gap in survival rates and improved treatment completion across the board.

Despite these gains, some disparities remained, particularly in the selection of treatment modalities for lung cancer, suggesting a need for further investigation [76].

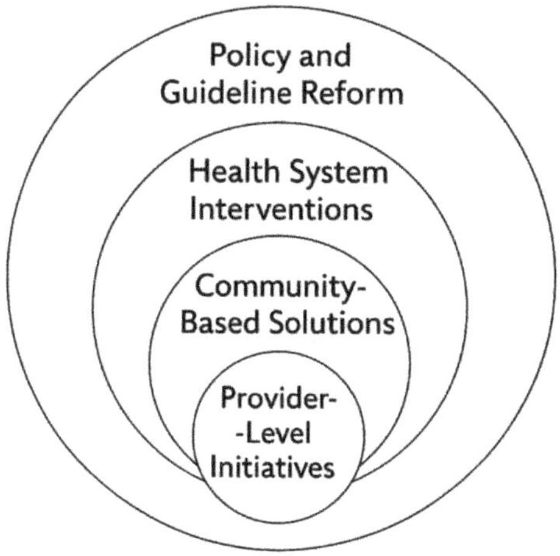
Policy and
Guideline Reform
Health System
Interventions
Community-
Based Solutions
Provider-
-Level
Initiatives

Figure 2. Intervention targets to address lung cancer care disparities.

Cultural barriers can be difficult to overcome at a provider level, but medical-adjacent support staff may help in this arena. One place to start is in the clinic, with clear communication between the patients and providers via the use of certified interpreters as well as written educational material available in the patient's primary language that is culturally appropriate [77–79]. Another possibility to improve care in this realm is leveraging the lay individuals in the community and trusted medical providers to help bridge knowledge gaps, alleviate patient concerns, and promote increased screening engagement and trust in the healthcare system [70,72]. Additionally, provider training on culturally competent care is critical to staff education [80].

Factors associated with low socioeconomic status that contribute to worse outcomes can be mitigated through several deliberate interventions. Local interventions to improve care compliance of patients with limited resources include transportation vouchers, free or discounted parking, appointments on weekends and evenings, care coordination (of labs, imaging, and provider visits) to minimize hospital trips, and appointments closer to home or virtual visits [77,81–90]. Other efforts that can mitigate access barriers that have shown some success are mobile screening clinics [91,92]. These programs deploy mobile low-dose CT units to community locations, offer on-site screenings to reduce travel burdens, and conduct targeted outreach to educate high-risk groups [91]. Recently proposed legislation supported by the Society of Thoracic Surgeons aims to expand the use of mobile lung cancer screening units. The bill establishes a competitive grant program within the health resources and services administration, emphasizing their role in reducing disparities and improving early detection for high-risk and underserved communities [92]. The use of patient navigators and social workers has been shown to help patients with limited health literacy complete medical recommendations [89]. State-funded screening programs can also help alleviate the cost associated with LCS [90].

Structural racism remains a difficult long-term problem. Implicit bias training and cultural communication training have been successful in improving care in other realms of healthcare [93,94]. Designing standardized staging and treatment protocols both nationally and locally at high-volume centers may minimize the effect of implicit bias. National- and local-level changes requiring equal representation in research at all levels of lung cancer will improve enrollment and participation of underrepresented groups in clinical trials and studies.

10. Conclusions

Addressing disparities in lung cancer care is essential to improving outcomes and achieving health equity for all patients. These disparities are driven by complex factors, including social determinants of health, systemic racism, and limited access to high-quality care. Targeted interventions, such as risk-based screening guidelines, culturally competent care, community-based initiatives, and policy reforms, are crucial to reducing these inequities. Prioritizing inclusivity, enhancing access to care, and implementing tailored strategies, such as real-time tracking tools, patient navigation, and mobile screening units, can help bridge gaps in care.

Author Contributions: Conceptualization, A.A.W.; methodology, A.A.W. and D.G.S.; investigation, D.G.S., J.M.P., Z.P., J.V., N.C., E.R., S.S. and J.M.; resources, A.A.W.; writing—original draft preparation, D.G.S., J.M.P., Z.P., J.V., N.C., E.R., S.S. and J.M.; writing—review and editing, A.A.W., S.P., and F.G.W.; supervision, A.A.W., S.P. and F.G.W. All authors have read and agreed to the published version of the manuscript.

Funding: This research received no external funding.

Data Availability Statement: No new data were created or analyzed in this study. Data sharing is not applicable to this article.

Conflicts of Interest: The authors declare no conflicts of interest.

Abbreviations

The following abbreviations are used in this manuscript:

SDOH	Social determinants of health
SES	Socioeconomic status
CT	Computed tomography
LCS	Lung cancer screening
USPSTF	United States Preventive Services Task Force
NLST	National Lung Screening Trial
NSCLC	Non-small-cell lung cancer
PET	Positron emission tomography
NCCN	National Comprehensive Cancer Network
CanCORS	Cancer Care Outcomes Research and Surveillance
SEER	Surveillance, Epidemiology, and End Results
EGFR	Epidermal growth factor receptor
ALK	Anaplastic lymphoma kinase
BGS	Broad-based genomic sequencing
RT	Radiation therapy
DLCO	Diffusing Capacity of the Lung for Carbon Monoxide
MIS	Minimally invasive surgery
STS	Society of Thoracic Surgeons
GTSD	General Thoracic Surgery Database
PFT	Pulmonary function test
CHWs	Community Health Workers

References

1. Haddad, D.N.; Sandler, K.L.; Henderson, L.M.; Rivera, M.P.; Aldrich, M.C. Disparities in Lung Cancer Screening: A Review. *Ann. Am. Thorac. Soc.* **2020**, *17*, 399–405. [CrossRef] [PubMed]
2. Siegel, R.L.; Giaquinto, A.N.; Jemal, A. Cancer Statistics, 2024. *CA Cancer J. Clin.* **2024**, *74*, 12–49. [CrossRef] [PubMed]

3. Natial Cancer Institute. Cancer of the Lung and Bronchus—Cancer Stat Facts. Available online: https://seer.cancer.gov/statfacts/html/lungb.html (accessed on 7 March 2025).
4. Dwyer, L.L.; Vadagam, P.; Vanderpoel, J.; Cohen, C.; Lewing, B.; Tkacz, J. Disparities in Lung Cancer: A Targeted Literature Review Examining Lung Cancer Screening, Diagnosis, Treatment, and Survival Outcomes in the United States. *J. Racial Ethn. Health Disparities* **2024**, *11*, 1489–1500. [CrossRef]
5. Karadzhov, G.; Albert, P.; Henry, K.; Abnet, C.; Lawrence, W.; Shiels, M.; Zhang, T.; Powell-Wiley, T.; Chen, Y. Cancer mortality and geographic inequalities: A detailed descriptive and spatial analysis of social determinants across US counties, 2018–2021. *Public Health* **2024**, *237*, 1–6. [CrossRef]
6. Annangi, S.; Nutalapati, S.; Foreman, M.G.; Pillai, R.; Flenaugh, E.L. Potential Racial Disparities Using Current Lung Cancer Screening Guidelines. *J. Racial Ethn. Health Disparities* **2019**, *6*, 22–26. [CrossRef] [PubMed]
7. American Lung Association. Lung Cancer Trends Brief. Available online: https://www.lung.org/research/trends-in-lung-disease/lung-cancer-trends-brief (accessed on 7 March 2025).
8. Brock, B.A.; Mir, H.; Flenaugh, E.L.; Oprea-Ilies, G.; Singh, R.; Singh, S. Social and Biological Determinants in Lung Cancer Disparity. *Cancers* **2024**, *16*, 612. [CrossRef]
9. Bonner, S.N.; Curley, R.; Love, K.; Akande, T.; Akhtar, A.; Erhunmwunsee, L. Structural Racism and Lung Cancer Risk: A Scoping Review. *JAMA Oncol.* **2024**, *10*, 122–128. [CrossRef]
10. Feagin, J.; Bennefield, Z. Systemic Racism and U.S. Health Care. *Soc. Sci. Med.* **2014**, *103*, 7–14. [CrossRef]
11. Pinsky, P.F.; Church, T.R.; Izmirlian, G.; Kramer, B.S. The National Lung Screening Trial: Results Stratified by Demographics, Smoking History, and Lung Cancer Histology. *Cancer* **2013**, *119*, 3976–3983. [CrossRef]
12. de Koning, H.J.; van der Aalst, C.M.; de Jong, P.A.; Scholten, E.T.; Nackaerts, K.; Heuvelmans, M.A.; Lammers, J.-W.J.; Weenink, C.; Yousaf-Khan, U.; Horeweg, N.; et al. Reduced Lung-Cancer Mortality with Volume CT Screening in a Randomized Trial. *N. Engl. J. Med.* **2020**, *382*, 503–513. [CrossRef]
13. Wolf, A.M.D.; Oeffinger, K.C.; Shih, T.Y.-C.; Walter, L.C.; Church, T.R.; Fontham, E.T.H.; Elkin, E.B.; Etzioni, R.D.; Guerra, C.E.; Perkins, R.B.; et al. Screening for Lung Cancer: 2023 Guideline Update from the American Cancer Society. *CA Cancer J. Clin.* **2024**, *74*, 50–81. [CrossRef] [PubMed]
14. Poon, C.; Wilsdon, T.; Sarwar, I.; Roediger, A.; Yuan, M. Why Is the Screening Rate in Lung Cancer Still Low? A Seven-Country Analysis of the Factors Affecting Adoption. *Front. Public Health* **2023**, *11*, 1264342. [CrossRef] [PubMed]
15. Shusted, C.S.; Evans, N.R.; Kane, G.C.; Juon, H.-S.; Barta, J.A. Analysis of Lung Cancer Screening by Race After USPSTF Expansion of Screening Eligibility in 2021. *JAMA Netw. Open* **2022**, *5*, e2217578. [CrossRef]
16. Lozier, J.W.; Fedewa, S.A.; Smith, R.A.; Silvestri, G.A. Lung Cancer Screening Eligibility and Screening Patterns Among Black and White Adults in the United States. *JAMA Netw. Open* **2021**, *4*, e2130350. [CrossRef] [PubMed]
17. Narayan, A.K.; Chowdhry, D.N.; Fintelmann, F.J.; Little, B.P.; Shepard, J.-A.O.; Flores, E.J. Racial and Ethnic Disparities in Lung Cancer Screening Eligibility. *Radiology* **2021**, *301*, 712–720. [CrossRef]
18. Choi, E.; Ding, V.Y.; Luo, S.J.; ten Haaf, K.; Wu, J.T.; Aredo, J.V.; Wilkens, L.R.; Freedman, N.D.; Backhus, L.M.; Leung, A.N.; et al. Risk Model–Based Lung Cancer Screening and Racial and Ethnic Disparities in the US. *JAMA Oncol.* **2023**, *9*, 1640–1648. [CrossRef]
19. Poulson, M.R.; Kenzik, K.M.; Singh, S.; Pavesi, F.; Steiling, K.; Litle, V.R.; Suzuki, K. Redlining, Structural Racism, and Lung Cancer Screening Disparities. *J. Thorac. Cardiovasc. Surg.* **2022**, *163*, 1920–1930.e2. [CrossRef]
20. Lake, M.; Shusted, C.S.; Juon, H.-S.; McIntire, R.K.; Zeigler-Johnson, C.; Evans, N.R.; Kane, G.C.; Barta, J.A. Black Patients Referred to a Lung Cancer Screening Program Experience Lower Rates of Screening and Longer Time to Follow-Up. *BMC Cancer* **2020**, *20*, 561. [CrossRef]
21. Navuluri, N.; Morrison, S.; Green, C.L.; Woolson, S.L.; Riley, I.L.; Cox, C.E.; Zullig, L.L.; Shofer, S. Racial Disparities in Lung Cancer Screening Among Veterans, 2013 to 2021. *JAMA Netw. Open* **2023**, *6*, e2318795. [CrossRef]
22. Núñez, E.R.; Caverly, T.J.; Zhang, S.; Glickman, M.E.; Qian, S.X.; Boudreau, J.H.; Slatore, C.G.; Miller, D.R.; Wiener, R.S. Adherence to Follow-up Testing Recommendations in US Veterans Screened for Lung Cancer, 2015–2019. *JAMA Netw. Open* **2021**, *4*, e2116233. [CrossRef]
23. Oshiro, C.E.S.; Frankland, T.B.; Mor, J.; Wong, C.P.; Martinez, Y.T.; Aruga, C.K.K.; Honda, S. Lung Cancer Screening by Race and Ethnicity in an Integrated Health System in Hawaii. *JAMA Netw. Open* **2022**, *5*, e2144381. [CrossRef] [PubMed]
24. Wilder, F.G.; Cangut, B.; Jindani, R.; Abioye, O.; Florez, N. Lung Cancer Screening among Minority Groups: Identifying Gaps in Screening and Opportunities for Intervention. *JTCVS Open* **2024**, *21*, 341–348. [CrossRef] [PubMed]
25. Sosa, E.; D'Souza, G.; Akhtar, A.; Sur, M.; Love, K.; Duffels, J.; Raz, D.J.; Kim, J.Y.; Sun, V.; Erhunmwunsee, L. Racial and Socioeconomic Disparities in Lung Cancer Screening in the United States: A Systematic Review. *CA Cancer J. Clin.* **2021**, *71*, 299–314. [CrossRef] [PubMed]
26. Raman, V.; Yong, V.; Erkmen, C.P.; Tong, B.C. Social Disparities in Lung Cancer Risk and Screening. *Thorac. Surg. Clin.* **2022**, *32*, 23–31. [CrossRef]

27. Schiffelbein, J.E.; Carluzzo, K.L.; Hasson, R.M.; Alford-Teaster, J.A.; Imset, I.; Onega, T. Barriers, Facilitators, and Suggested Interventions for Lung Cancer Screening Among a Rural Screening-Eligible Population. *J. Prim. Care Community Health* **2020**, *11*, 2150132720930544. [CrossRef]
28. Jonnalagadda, S.; Bergamo, C.; Lin, J.J.; Lurslurchachai, L.; Diefenbach, M.; Smith, C.; Nelson, J.E.; Wisnivesky, J.P. Beliefs and Attitudes about Lung Cancer Screening among Smokers. *Lung Cancer* **2012**, *77*, 526–531. [CrossRef]
29. Carter-Harris, L.; Ceppa, D.P.; Hanna, N.; Rawl, S.M. Lung Cancer Screening: What Do Long-Term Smokers Know and Believe? *Health Expect.* **2017**, *20*, 59–68. [CrossRef]
30. Carter-Harris, L.; Hermann, C.P.; Schreiber, J.; Weaver, M.T.; Rawl, S.M. Lung Cancer Stigma Predicts Timing of Medical Help-Seeking Behavior. *Oncol. Nurs. Forum* **2014**, *41*, E203–E210. [CrossRef]
31. Goldstraw, P.; Crowley, J.; Chansky, K.; Giroux, D.J.; Groome, P.A.; Rami-Porta, R.; Postmus, P.E.; Rusch, V.; Sobin, L.; International Association for the Study of Lung Cancer International Staging Committee; et al. The IASLC Lung Cancer Staging Project: Proposals for the Revision of the TNM Stage Groupings in the Forthcoming (Seventh) Edition of the TNM Classification of Malignant Tumours. *J. Thorac. Oncol.* **2007**, *2*, 706–714. [CrossRef]
32. Gould, M.K.; Schultz, E.M.; Wagner, T.H.; Xu, X.; Ghaus, S.J.; Wallace, R.B.; Provenzale, D.; Au, D.H. Disparities in Lung Cancer Staging with Positron Emission Tomography in the Cancer Care Outcomes Research and Surveillance (CanCORS) Study. *J. Thorac. Oncol.* **2011**, *6*, 875–883. [CrossRef]
33. National Comprehensive Cancer Network. NCCN Clinical Practice Guidelines in Oncology: Non-Small Cell Lung Cancer. Available online: https://www.nccn.org/guidelines/guidelines-detail?category=1&id=1450 (accessed on 16 July 2024).
34. Morgan, R.L.; Karam, S.D.; Bradley, C.J. Ethnic Disparities in Imaging Utilization at Diagnosis of Non-Small Cell Lung Cancer. *J. Natl. Cancer Inst.* **2020**, *112*, 1204–1212. [CrossRef]
35. Anand, S.; Vikramdeo, K.S.; Singh, S.; Singh, A.P.; Dasgupta, S. Racial Disparities in the Genetic Landscape of Lung Cancer. *Cancer Health Disparities* **2022**, *6*, 210. [PubMed]
36. Roberts, T.J.; Kehl, K.L.; Brooks, G.A.; Sholl, L.; Wright, A.A.; Landrum, M.B.; Keating, N.L. Practice-Level Variation in Molecular Testing and Use of Targeted Therapy for Patients With Non-Small Cell Lung Cancer and Colorectal Cancer. *JAMA Netw. Open* **2023**, *6*, e2310809. [CrossRef] [PubMed]
37. Tuminello, S.; Turner, W.M.; Untalan, M.; Ivic-Pavlicic, T.; Flores, R.; Taioli, E. Racial and Socioeconomic Disparities in Non-Small Cell Lung Cancer Molecular Diagnostics Uptake. *J. Natl. Cancer Inst.* **2025**, *117*, 112–119. [CrossRef] [PubMed]
38. Lynch, J.A.; Berse, B.; Rabb, M.; Mosquin, P.; Chew, R.; West, S.L.; Coomer, N.; Becker, D.; Kautter, J. Underutilization and Disparities in Access to EGFR Testing among Medicare Patients with Lung Cancer from 2010–2013. *BMC Cancer* **2018**, *18*, 306. [CrossRef]
39. Illei, P.B.; Wong, W.; Wu, N.; Chu, L.; Gupta, R.; Schulze, K.; Gubens, M.A. ALK Testing Trends and Patterns Among Community Practices in the United States. *JCO Precis. Oncol.* **2018**, *2*, 1–11. [CrossRef]
40. Kehl, K.L.; Lathan, C.S.; Johnson, B.E.; Schrag, D. Race, Poverty, and Initial Implementation of Precision Medicine for Lung Cancer. *J. Natl. Cancer Inst.* **2019**, *111*, 431–434. [CrossRef]
41. Larson, K.L.; Huang, B.; Chen, Q.; Tucker, T.; Schuh, M.; Arnold, S.M.; Kolesar, J.M. EGFR Testing and Erlotinib Use in Non-Small Cell Lung Cancer Patients in Kentucky. *PLoS ONE* **2020**, *15*, e0237790. [CrossRef]
42. Cheng, H.; Hosgood, H.D.; Deng, L.; Ye, K.; Su, C.; Sharma, J.; Yang, Y.; Halmos, B.; Perez-Soler, R. Survival Disparities in Black Patients With EGFR-Mutated Non-Small-Cell Lung Cancer. *Clin. Lung Cancer* **2020**, *21*, 177–185. [CrossRef]
43. Begnaud, A.; Yang, P.; Robichaux, C.; Rubin, N.; Kratzke, R.; Melzer, A.; Aliferis, C.; Jacobson, P. Evidence That Established Lung Cancer Mortality Disparities in American Indians Are Not Due to Lung Cancer Genetic Testing and Targeted Therapy Disparities. *Clin. Lung Cancer* **2020**, *21*, e164–e168. [CrossRef]
44. Riaz, F.; Presley, C.J.; Chiang, A.C.; Longtine, J.A.; Soulos, P.R.; Adelson, K.B.; Herbst, R.S.; Nussbaum, N.C.; Sorg, R.A.; Abernethy, A.P.; et al. Disparities in Broad-Based Genomic Sequencing for Patients with Advanced Non-Small Cell Lung Cancer. *J. Geriatr. Oncol.* **2019**, *10*, 669–672. [CrossRef] [PubMed]
45. Wu, N.; Ge, W.; Quek, R.G.; Gleeson, M.; Pouliot, J.-F.; Dietz, H.; Jalbert, J.J.; Harnett, J.; Antonia, S.J. Trends in Real-World Biomarker Testing and Overall Survival in US Patients with Advanced Non-Small-Cell Lung Cancer. *Future Oncol.* **2022**, *18*, 4385–4397. [CrossRef] [PubMed]
46. Meernik, C.; Raveendran, Y.; Kolarova, M.; Rahman, F.; Olunuga, E.; Hammond, E.; Shivaramakrishnan, A.; Hendren, S.; Bosworth, H.B.; Check, D.K.; et al. Racial and Ethnic Disparities in Genomic Testing among Lung Cancer Patients: A Systematic Review. *J. Natl. Cancer Inst.* **2024**, *116*, 812–828. [CrossRef]
47. Mitchell, K.A.; Zingone, A.; Toulabi, L.; Boeckelman, J.; Ryan, B.M. Comparative Transcriptome Profiling Reveals Coding and Noncoding RNA Differences in NSCLC from African Americans and European Americans. *Clin. Cancer Res.* **2017**, *23*, 7412–7425. [CrossRef]

48. Campbell, J.D.; Lathan, C.; Sholl, L.; Ducar, M.; Vega, M.; Sunkavalli, A.; Lin, L.; Hanna, M.; Schubert, L.; Thorner, A.; et al. Comparison of Prevalence and Types of Mutations in Lung Cancers Among Black and White Populations. *JAMA Oncol.* **2017**, *3*, 801–809. [CrossRef]
49. Wendler, D.; Kington, R.; Madans, J.; Van Wye, G.; Christ-Schmidt, H.; Pratt, L.A.; Brawley, O.W.; Gross, C.P.; Emanuel, E. Are Racial and Ethnic Minorities Less Willing to Participate in Health Research? *PLoS Med.* **2006**, *3*, e19. [CrossRef] [PubMed]
50. Kanuparthy, M.; Kanuparthy, S.; Harris, D.D.; Broadwin, M.; Stone, C.; Abbas, A.E.; Sellke, F.W. Gender, Race, and Ethnicity in Lung Cancer Clinical Trial Participation: Analysis of 253,845 Patients from 2002 to 2021. *J. Thorac. Cardiovasc. Surg.* **2024**. *Published online.* [CrossRef]
51. Kwak, M.; Bassiri, A.; Jiang, B.; Sinopoli, J.; Tapias-Vargas, L.; Linden, P.A.; Towe, C.W. National Enrollment of Lung Cancer Clinical Trials Is Disproportionate Based on Race and Health Care Access. *J. Thorac. Cardiovasc. Surg.* **2024**, *168*, 1235–1242. [CrossRef]
52. Wheeler, M.; Karanth, S.; Divaker, J.; Yoon, H.-S.; Yang, J.J.; Ratcliffe, M.; Blair, M.; Mehta, H.J.; Rackauskas, M.; Braithwaite, D. Participation in Non-Small Cell Lung Cancer Clinical Trials in the United States by Race/Ethnicity. *Clin. Lung Cancer* **2025**, *26*, 52–57.e2. [CrossRef]
53. Farjah, F.; Wood, D.E.; Yanez, N.D.; Vaughan, T.L.; Symons, R.G.; Krishnadasan, B.; Flum, D.R. Racial Disparities among Patients with Lung Cancer Who Were Recommended Operative Therapy. *Arch. Surg.* **2009**, *144*, 14–18. [CrossRef]
54. Wolf, A.; Alpert, N.; Tran, B.V.; Liu, B.; Flores, R.; Taioli, E. Persistence of Racial Disparities in Early-Stage Lung Cancer Treatment. *J. Thorac. Cardiovasc. Surg.* **2019**, *157*, 1670–1679.e4. [CrossRef]
55. Holmes, J.A.; Chen, R.C. Racial Disparities in Time From Diagnosis to Treatment for Stage I Non–Small Cell Lung Cancer. *JNCI Cancer Spectr.* **2018**, *2*, pky007. [CrossRef] [PubMed]
56. Annesi, C.A.; Poulson, M.R.; Mak, K.S.; Tapan, U.; Dechert, T.A.; Litle, V.R.; Suzuki, K. The Impact of Residential Racial Segregation on Non-Small Cell Lung Cancer Treatment and Outcomes. *Ann. Thorac. Surg.* **2022**, *113*, 1291–1298. [CrossRef]
57. Lutfi, W.; Martinez-Meehan, D.; Sultan, I.; Evans, N.; Dhupar, R.; Luketich, J.D.; Christie, N.A.; Okusanya, O.T. Racial Disparities in Local Therapy for Early Stage Non-Small-Cell Lung Cancer. *J. Surg. Oncol.* **2020**, *122*, 1815–1820. [CrossRef] [PubMed]
58. Bonner, S.N.; He, C.; Clark, M.; Adams, K.; Orelaru, F.; Popoff, A.; Chang, A.; Wakeam, E.; Lagisetty, K. Understanding Racial Differences in Lung Cancer Surgery Through a Statewide Quality Collaborative. *Ann. Surg. Oncol.* **2023**, *30*, 517–526. [CrossRef] [PubMed]
59. Taioli, E.; Liu, B.; Nicastri, D.G.; Lieberman-Cribbin, W.; Leoncini, E.; Flores, R.M. Personal and Hospital Factors Associated with Limited Surgical Resection for Lung Cancer, in-Hospital Mortality and Complications in New York State. *J. Surg. Oncol.* **2017**, *116*, 471–481. [CrossRef]
60. Taioli, E.; Flores, R. Appropriateness of Surgical Approach in Black Patients with Lung Cancer-15 Years Later, Little Has Changed. *J. Thorac. Oncol.* **2017**, *12*, 573–577. [CrossRef]
61. Ezer, N.; Mhango, G.; Bagiella, E.; Goodman, E.; Flores, R.; Wisnivesky, J.P. Racial Disparities in Resection of Early Stage Non-Small Cell Lung Cancer: Variability Among Surgeons. *Med. Care* **2020**, *58*, 392–398. [CrossRef]
62. Halloran, S.J.; Alvarado, C.E.; Sarode, A.L.; Jiang, B.; Sinopoli, J.; Linden, P.A.; Towe, C.W. Disparities in Access to Thoracic Surgeons among Patients Receiving Lung Lobectomy in the United States. *Curr. Oncol.* **2023**, *30*, 2801–2811. [CrossRef]
63. Watkins, A.A.; Parsons, N.; Shehata, D.G.; Vigna, C.; Lagisetty, K.; Bonner, S.; Lopez, E.; Wilder, F.G.; Stock, C.T.; Moffatt-Bruce, S.; et al. Race, Ethnicity, and Payor Status Impact the Surgical Approach and Postoperative Outcomes of Lung Cancer Amongst Patients within The Society of Thoracic Surgeons General Thoracic Surgery Database. *Ann. Surg.* **2025**. [CrossRef]
64. Jones, C.C.; Mercaldo, S.F.; Blume, J.D.; Wenzlaff, A.S.; Schwartz, A.G.; Chen, H.; Deppen, S.A.; Bush, W.S.; Crawford, D.C.; Chanock, S.J.; et al. Racial Disparities in Lung Cancer Survival: The Contribution of Stage, Treatment, and Ancestry. *J. Thorac. Oncol.* **2018**, *13*, 1464–1473. [CrossRef] [PubMed]
65. Weksler, B.; Kosinski, A.S.; Burfeind, W.R.; Silvestry, S.C.; Sullivan, J.; D'Amico, T.A. Racial and Ethnic Differences in Lung Cancer Surgical Stage: An STS Database Study. *Thorac. Cardiovasc. Surg.* **2015**, *63*, 538–543. [CrossRef]
66. Shi, H.; Seegobin, K.; Heng, F.; Zhou, K.; Chen, R.; Qin, H.; Manochakian, R.; Zhao, Y.; Lou, Y. Genomic Landscape of Lung Adenocarcinomas in Different Races. *Front. Oncol.* **2022**, *12*, 946625. [CrossRef] [PubMed]
67. Monestime, S.; Rigney, M.; Phipps, N.; Carlson, C.; Alongi, T.; Redding, M.; King, J.C. Health Inequities across the Lung Cancer Care Continuum in Ten Marginalized Populations: A Narrative Review. *J. Thorac. Dis.* **2023**, *15*, 6345–6361. [CrossRef] [PubMed]
68. Bhakta, N.R.; Bime, C.; Kaminsky, D.A.; McCormack, M.C.; Thakur, N.; Stanojevic, S.; Baugh, A.D.; Braun, L.; Lovinsky-Desir, S.; Adamson, R.; et al. Race and Ethnicity in Pulmonary Function Test Interpretation: An Official American Thoracic Society Statement. *Am. J. Respir. Crit. Care Med.* **2023**, *207*, 978–995. [CrossRef]
69. Richmond, J.; Fernandez, J.R.; Bonnet, K.; Sellers, A.; Schlundt, D.G.; Forde, A.T.; Wilkins, C.H.; Aldrich, M.C. Patient lung cancer screening decisions and environmental and psychosocial factors. *JAMA Netw. Open* **2024**, *7*, e2412880. [CrossRef]

70. Hand, T.; Rosseau, N.A.; Stiles, C.E.; Sheih, T.; Ghandakly, E.; Oluwasanu, M.; Olopade, O.I. The Global Role, Impact, and Limitations of Community Health Workers (CHWs) in Breast Cancer Screening: A Scoping Review and Recommendations to Promote Health Equity for All. *Glob. Health Action* **2021**, *14*, 1883336. [CrossRef]
71. Social Determinants of Health Framework and Resource Guide. Available online: https://www.ontariohealth.ca/system-planning/social-determinants-of-health-framework-and-resource-guide (accessed on 21 February 2025).
72. Elder, J.P.; Haughton, J.; Perez, L.G.; Martínez, M.E.; De la Torre, C.L.; Slymen, D.J.; Arredondo, E.M. Promoting Cancer Screening among Churchgoing Latinas: Fe En Acción/Faith in Action. *Health Educ. Res.* **2017**, *32*, 163–173. [CrossRef]
73. Niranjan, S.J.; Opoku-Agyeman, W.; Hardy, C.M.; Bowman, T.; Vedre-Kyanam, A.; Hearld, K.R.; Dransfield, M.T.; Baskin, M.L. Using Community Health Advisors to Increase Lung Cancer Screening Awareness in the Black Belt: A Pilot Study. *J. Cancer Educ.* **2023**, *38*, 1286–1295. [CrossRef]
74. Social Determinants of Health. Available online: https://odphp.health.gov/healthypeople/priority-areas/social-determinants-health (accessed on 21 February 2025).
75. Manning, M.; Yongue, C.; Garikipati, A.; Cykert, S.; Eng, E.; Schaal, J.; Lightfoot, A.; Jones, N.; Robertson, L. Overall Survival From a Prospective Multi-Institutional Trial to Resolve Black-White Disparities in the Treatment of Early Stage Breast and Lung Cancer. *Int. J. Radiat. Oncol. Biol. Phys.* **2021**, *111*, S28. [CrossRef]
76. Potter, A.L.; Xu, N.N.; Senthil, P.; Srinivasan, D.; Lee, H.; Gazelle, G.S.; Chelala, L.; Zheng, W.; Fintelmann, F.J.; Sequist, L.V.; et al. Pack-Year Smoking History: An Inadequate and Biased Measure to Determine Lung Cancer Screening Eligibility. *J. Clin. Oncol.* **2024**, *42*, 2026–2037. [CrossRef] [PubMed]
77. Wang, G.X.; Baggett, T.P.; Pandharipande, P.V.; Park, E.R.; Percac-Lima, S.; Shepard, J.-A.O.; Fintelmann, F.J.; Flores, E.J. Barriers to Lung Cancer Screening Engagement from the Patient and Provider Perspective. *Radiology* **2019**, *290*, 278–287. [CrossRef]
78. Jun, J.; Nan, X. Determinants of Cancer Screening Disparities Among Asian Americans: A Systematic Review of Public Health Surveys. *J. Cancer Educ.* **2018**, *33*, 757–768. [CrossRef]
79. Liss, D.T.; Baker, D.W. Understanding Current Racial/Ethnic Disparities in Colorectal Cancer Screening in the United States: The Contribution of Socioeconomic Status and Access to Care. *Am. J. Prev. Med.* **2014**, *46*, 228–236. [CrossRef] [PubMed]
80. White, P.M.; Itzkowitz, S.H. Barriers Driving Racial Disparities in Colorectal Cancer Screening in African Americans. *Curr. Gastroenterol. Rep.* **2020**, *22*, 41. [CrossRef] [PubMed]
81. Abraído-Lanza, A.F.; Viladrich, A.; Flórez, K.R.; Céspedes, A.; Aguirre, A.N.; De La Cruz, A.A. Commentary: Fatalismo Reconsidered: A Cautionary Note for Health-Related Research and Practice with Latino Populations. *Ethn. Dis.* **2007**, *17*, 153–158.
82. Griggs, J.; Maingi, S.; Blinder, V.; Denduluri, N.; Khorana, A.A.; Norton, L.; Francisco, M.; Wollins, D.S.; Rowland, J.H. American Society of Clinical Oncology Position Statement: Strategies for Reducing Cancer Health Disparities Among Sexual and Gender Minority Populations. *J. Clin. Oncol.* **2017**, *35*, 2203–2208. [CrossRef]
83. Delmerico, J.; Hyland, A.; Celestino, P.; Reid, M.; Cummings, K.M. Patient Willingness and Barriers to Receiving a CT Scan for Lung Cancer Screening. *Lung Cancer* **2014**, *84*, 307–309. [CrossRef]
84. Ali, N.; Lifford, K.J.; Carter, B.; McRonald, F.; Yadegarfar, G.; Baldwin, D.R.; Weller, D.; Hansell, D.M.; Duffy, S.W.; Field, J.K.; et al. Barriers to Uptake among High-Risk Individuals Declining Participation in Lung Cancer Screening: A Mixed Methods Analysis of the UK Lung Cancer Screening (UKLS) Trial. *BMJ Open* **2015**, *5*, e008254. [CrossRef]
85. Quaife, S.L.; Marlow, L.A.V.; McEwen, A.; Janes, S.M.; Wardle, J. Attitudes towards Lung Cancer Screening in Socioeconomically Deprived and Heavy Smoking Communities: Informing Screening Communication. *Health Expect.* **2017**, *20*, 563–573. [CrossRef]
86. Whorms, D.S.; Narayan, A.K.; Pourvaziri, A.; Miles, R.C.; Glover, M.; Herrington, J.; Saini, S.; Brink, J.A.; Flores, E.J. Analysis of the Effects of a Patient-Centered Rideshare Program on Missed Appointments and Timeliness for MRI Appointments at an Academic Medical Center. *J. Am. Coll. Radiol.* **2021**, *18*, 240–247. [CrossRef] [PubMed]
87. Wang, G.X.; Pizzi, B.T.; Miles, R.C.; Dontchos, B.N.; LaPointe, A.P.; Lehman, C.D.; Narayan, A.K. Implementation and Utilization of a "Pink Card" Walk-In Screening Mammography Program Integrated With Physician Visits. *J. Am. Coll. Radiol.* **2020**, *17*, 1602–1608. [CrossRef] [PubMed]
88. Lee, C. Screening for Lung Cancer: Effective Recruitment Methods. *AJR Am. J. Roentgenol.* **2018**, *210*, 514–517. [CrossRef] [PubMed]
89. Percac-Lima, S.; Ashburner, J.M.; Rigotti, N.A.; Park, E.R.; Chang, Y.; Kuchukhidze, S.; Atlas, S.J. Patient Navigation for Lung Cancer Screening among Current Smokers in Community Health Centers a Randomized Controlled Trial. *Cancer Med.* **2018**, *7*, 894–902. [CrossRef]
90. Eberth, J.M.; Thibault, A.; Caldwell, R.; Josey, M.J.; Qiang, B.; Pena, E.; LaFrance, D.; Berger, F.G. A Statewide Program Providing Colorectal Cancer Screening to the Uninsured of South Carolina. *Cancer* **2018**, *124*, 1912–1920. [CrossRef]
91. Peregrin, T. Reinventing the Wheel: Mobile Cancer Screening Saves Lives, Provides Equitable Preventative Care. Available online: https://www.facs.org/for-medical-professionals/news-publications/news-and-articles/bulletin/2022/september-2022-volume-107-issue-9/reinventing-the-wheel-mobile-cancer-screening-saves-lives-provides-equitable-preventative-care/ (accessed on 2 January 2025).

92. Brandt, D. Proposed Law Seeks to Bring Mobile Lung Cancer Screenings Closer to Communities. Available online: https://www.sts.org/blog/proposed-law-seeks-bring-mobile-lung-cancer-screenings-closer-communities (accessed on 2 January 2025).
93. Gopal, D.P.; Chetty, U.; O'Donnell, P.; Gajria, C.; Blackadder-Weinstein, J. Implicit Bias in Healthcare: Clinical Practice, Research and Decision Making. *Future Healthc. J.* **2021**, *8*, 40–48. [CrossRef]
94. Cooper, L.A.; Saha, S.; van Ryn, M. Mandated Implicit Bias Training for Health Professionals-A Step Toward Equity in Health Care. *JAMA Health Forum* **2022**, *3*, e223250. [CrossRef]

cancers MDPI

Review

The Surgical Renaissance: Advancements in Video-Assisted Thoracoscopic Surgery and Robotic-Assisted Thoracic Surgery and Their Impact on Patient Outcomes

Jennifer M. Pan [1], Ammara A. Watkins [2], Cameron T. Stock [2], Susan D. Moffatt-Bruce [2] and Elliot L. Servais [2,*]

[1] Division of General Surgery, Beth Israel Deaconess Medical Center, Boston, MA 02215, USA
[2] Division of Cardiothoracic Surgery, Lahey Hospital and Medical Center, Burlington, MA 01805, USA
* Correspondence: elliot.servais@lahey.org

Simple Summary: Lung cancer treatment often involves surgical resection. Traditional resection involves a large thoracotomy incision to access the chest cavity. However, thoracotomy has become less common since the introduction of minimally invasive surgery (MIS). Minimally invasive surgery includes video-assisted thoracoscopic surgery (VATS) and robotic-assisted thoracic surgery (RATS) and involves small incisions to accomplish the same operation. MIS techniques have improved patient outcomes compared to thoracotomy. Patients recover faster in the hospital, have fewer complications and less pain, and return to baseline function faster. These techniques have now become the standard of care for lung cancer resection.

Abstract: Minimally invasive thoracic surgery has advanced the treatment of lung cancer since its introduction in the 1990s. Video-assisted thoracoscopic surgery (VATS) and robotic-assisted thoracic surgery (RATS) offer the advantage of smaller incisions without compromising patient outcomes. These techniques have been shown to be safe and effective in standard pulmonary resections (lobectomy and sub-lobar resection) and in complex pulmonary resections (sleeve resection and pneumonectomy). Furthermore, several studies show these techniques enhance patient outcomes from early recovery to improved quality of life (QoL) and excellent oncologic results. The rise of RATS has yielded further operative benefits compared to thoracoscopic surgery. The wristed instruments, neutralization of tremor, dexterity, and magnification allow for more precise and delicate dissection of tissues and vessels. This review summarizes of the advancements in minimally invasive thoracic surgery and the positive impact on patient outcomes.

Keywords: VATS; lung cancer; RATS; minimally invasive surgery; thoracic outcomes

1. Introduction of Minimally Invasive Lung Resection

Surgery remains a cornerstone therapy in lung cancer. Pulmonary resection is the mainstay treatment for early-stage lung cancer [1]. As the pharmacologic treatment of lung cancer improves, surgery in locally advanced-stage lung cancer has become more feasible [2–4]. With this, there have been dramatic advancements in operative techniques and modalities for lung resection. As minimally invasive surgery (MIS) has grown in popularity in other fields, it has also been eagerly adopted by thoracic surgeons. MIS was first introduced in the 1990s. The first video-assisted thoracoscopic surgery (VATS) cases were described in the literature over thirty years ago [5]. Since then, multiple studies have examined and established the feasibility, safety, and advantages of VATS. In the early 2000s, robotic-assisted thoracoscopic surgery (RATS) was introduced. The first case series demonstrated the flexibility of the robotic platform to perform lobectomies, tumor resections, enucleations, and even bulla stitching [6].

The field of thoracic surgery has transformed since the introduction of minimally invasive surgery. Open thoracotomy was previously regarded as the gold standard in lung cancer treatment [7]. Over the past few decades, VATS and robotic thoracic surgery have consistently demonstrated improved patient outcomes, from fewer postoperative complications to shorter hospital stays and appropriate oncologic safety [8]. The improvements in patient outcomes have resulted in a change in the standard of care. The adoption of minimally invasive surgery has increased tremendously over the past decade [9,10]. Minimally invasive resections have become the standard of care in lung cancer treatment [8]. In fact, according to a 2023 review of the Society of Thoracic Surgeons General Thoracic Surgery Database (STS-GTSD), over 80% of lobectomies, segmentectomies, and wedge resections were performed via a minimally invasive approach (Figure 1) [9].

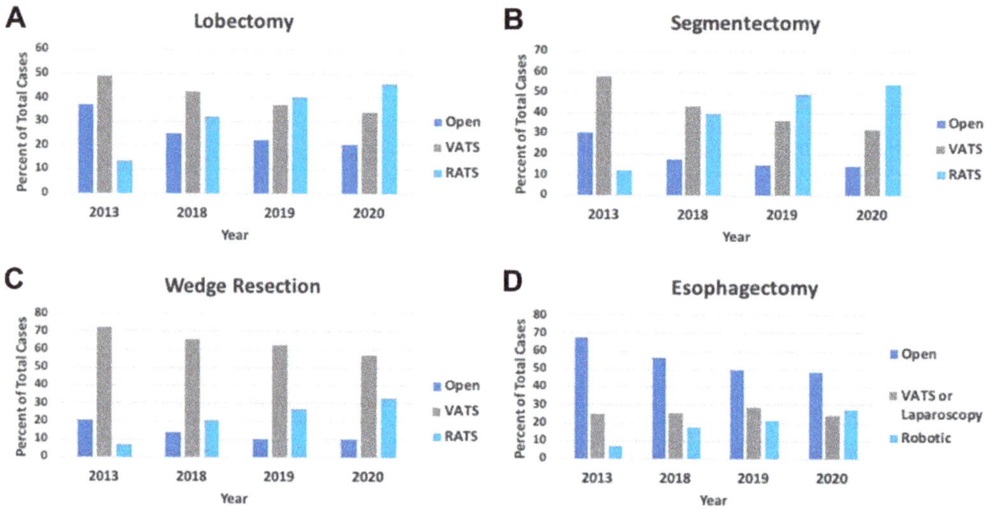

Figure 1. Distribution of cases and modalities over time. Modalities were thoracotomy (dark blue bars), VATS (grey bars), and RATS (blue bars). ([2022] Servais et al. Reproduced with permission from the authors [9]).

The objective of this review is to summarize the advancements in minimally invasive techniques for lung cancer and the impact on patient outcomes.

2. Video-Assisted Thoracoscopic Surgery for Lung Cancer

Since the introduction of VATS, numerous studies have demonstrated either equivalent or improved outcomes compared to thoracotomy. VATS has been shown to be noninferior or better for patients in several realms, particularly in early-stage lung cancer. The CALGB309802 study was one of the first prospective studies to examine the outcomes of patients who underwent a VATS approach. They established that VATS lobectomy outcomes were comparable to those after a thoracotomy [11]. Multiple studies have found no significant difference in operative time [12–15]. The majority of comparative studies of open and VATS lobectomy for early-stage lung cancer reported significantly lower intraoperative blood loss during VATS [16]. Yan et al. also reviewed median chest tube duration by approach. While chest tube duration was lower after VATS lobectomy, they were unable to draw statistical significance [16]. In another meta-analysis, Whitson et al. concluded that chest drain duration was significantly shorter after VATS than thoracotomy. In other postoperative outcomes, VATS has been established to be as safe as open thoracotomy [12]. The VIOLET trial, a recent randomized controlled trial (RCT), investigated postoperative outcomes in patients who underwent VATS or open lobectomies. There was no difference in serious adverse events between the two groups. While the VATS group had a higher rate of prolonged air leaks and bleeding, they had a shorter hospital course, a lower readmission rate, and less overall pain [15]. In another RCT, Long et al. randomized patients with early NSCLC to undergo lobectomy via VATS or thoracotomy (Clinicaltrials.gov NCT01102517). The operative time was significantly shorter, and blood loss was significantly lower after VATS. There was no difference in postoperative complications [17]. Multiple observational studies have found either an equivalent or lower rate of prolonged air leaks and other postoperative complications after VATS surgery [12,14,16,18–20]. Patients who underwent VATS lobectomy in the VIOLET trial had a shorter length of hospital stay, which is consistent with prior existing studies and meta-analyses [12–15,18,21,22].

VATS lobectomy for lung cancer has demonstrated equivalent or improved oncologic and survival outcomes compared to open lobectomy [13,14,16,18,20,21,23]. The recurrence rates of VATS are comparable to those of open thoracotomy [15,24]. In a meta-analysis, locoregional recurrence was similar between the two, but systemic recurrence was significantly lower for VATS [16]. The disease-free and overall survival rate between VATS and open is comparable [11,12,15,18,24]. The quality of lymph node dissection via VATS has been a much-debated topic. In a landmark trial, Z0030, no statistical differences were seen in the completeness of lymphadenectomy between VATS and thoracotomy approaches [25]. In fact, several studies have shown that an appropriate lymphadenectomy can be performed via a VATS approach for both total lymph node harvest and lymph node station sampling [14,15,18,19,24]. VATS is associated with a lower rate of upstaging by pathologic stage [26,27]. Patients who undergo VATS have been found to undergo more of their planned chemotherapy regimen with less of a need for reduced doses [28]. While there is a lower rate of upstaging, VATS has actually demonstrated either equivalent or improved survival compared to thoracotomy [26,27,29].

With modern advances in neoadjuvant treatment, more locally advanced and even late-stage lung cancer patients are now able to undergo oncologic lung resection. While there are no randomized control trials comparing VATS to open in these patients, several studies have shown similar outcomes between VATS and thoracotomy following induction therapy. In a retrospective review of patients who underwent neoadjuvant chemotherapy, VATS patients were sicker at baseline, with higher clinical stage, age, coronary disease, and chronic pulmonary disease. Despite having more comorbidities, VATS had improved 3-year survival compared to open [30]. Disease-free survival and recurrence rates were not significantly different [30–32]. In a review of the National Cancer Database (NCDB) of later-stage NSCLC patients, VATS and open had comparable resection outcomes, lymphadenectomy, and complication rates and similar overall survival. Patients after VATS had a shorter chest tube duration and length of stay [31]. Patients who underwent induction therapy did have a higher rate of conversion to open, with reasons being fibrotic tissue or nodes, adhesions, bleeding, or extensive involvement of the vasculature [4,33].

The advantages of VATS led to a shift in the 2000s, with increased use of VATS for lung cancer treatment. It became the new standard of care, particularly for early-stage NSCLC, with clear evidence showing similar or improved patient outcomes, from perioperative recovery to oncologic outcomes [34,35].

3. Robotic-Assisted Thoracic Surgery for Lung Cancer

Since the introduction of robotic surgery, RATS has become the most common approach for anatomic lung resections [9]. There are many advantages to the robotic platform compared to open and VATS. Minimally invasive approaches allow for dexterity and magnification. Compared to VATS, the robotic platform enhances maneuverability with wristed instruments, eliminates physiologic tremor, and provides three-dimensional visualization of the field. The robotic platform also routinely utilizes insufflation, which also improves visualization [36].

3.1. Robotic and Open Thoracotomy Outcomes

Robotic-assisted lung resection confers improved outcomes compared to thoracotomy [37–41]. In a large database study of the State Inpatient Database, Kent et al. compared the outcomes of thoracotomy compared to minimally invasive techniques. Patients who underwent robotic-assisted resection had significantly lower mortality, length of stay, and overall complication rates compared to thoracotomy [42]. In an analysis of the Premier Healthcare Database, the robotic approach was associated with longer operative times (275.5 vs. 235.3 min, $p < 0.0001$) but significantly fewer postoperative complications, shorter hospital stay, and higher rates of discharge home. Patients after RATS had less postoperative bleeding and fewer respiratory complications, including pneumonia and the need for mechanical ventilation [43]. These trends were also demonstrated by Nguyen et al., who compared open and robotic cases between 2013 and 2015 [44]. A meta-analysis of minimally invasive and open lobectomies found the same benefits of robotic-assisted surgery. Robotic-assisted lobectomy had a significant reduction in blood loss, chest tube duration, 30-day mortality, and overall complication rates, particularly pulmonary complications [45].

The improved outcomes are consistent in even later-stage disease. Zirafa et al. compared the post-surgical outcomes of locally advanced NSCLC. The operative time for robotic-assisted surgery was longer than open thoracotomy. Notably, the robot operative time did decrease over time and with the introduction of the da Vinci Xi system (Intuitive Surgical, Sunnyvale, CA, USA). Reasons may be due to improved surgeon and staff experience. The length of hospital stay and postoperative complication rates were lower in the robotic-assisted group [46]. In another analysis of patients with clinical T4 disease within the National Cancer Database, patients who underwent MIS resection had a shorter hospital stay. There were no differences in short-term mortality or overall survival [47].

Compared to open lobectomy, RATS lobectomy shows improvement in postoperative outcomes. Robotic resection is effective even for later-stage lung cancers, with similar outcomes to open approaches.

3.2. RATS and VATS Outcomes

RATS has similar or improved outcomes to VATS surgery [43,48–50]. Agzarian et al. performed a systematic review of the two approaches. While the operative time for VATS was shorter than for RATS, there were no differences in perioperative outcomes, such as blood loss, prolonged air leak, chest tube duration, and length of stay [51]. In a more recent multi-center analysis of lobectomy cases, the operative time of a RATS lobectomy was significantly shorter than for VATS or open lobectomy. Additionally, patients who underwent a robotic-assisted surgery had lower transfusion rates and shorter hospital stays compared to those who underwent VATS [41]. The shorter robotic operative time was attributed to increased familiarity and experience with robotic-assisted surgery by the operative staff.

Louie et al. found that patients who underwent robotic-assisted lobectomies had more comorbidities than those who underwent VATS. Patients who underwent robotic-assisted lung resection were more likely to be older and have a lower performance status, cardiac disease, and higher body mass index (BMI) [52]. Despite these differences, surgical outcomes were comparable, suggesting that robotic-assisted lobectomy may be preferable in older patients with comorbidities. A randomized controlled trial comparing RATS and VATS (ROMAN) found no difference in the duration of surgery, perioperative complications, or postoperative stay. The robotic approach yielded a more comprehensive sampling of lymph nodes [53]. In a more recent meta-analysis comparing minimally invasive pulmonary resections, perioperative morbidity was similar, but 30-day mortality was significantly lower after a robotic lobectomy or segmentectomy. They also identified a significantly lower conversion to open rate with the robotic approach [54]. Servais et al. analyzed the STS-GTSD for rates of conversion to thoracotomy (Table 1). RATS had a significantly lower rate of conversion compared to VATS (6.0% vs. 11.0%, $p < 0.001$). While conversion to open from RATS occurred more emergently and for vascular reasons, there was no difference in mortality [55]. Robotic-assisted lobectomy yields comparable, if not improved, intraoperative and postoperative outcomes compared to VATS.

Table 1. Outcomes of centers with low, medium, and high volumes of VATS or RATS lobectomy. ([2022] Servais et al. Reproduced with permission from authors [55]).

	Participant Center Volume Tertile			
	Low	Medium	High	*p*
VATS	n = 2092	n = 6569	n = 19,034	
Mortality, %	1.15	0.84	0.86	0.38
Major complication, %	7.90	7.19	6.25	0.002
Conversion to open, %	27.33	10.56	7.23	<0.001
RATS	n = 5683	n = 5599	n = 9107	
Mortality, %	0.83	0.80	0.96	0.56
Major complication, %	7.40	7.13	6.42	<0.001
Conversion to open, %	9.72	9.48	7.02	<0.001

RATS, robotic-assisted thoracoscopic surgery; VATS, video-assisted thoracoscopic surgery.

4. Oncologic Outcomes

The quality of lymph node sampling and dissection has been shown to impact survival in patients with NSCLC [25,56,57]. The extent of lymph node sampling is an important operative quality metric. Oncologic impact after surgery is a vital measure of patient outcomes. The quality of minimally invasive lymph node evaluation has been reviewed extensively. Robot-assisted dissection results in improved nodal harvest compared to thoracotomy [38,58–60]. Wilson et al. conducted a multi-institutional review of early-stage NSCLC patients who underwent resection. The rate of overall robotic nodal upstaging was 10.9%. When separated by T stage, the rate of upstaging was comparable to that of thoracotomy and superior to VATS [58]. Higher rates of nodal harvest were also seen in a retrospective analysis of open, VATS, and RATS cases. Robotic nodal dissection yielded more overall nodes and more hilar lymph nodes compared to open and VATS [59]. A large retrospective review of stage I NSCLC found that more lymph node stations were dissected with the robotic approach than the open approach or VATS. While upstaging rates were not examined, the robotic group had a higher proportion of pathological N1 nodes [60]. The ROMAN RCT of early NSCLC found that the robotic approach was superior in dissection of both hilar and mediastinal lymph nodes compared to VATS in early-stage disease [53]. The improved lymph node outcomes with the robotic approach may be a result of improved visualization of the field and articulation of the instruments to allow for specific and delicate dissection.

Robotic-assisted surgery for lung cancer has equivalent overall survival and disease-free outcomes to open and VATS approaches [60–63]. Park et al. reported in a multi-center study of robotic lobectomies for stage I-III NSCLC an overall 1-year and 5-year survival rate of 98% and 80%, respectively, with comparable stage-specific survival to prior VATS data [64]. When comparing survival and recurrence outcomes for open, VATS, and RATS lobectomies for stage I-IIIa, there were no statistically significant differences between the three approaches [65]. These results were also demonstrated in a meta-analysis comparing the three modalities [45]. In patients with cT4 NSCLC, survival up to 84 months was similar between MIS and open resection. At five years, the survival rate after MIS was 53.4%, and after open, it was 51.2%, but this was not statistically significant [47]. Zirafa et al. compared outcomes after open and robotic resection for locally advanced lung cancer. They found that the overall 5-year survival was 34.3% and 31.0% for the robotic and open group, respectively. Progression of disease was found in 65.6% of patients and 68.6% of patients treated with robotic and open surgery, respectively. These differences were not statistically significant [46]. Between the MIS techniques, a recent meta-analysis identified similar overall survival; however, patients treated with robotic resection had a longer disease-free survival [66].

5. Quality of Life

Thoracotomy incisions are painful, and they can impede patient recovery. Patients who undergo a minimally invasive approach consistently have short hospital stays and more discharges to home [67]. The use of a rib spreader during VATS surgery leads to more pain medication use with slower recovery [68]. Early analysis of VATS and thoracotomy outcomes demonstrated that patients who underwent VATS had more independence at time of hospital discharge, less pain, faster return to work, and higher rates of initiating adjuvant chemotherapy [67]. The VIOLET trial found that patients who were randomized to VATS had improved physical function at five weeks compared to open thoracotomy. The thoracotomy group took an average of six months to achieve the same level of physical fitness that the VATS group achieved at five weeks after resection. Patients who underwent VATS also had less overall pain by postoperative day two. VATS patients continued to report lower pain scores up to a year after their operation [15]. In a randomized controlled trial, patients undergoing lobectomy for stage I NSCLC were randomly assigned to VATS or anterolateral thoracotomy (Clinicaltrials.gov NCT01278888). Patients who underwent VATS had significantly lower pain scores within 24 h of surgery. The difference in pain levels was sustained throughout the year after surgery. Quality of life (QoL) and emotional function were significantly improved in patients who were treated with VATS [22].

Cerfolio et al. analyzed his initial cohort of robotic resections and found significantly improved mental and physical QoL scores and lower pain scores at 3-week follow-up compared to thoracotomy [69]. Quality of life questionnaires were given to patients undergoing robotic, VATS, and open pulmonary resection. Patients treated with RATS resection had the highest measures of functional QoL and the fewest number of symptoms [70]. Lacroix et al. analyzed patients who underwent robotic or open lobectomy. The patients who underwent robotic lobectomy were given a weaker postoperative pain control protocol. They found no difference in pain between the two cohorts. At one month, patients who underwent RATS lobectomy had less pain and improved pulmonary function tests compared to the open group [71]. In a review of the SEER database of opioid use, open resection had increased persistent opioid use after surgery compared to RATS and VATS. Interestingly, this was only observed in opioid-naive patients. There was no difference in persistent opioid use in chronic-opioid-use patients [72]. Kwon et al. reviewed pain scores in 498 patients who underwent pulmonary resection. There was a significant improvement in acute pain in patients who underwent minimally invasive surgery compared to open surgery. VATS and RATS lung resections resulted in less pain, faster recovery, and improved QoL [73].

6. Cost

The cost of robotic surgery has been a concern, especially considering the upfront costs and system maintenance of a robotic system [74–76]. In 2006, Park et al. cited an initial purchase cost of USD 1 million with an annual maintenance cost of USD 100,000 and a technical cost of USD 730 on average per case [74]. In a cost comparison of open, VATS, and robotic surgery for lung cancer, the costs of open compared to robotic cases were not statistically significant. However, robotic cases on average were USD 3182 more than VATS ($p < 0.001$). A reduction of robotic operating time by 68 min or a reduction of a hospital stay by 1.86 days would eliminate the statistically significant difference in cost between VATS and RATS cases [77].

The cost trends of robotic-assisted lung resection have changed over time as more centers now own robotic systems and are performing robotic-assisted cases. In a review of the Premier database from 2009 to 2011, average robotic-assisted operation costs were significantly more expensive than VATS without any significant differences in length of stay or adverse events [78]. However, in a review of the Premier Healthcare Database from 2008 to 2015, the costs were more comparable. The authors divided the review period into an early (2008–2012) and late period (2013–2015). Hospitals with an annual case volume of >25 lobectomies during the late period had comparable costs among RATS, VATS, and open lobectomies. Additionally, during the late period, robotic-assisted lobectomies had significantly improved outcomes and shorter length of stay [44]. With the increase in robotic cases and training programs, familiarity and experience in performing robotic-assisted lung resections have improved. Kneuertz et al. reviewed their cost data from 2012 to 2017. Robotic operative times were significantly shorter than VATS and equivalent to open times. Overall costs for VATS and robotic-assisted surgery were comparable. The initial operative costs of open surgery were significantly lower than those of RATS, but those costs were recuperated in the postoperative period [79]. Alwatari et al. reviewed the National Inpatient Database of lung resections and found that, overall, robotic resections had increased hospital costs. However, there was no analysis based on hospital volume of robotic cases [50]. In an analysis of the Nationwide Readmissions Database, Verma et al. stratified cost and outcomes by hospital volume. They found that high-volume hospitals had lower overall costs when performing robotic lobectomy [80]. This may reflect the impact of more experienced teams with streamlined operating systems. A recent RCT (RAVAL) comparing RATS to VATS lobectomies found that the incremental cost-effectiveness ratio (ICER) for robotic surgery was within the favorable limits despite increased costs compared to VATS. Given this, the authors concluded that robotic-assisted lobectomy was cost-effective compared to VATS [81].

A major contributor to the cost of robotic-assisted surgery is the operative time and maintenance. While the operative time does not always reflect the quality of the operation or post-surgical outcomes, it is a metric that impacts the total case number, patients treated, and hospital cost. As the volume and RATS experience of centers increase, operative time decreases, enabling the treatment of more patients. Lastly, newer robotic-system-acquisition models, such as leasing or "pay-per-use" contracts, have significantly changed the cost algorithms.

7. Segmentectomy and Complex Pulmonary Resections

The standard of care for early NSCLC has historically been lobectomy [7]. Recently, two RCTs have compared sublobar resection to lobectomy for early NSCLC. In JCOG0802, 1106 patients were randomized to undergo a lobectomy or segmentectomy for Stage IA disease. Both the five-year overall survival and relapse-free survival of the segmentectomy group were noninferior to the lobectomy group. Despite similar survival rates, recurrence rates in the segmentectomy group were higher. The segmentectomy group had significantly improved FEV1 at the 1-year follow-up, despite not reaching the minimum threshold for clinical significance [82]. CALGB 140503 randomized 697 patients with Stage IA NSCLC to undergo either a lobectomy or sublobar resection. Sublobar resection, including wedge resection and segmentectomy, was noninferior to lobectomy for overall survival and disease-free survival [83].

With the acceptance of segmentectomy for lung cancer and the adoption of minimally invasive surgery, the outcomes for minimally invasive segmentectomy have significantly improved [84]. Thoracoscopic segmentectomy has similar nodal evaluation, postoperative complication rates, recurrence rates, and survival to thoracoscopic lobectomy [85–88]. Compared to open segmentectomy, the VATS approach has shown equivalent lymphadenectomy, decreased pulmonary complications, and improved disease-free and overall survival [89]. Robotic segmentectomy has been shown to be a safe operation with appropriate oncologic resection and survival [87,88,90–93]. In a review of early-stage NSCLC patients from the NCDB, patients who underwent minimally invasive segmentectomy had a shorter length of stay and similar nodal upstaging and long-term survival when compared to open segmentectomy [94]. Watkins et al. performed an analysis of the STS-GSTD from 2013 to 2021 of elective segmentectomies for NSCLC. Segmentectomy volume significantly impacted the choice of surgical approach (RATS, VATS, or open). High-volume centers (>16 cases per year) utilized RATS significantly more than medium- (4–16 cases per year) or low-volume (<4 cases per year) centers. RATS had greater nodal sampling, but N1 upstaging was more common in the open group. RATS had a significantly lower rate of conversion to open compared to VATS. MIS approaches had fewer postoperative complications and a significantly shower hospital stay compared to open [95].

Minimally invasive techniques have been established to be safe in complex pulmonary resections for lung cancer [96–100]. The improvements in patient outcomes after minimally invasive surgery are also seen in complex pulmonary resections. A review of the NCDB found that patients who underwent pneumonectomies via MIS had similar complication rates, perioperative mortality rates, and improved lymphadenectomy when compared to the open group [101]. In a comparison of open and MIS sleeve lobectomies, patients in the robotic group had a shorter operative time, similar complication rates, and improved survival rates compared to the open group. There was no difference in disease-free survival among the three techniques [102]. The patient outcome advantages of the VATS and RATS approaches are seen across simple lobectomies and segmentectomies to more complex pulmonary resections.

8. Advancements in VATS and RATS

Since the introduction of VATS over thirty years ago, the idea of uniportal VATS (U-VATS) has surfaced. Rather than the traditional three- or four-port technique, uniportal surgery consists of a single incision, typically 4 cm or less [103]. The theoretical benefit of the uniport is the parallel instrumentation with the camera [104]. In a retrospective analysis of uniportal and multiportal VATS in North America, U-VATS was found to have a significantly shorter operative time, less blood loss, shorter chest tube duration, and a shorter length of stay. The rates of conversion to thoracotomy were not statistically different. Furthermore, there was no difference in the number of stations dissected, nodal upstaging, or margin positivity. The postoperative complications were also comparable [105]. Similar findings of shorter chest tube drainage and hospital stay were also seen in a systematic review comparing U-VATS and multiportal VATS [106]. Uniportal robotic-assisted lung resection is also feasible and safe, but it has been less studied [107–109]. In a smaller multi-center study, Manolache et al. compared uniportal RATS to multiport RATS. They found that uniportal RATS was used to perform significantly more segmentectomies. There was no conversion to open in the uniportal group. The operative time and length of stay were lower for uniportal RATS. There was no difference in 30-day mortality [108]. We anticipate significant growth in robotic uniportal thoracic surgery in the near future with the impending FDA approval of the robotic single-port system (SP, Intuitive Surgical, Sunnyvale, CA, USA).

One of the disadvantages of VATS is the lack of 3D visualization of the tissue. There is a loss of depth, thus making it harder to distinguish the proper planes. 3D technology has been introduced for VATS. Operating staff wear 3D glasses and use a specific 3D camera for VATS. Bagan et al. compared this technology with traditional 2D VATS. They found that blood loss, morbidity, duration of chest tube, and lymph node dissection were comparable. The operating time was significantly reduced in the 3D VATS cohort [110]. While 3D VATS has been shown to be feasible, there remain limited data on its use.

For the identification of vasculature, planes, and tumors, the da Vinci robotic systems (Intuitive Surgical, Sunnyvale, CA, USA) have an intraoperative near-infrared fluorescence (Firefly) that can be used with indocyanine green (ICG). ICG can help identify aberrant vasculature, intersegmental planes, and small or deep tumors [111]. Pardolesi et al. demonstrated the delineation of intersegmental planes following ICG peripheral injection [112]. ICG can also be injected into specific lesions for identification. Geraci et al. described a method for using bronchoscopy preoperatively to identify and inject ICG into the target lesion. Peripheral ICG was also used to identify the planes. Using the Firefly, 86% of the 93 nodules were identified intraoperatively, and all patients had an R0 resection [113].

Another innovative method for the identification of nodules, particularly those with ground-glass opacities, is a fluorescent tracer (OTL38). OTL38 is a folate-receptor targeted fluorescent tracer that accumulates in malignant tissue and is visualized at specific wavelengths. It has been previously studied in VATS surgery with the use of a specific thoracoscope designed to detect the tracer (VATS-IMI) [114]. A "Sensitive Firefly" vision mode was created for the da Vinci platform in a pilot study of patients who received OTL38. The vision mode was specifically designed to identify tumor-specific fluorescence. The VATS-IMI thoracoscope was used afterwards to serve as a control for the "Sensitive Firefly" mode. The standard robotic white-light scope was able to identify seven out of ten of the pleural nodules based on standard signs of pleural puckering or distortion. The "Sensitive Firefly" and VATS-IMI scope were able to identify all ten of the nodules. There was no significant difference in the mean fluorescence intensity of the tumor, the mean fluorescence intensity of the background parenchyma, or the mean signal-to-background ratio between the "Sensitive Firefly" and VATS-IMI [115]. This is a powerful tool for surgeons, especially with the lack of haptic feedback of the robotic platform, to remove smaller and deeper nodules.

One of the challenges in segmental lung resection is the variation in vascular anatomy and the identification of intersegmental planes. The concept of 3D-CT technology for preoperative planning has gained more traction [116–118]. Ujiie et al. have described the use of a preoperative planning system to map out 3D lung anatomy prior to surgical resection. This 3D model was integrated into the robotic platform for the surgeon to view via the console during the case to allow for identification of aberrant vascular anatomy [119].

Innovations in surgical technology can assist in preoperative planning and improve the precision and outcomes of minimally invasive surgery.

9. Conclusions

The development of minimally invasive surgery has greatly advanced lung cancer treatment. VATS and RATS lung resection have consistently demonstrated enhanced patient outcomes compared to open lung resection via thoracotomy. Patients treated with minimally invasive techniques have fewer postoperative complications, improved pulmonary recovery, shorter hospital stays, less pain, and improved quality of life. Additionally, MIS for lung cancer has comparable oncologic outcomes related to overall survival, disease-free survival, and quality of lymphadenectomy. These improvements have led to a shift in standard-of-care treatment of lung cancer. With the rise of uniportal surgery, patient recovery may be even faster without compromising other outcomes. Advanced imaging techniques can offer improved identification of lesions or aberrant vasculature and allow for more tissue-sparing resections.

As minimally invasive surgery technology continues to evolve, the treatment of lung cancer will also evolve towards less invasive, safer, and more effective lung cancer operations.

Author Contributions: Conceptualization, all authors; writing—original draft preparation, J.M.P.; writing—review and editing, all authors; supervision, E.L.S. All authors have read and agreed to the published version of the manuscript.

Funding: This research received no external funding.

Conflicts of Interest: Servais is a consultant for Intuitive Surgical.

References

1. Riely, G.J.; Wood, D.E.; Ettinger, D.S.; Aisner, D.L.; Akerley, W.; Bauman, J.R.; Bharat, A.; Bruno, D.S.; Chang, J.Y.; Chiriea, L.R.; et al. NCCN Clinical Practice Guidelines in Oncology: Non-Small Cell Lung Cancer. *J. Natl. Compr. Cancer Netw.* **2024**, *22*, 249–274. [CrossRef] [PubMed]
2. Aguado, C.; Chara, L.; Antoñanzas, M.; Matilla Gonzalez, J.M.; Jiménez, U.; Hernanz, R.; Mielgo-Rubio, X.; Trujillo-Reyes, J.C.; Couñago, F. Neoadjuvant Treatment in Non-Small Cell Lung Cancer: New Perspectives with the Incorporation of Immunotherapy. *World J. Clin. Oncol.* **2022**, *13*, 314–322. [CrossRef] [PubMed]
3. Fang, L.; Wang, L.; Wang, Y.; Lv, W.; Hu, J. Video Assisted Thoracic Surgery vs. Thoracotomy for Locally Advanced Lung Squamous Cell Carcinoma after Neoadjuvant Chemotherapy. *J. Cardiothorac. Surg.* **2018**, *13*, 128. [CrossRef] [PubMed]
4. Sedighim, S.; Frank, M.I.; Heutlinger, O.; Lee, C.; Hachey, S.J.; Keshava, H.B. A Systematic Review of Short-Term Outcomes of Minimally Invasive Thoracoscopic Surgery for Lung Cancer after Neoadjuvant Systemic Therapy. *Cancers* **2023**, *15*, 3908. [CrossRef]

5. Lewis, R.J.; Caccavale, R.J.; Sisler, G.E.; Mackenzie, J.W. One Hundred Consecutive Patients Undergoing Video-Assisted Thoracic Operations. *Ann. Thorac. Surg.* **1992**, *54*, 421–426. [CrossRef]
6. Melfi, F.M.A.; Menconi, G.F.; Mariani, A.M.; Angeletti, C.A. Early Experience with Robotic Technology for Thoracoscopic Surgery. *Thorac. Surg.* **2002**, *21*, 864–868. [CrossRef]
7. Rubinstein, L.V. Randomized Trial of Lobectomy versus Limited Resection for T1 N0 non-Small Cell Lung Cancer. *Ann. Thorac. Surg.* **1995**, *60*, 615–623.
8. Demmy, T.L.; Yendamuri, S.; D'Amico, T.A.; Burfeind, W.R. Oncologic Equivalence of Minimally Invasive Lobectomy: The Scientific and Practical Arguments. *Ann. Thorac. Surg.* **2018**, *106*, 609–617. [CrossRef]
9. Servais, E.L.; Blasberg, J.D.; Brown, L.M.; Towe, C.W.; Seder, C.W.; Onaitis, M.W.; Block, M.I.; David, E.A. The Society of Thoracic Surgeons General Thoracic Surgery Database: 2022 Update on Outcomes and Research. *Ann. Thorac. Surg.* **2023**, *115*, 43–49. [CrossRef]
10. Mitzman, B.; Wang, X.; Haaland, B.; Varghese, T.K. Trends and Factors Affecting Approach Choice to Pulmonary Resection. *J. Surg. Oncol.* **2022**, *126*, 599–608. [CrossRef]
11. Swanson, S.J.; Herndon, J.E.; D'Amico, T.A.; Demmy, T.L.; McKenna, R.J.; Green, M.R.; Sugarbaker, D.J. Video-Assisted Thoracic Surgery Lobectomy: Report of CALGB 39802—A Prospective, Multi-Institution Feasibility Study. *J. Clin. Oncol.* **2007**, *25*, 4993–4997. [CrossRef] [PubMed]
12. Whitson, B.A.; Andrade, R.S.; Boettcher, A.; Bardales, R.; Kratzke, R.A.; Dahlberg, P.S.; Maddaus, M.A. Video-Assisted Thoracoscopic Surgery Is More Favorable than Thoracotomy for Resection of Clinical Stage I Non-Small Cell Lung Cancer. *Ann. Thorac. Surg.* **2007**, *83*, 1965–1970. [CrossRef]
13. Handy, J.R., Jr.; Asaph, J.W.; Douville, E.C.; Ott, G.Y.; Grunkemeier, G.L.; Wu, Y. Does Video-Assisted Thoracoscopic Lobectomy for Lung Cancer Provide Improved Functional Outcomes Compared with Open Lobectomy? *Eur. J. Cardiothorac. Surg.* **2009**, *37*, 451–455. [CrossRef]
14. Scott, W.J.; Allen, M.S.; Darling, G.; Meyers, B.; Decker, P.A.; Putnam, J.B.; Mckenna, R.W.; Landrenau, R.J.; Jones, D.R.; Inculet, R.I.; et al. Video-Assisted Thoracic Surgery versus Open Lobectomy for Lung Cancer: A Secondary Analysis of Data from the American College of Surgeons Oncology Group Z0030 Randomized Clinical Trial. *J. Thorac. Cardiovasc. Surg.* **2010**, *139*, 976–983. [CrossRef]
15. Lim, E.; Batchelor, T.J.P.; Dunning, J.; Shackcloth, M.; Anikin, V.; Naidu, B.; Belcher, E.; Loubani, M.; Zamvar, V.; Harris, R.A.; et al. Video-Assisted Thoracoscopic or Open Lobectomy in Early-Stage Lung Cancer. *NEJM Evid.* **2022**, *1*, EVIDoa2100016. [CrossRef] [PubMed]
16. Yan, T.D.; Black, D.; Bannon, P.G.; McCaughan, B.C. Systematic Review and Meta-Analysis of Randomized and Nonrandomized Trials on Safety and Efficacy of Video-Assisted Thoracic Surgery Lobectomy for Early-Stage Non–Small-Cell Lung Cancer. *J. Clin. Oncol.* **2009**, *27*, 2553–2562. [CrossRef] [PubMed]
17. Long, H.; Tan, Q.; Luo, Q.; Wang, Z.; Jiang, G.; Situ, D.; Lin, Y.; Su, X.; Liu, Q.; Rong, T. Thoracoscopic Surgery versus Thoracotomy for Lung Cancer: Short-Term Outcomes of a Randomized Trial. *Ann. Thorac. Surg.* **2018**, *105*, 386–392. [CrossRef]
18. Nwogu, C.E.; D'Cunha, J.; Pang, H.; Gu, L.; Wang, X.; Richards, W.G.; Veit, L.J.; Demmy, T.L.; Sugarbaker, D.J.; Kohman, L.J.; et al. VATS Lobectomy Has Better Perioperative Outcomes than Open Lobectomy: CALGB 31001, an Ancillary Analysis of CALGB 140202 (Alliance). *Ann. Thorac. Surg.* **2015**, *99*, 399–405. [CrossRef]
19. Whitson, B.A.; Groth, S.S.; Duval, S.J.; Swanson, S.J.; Maddaus, M.A. Surgery for Early-Stage Non-Small Cell Lung Cancer: A Systematic Review of the Video-Assisted Thoracoscopic Surgery versus Thoracotomy Approaches to Lobectomy. *Ann. Thorac. Surg.* **2008**, *86*, 2008–2018. [CrossRef]
20. Falcoz, P.-E.; Puyraveau, M.; Thomas, P.-A.; Decaluwe, H.; Hürtgen, M.; Petersen, R.H.; Hansen, H.; Brunelli, A. Video-Assisted Thoracoscopic Surgery versus Open Lobectomy for Primary Non-Small-Cell Lung Cancer: A Propensity-Matched Analysis of Outcome from the European Society of Thoracic Surgeon Database. *Eur. J. Cardiothorac. Surg.* **2016**, *49*, 602–609. [CrossRef]
21. Flores, R.M.; Park, B.J.; Dycoco, J.; Aronova, A.; Hirth, Y.; Rizk, N.P.; Bains, M.; Downey, R.J.; Rusch, V.W. Lobectomy by Video-Assisted Thoracic Surgery (VATS) versus Thoracotomy for Lung Cancer. *J. Thorac. Cardiovasc. Surg.* **2009**, *138*, 11–18. [CrossRef] [PubMed]
22. Bendixen, M.; Jørgensen, O.D.; Kronborg, C.; Andersen, C.; Licht, P.B. Postoperative Pain and Quality of Life after Lobectomy via Video-Assisted Thoracoscopic Surgery or Anterolateral Thoracotomy for Early Stage Lung Cancer: A Randomised Controlled Trial. *Lancet Oncol.* **2016**, *17*, 836–844. [CrossRef]
23. Wolf, A.; Liu, B.; Leoncini, E.; Nicastri, D.; Lee, D.-S.; Taioli, E.; Flores, R. Outcomes for Thoracoscopy versus Thoracotomy Not Just Technique Dependent: A Study of 9,787 Patients. *Ann. Thorac. Surg.* **2018**, *105*, 886–891. [CrossRef]
24. Sugi, K.; Kaneda, Y.; Esato, K. Video-assisted Thoracoscopic Lobectomy Achieves a Satisfactory Long-term Prognosis in Patients with Clinical Stage IA Lung Cancer. *World J. Surg.* **2000**, *24*, 27–31. [CrossRef] [PubMed]
25. Darling, G.E.; Allen, M.S.; Decker, P.A.; Ballman, K.; Malthaner, R.A.; Inculet, R.I.; Jones, D.R.; McKenna, R.J.; Landreneau, R.J.; Rusch, V.W.; et al. Randomized Trial of Mediastinal Lymph Node Sampling versus Complete Lymphadenectomy during Pulmonary Resection in the Patient with N0 or N1 (Less than Hilar) Non–Small Cell Carcinoma: Results of the American College of Surgery Oncology Group Z0030 Trial. *J. Thorac. Cardiovasc. Surg.* **2011**, *141*, 662–670. [CrossRef]
26. Martin, J.T.; Durbin, E.B.; Chen, L.; Gal, T.; Mahan, A.; Ferraris, V.; Zwischenberger, J. Nodal Upstaging during Lung Cancer Resection Is Associated with Surgical Approach. *Ann. Thorac. Surg.* **2016**, *101*, 238–245. [CrossRef] [PubMed]

27. Licht, P.B.; Jørgensen, O.D.; Ladegaard, L.; Jakobsen, E. A National Study of Nodal Upstaging after Thoracoscopic versus Open Lobectomy for Clinical Stage I Lung Cancer. *Ann. Thorac. Surg.* **2013**, *96*, 943–950. [CrossRef] [PubMed]
28. Petersen, R.P.; Pham, D.; Burfeind, W.R.; Hanish, S.I.; Toloza, E.M.; Harpole, D.H.; D'Amico, T.A. Thoracoscopic Lobectomy Facilitates the Delivery of Chemotherapy after Resection for Lung Cancer. *Ann. Thorac. Surg.* **2007**, *83*, 1245–1250. [CrossRef] [PubMed]
29. Berry, M.F.; D'Amico, T.A.; Onaitis, M.W.; Kelsey, C.R. Thoracoscopic Approach to Lobectomy for Lung Cancer Does Not Compromise Oncologic Efficacy. *Ann. Thorac. Surg.* **2014**, *98*, 197–202. [CrossRef]
30. Yang, C.-F.J.; Meyerhoff, R.R.; Mayne, N.R.; Singhapricha, T.; Toomey, C.B.; Speicher, P.J.; Hartwig, M.G.; Tong, B.C.; Onaitis, M.W.; Harpole, D.H.; et al. Long-Term Survival Following Open versus Thoracoscopic Lobectomy after Preoperative Chemotherapy for Non-Small Cell Lung Cancer. *Eur. J. Cardiothorac. Surg.* **2016**, *49*, 1615–1623. [CrossRef]
31. Yang, C.-F.J.; Nwosu, A.; Mayne, N.R.; Wang, Y.; Raman, V.; Meyerhoff, R.R.; D'Amico, T.A.; Berry, M.F. A Minimally Invasive Approach to Lobectomy after Induction Therapy Does Not Compromise Survival. *Ann. Thorac. Surg.* **2020**, *109*, 1503–1511. [CrossRef] [PubMed]
32. Suh, J.W.; Park, S.Y.; Lee, C.Y.; Lee, J.G.; Kim, D.J.; Paik, H.C.; Chung, K.Y. Feasibility and Surgical Outcomes of Video-assisted Thoracoscopic Pulmonary Resection in Patients with Advanced-stage Lung Cancer after Neoadjuvant Chemoradiotherapy. *Thorac. Cancer* **2019**, *10*, 1241–1247. [CrossRef]
33. Hireche, K.; Lounes, Y.; Bacri, C.; Solovei, L.; Marty-Ané, C.; Canaud, L.; Alric, P. VATS versus Open Lobectomy Following Induction Therapy for Stage III NSCLC: A Propensity Score-Matched Analysis. *Cancers* **2023**, *15*, 414. [CrossRef] [PubMed]
34. Howington, J.A.; Blum, M.G.; Chang, A.C.; Balekian, A.A.; Murthy, S.C. Treatment of Stage I and II Non-Small Cell Lung Cancer. *Chest* **2013**, *143*, e278S–e313S. [CrossRef] [PubMed]
35. Detterbeck, F.C.; Lewis, S.Z.; Diekemper, R.; Addrizzo-Harris, D.; Alberts, W.M. Executive Summary. *Chest* **2013**, *143*, 7S–37S. [CrossRef]
36. Lazar, J.F.; Hwalek, A.E. A Review of Robotic Thoracic Surgery Adoption and Future Innovations. *Thorac. Surg. Clin.* **2023**, *33*, 1–10. [CrossRef]
37. Adams, R.D.; Bolton, W.D.; Stephenson, J.E.; Henry, G.; Robbins, E.T.; Sommers, E. Initial Multicenter Community Robotic Lobectomy Experience: Comparisons to a National Database. *Ann. Thorac. Surg.* **2014**, *97*, 1893–1900. [CrossRef]
38. Nelson, D.B.; Mehran, R.J.; Mitchell, K.G.; Rajaram, R.; Correa, A.M.; Bassett, R.L.; Antonoff, M.B.; Hofstetter, W.L.; Roth, J.A.; Sepesi, B.; et al. Robotic-Assisted Lobectomy for Non-Small Cell Lung Cancer: A Comprehensive Institutional Experience. *Ann. Thorac. Surg.* **2019**, *108*, 370–376. [CrossRef]
39. Veluswamy, R.R.; Whittaker Brown, S.-A.; Mhango, G.; Sigel, K.; Nicastri, D.G.; Smith, C.B.; Bonomi, M.; Galsky, M.D.; Taioli, E.; Neugut, A.I.; et al. Comparative Effectiveness of Robotic-Assisted Surgery for Resectable Lung Cancer in Older Patients. *Chest* **2020**, *157*, 1313–1321. [CrossRef]
40. Zhang, O.; Alzul, R.; Carelli, M.; Melfi, F.; Tian, D.; Cao, C. Complications of Robotic Video-Assisted Thoracoscopic Surgery Compared to Open Thoracotomy for Resectable Non-Small Cell Lung Cancer. *J. Pers. Med.* **2022**, *12*, 1311. [CrossRef]
41. Kent, M.S.; Hartwig, M.G.; Vallières, E.; Abbas, A.E.; Cerfolio, R.J.; Dylewski, M.R.; Fabian, T.; Herrera, L.J.; Jett, K.G.; Lazzaro, R.S.; et al. Pulmonary Open, Robotic and Thoracoscopic Lobectomy (PORTaL) Study: An Analysis of 5721 Cases. *Ann. Surg.* 2021; *publish ahead of print*. [CrossRef]
42. Kent, M.; Wang, T.; Whyte, R.; Curran, T.; Flores, R.; Gangadharan, S. Open, Video-Assisted Thoracic Surgery, and Robotic Lobectomy: Review of a National Database. *Ann. Thorac. Surg.* **2014**, *97*, 236–244. [CrossRef] [PubMed]
43. Oh, D.S.; Reddy, R.M.; Gorrepati, M.L.; Mehendale, S.; Reed, M.F. Robotic-Assisted, Video-Assisted Thoracoscopic and Open Lobectomy: Propensity-Matched Analysis of Recent Premier Data. *Ann. Thorac. Surg.* **2017**, *104*, 1733–1740. [CrossRef]
44. Nguyen, D.M.; Sarkaria, I.S.; Song, C.; Reddy, R.M.; Villamizar, N.; Herrera, L.J.; Shi, L.; Liu, E.; Rice, D.; Oh, D.S. Clinical and Economic Comparative Effectiveness of Robotic-Assisted, Video-Assisted Thoracoscopic, and Open Lobectomy. *J. Thorac. Dis.* **2020**, *12*, 296–306. [CrossRef] [PubMed]
45. Aiolfi, A.; Nosotti, M.; Micheletto, G.; Khor, D.; Bonitta, G.; Perali, C.; Marin, J.; Biraghi, T.; Bona, D. Pulmonary Lobectomy for Cancer: Systematic Review and Network Meta-Analysis Comparing Open, Video-Assisted Thoracic Surgery, and Robotic Approach. *Surgery* **2021**, *169*, 436–446. [CrossRef] [PubMed]
46. Zirafa, C.C.; Romano, G.; Sicolo, E.; Bagalà, E.; Manfredini, B.; Alì, G.; Castaldi, A.; Morganti, R.; Davini, F.; Fontanini, G.; et al. Robotic versus Open Surgery in Locally Advanced Non-Small Cell Lung Cancer: Evaluation of Surgical and Oncological Outcomes. *Curr. Oncol.* **2023**, *30*, 9104–9115. [CrossRef] [PubMed]
47. Rodriguez-Quintero, J.H.; Elbahrawy, M.M.; Montal, A.M.; Jindani, R.; Vimolratana, M.; Kamel, M.K.; Stiles, B.M.; Chudgar, N.P. Minimally Invasive Surgery for Clinical T4 Non-Small-Cell Lung Cancer: National Trends and Outcomes. *Eur. J. Cardiothorac. Surg.* **2024**, *65*, ezae009. [CrossRef]
48. Louie, B.E.; Farivar, A.S.; Aye, R.W.; Vallières, E. Early Experience with Robotic Lung Resection Results in Similar Operative Outcomes and Morbidity When Compared with Matched Video-Assisted Thoracoscopic Surgery Cases. *Ann. Thorac. Surg.* **2012**, *93*, 1598–1605. [CrossRef]
49. Reddy, R.M.; Gorrepati, M.L.; Oh, D.S.; Mehendale, S.; Reed, M.F. Robotic-Assisted versus Thoracoscopic Lobectomy Outcomes from High-Volume Thoracic Surgeons. *Ann. Thorac. Surg.* **2018**, *106*, 902–908. [CrossRef]

50. Alwatari, Y.; Khoraki, J.; Wolfe, L.G.; Ramamoorthy, B.; Wall, N.; Liu, C.; Julliard, W.; Puig, C.A.; Shah, R.D. Trends of Utilization and Perioperative Outcomes of Robotic and Video-Assisted Thoracoscopic Surgery in Patients with Lung Cancer Undergoing Minimally Invasive Resection in the United States. *JTCVS Open* **2022**, *12*, 385–398. [CrossRef]
51. Agzarian, J.; Fahim, C.; Shargall, Y.; Yasufuku, K.; Waddell, T.K.; Hanna, W.C. The Use of Robotic-Assisted Thoracic Surgery for Lung Resection: A Comprehensive Systematic Review. *Semin. Thorac. Cardiovasc. Surg.* **2016**, *28*, 182–192. [CrossRef]
52. Louie, B.E.; Wilson, J.L.; Kim, S.; Cerfolio, R.J.; Park, B.J.; Farivar, A.S.; Vallières, E.; Aye, R.W.; Burfeind, W.R.; Block, M.I. Comparison of Video-Assisted Thoracoscopic Surgery and Robotic Approaches for Clinical Stage I and Stage II Non-Small Cell Lung Cancer Using The Society of Thoracic Surgeons Database. *Ann. Thorac. Surg.* **2016**, *102*, 917–924. [CrossRef] [PubMed]
53. Veronesi, G.; Abbas, A.E.-S.; Muriana, P.; Lembo, R.; Bottoni, E.; Perroni, G.; Testori, A.; Dieci, E.; Bakhos, C.T.; Car, S.; et al. Perioperative Outcome of Robotic Approach versus Manual Videothoracoscopic Major Resection in Patients Affected by Early Lung Cancer: Results of a Randomized Multicentric Study (ROMAN Study). *Front. Oncol.* **2021**, *11*, 726408. [CrossRef]
54. Liang, H.; Liang, W.; Zhao, L.; Chen, D.; Zhang, J.; Zhang, Y.; Tang, S.; He, J. Robotic versus Video-Assisted Lobectomy/Segmentectomy for Lung Cancer: A Meta-Analysis. *Ann. Surg.* **2018**, *268*, 254–259. [CrossRef]
55. Servais, E.L.; Miller, D.L.; Thibault, D.; Hartwig, M.G.; Kosinski, A.S.; Stock, C.T.; Price, T.; Quadri, S.M.; D'Agostino, R.S.; Burfeind, W.R. Conversion to Thoracotomy during Thoracoscopic vs Robotic Lobectomy: Predictors and Outcomes. *Ann. Thorac. Surg.* **2022**, *114*, 409–417. [CrossRef]
56. Keller, S.M.; Adak, S.; Wagner, H.; Johnson, D.H. Mediastinal Lymph Node Dissection Improves Survival in Patients with Stages II and IIIa Non-Small Cell Lung Cancer. *Ann. Thorac. Surg.* **2000**, *70*, 358–365. [CrossRef] [PubMed]
57. Nissen, A.P.; Vreeland, T.J.; Teshome, M.; Archer, M.A.; Francescatti, A.B.; Katz, M.H.G.; Hunt, K.K.; Zheng, L.; Mullett, T.W. American College of Surgeons Commission on Cancer Standard for Curative-Intent Pulmonary Resection. *Ann. Thorac. Surg.* **2022**, *113*, 5–8. [CrossRef] [PubMed]
58. Wilson, J.L.; Louie, B.E.; Cerfolio, R.J.; Park, B.J.; Vallières, E.; Aye, R.W.; Abdel-Razek, A.; Bryant, A.; Farivar, A.S. The Prevalence of Nodal Upstaging during Robotic Lung Resection in Early Stage Non-Small Cell Lung Cancer. *Ann. Thorac. Surg.* **2014**, *97*, 1901–1907. [CrossRef]
59. Toker, A.; Özyurtkan, M.O.; Demirhan, Ö.; Ayalp, K.; Kaba, E.; Uyumaz, E. Lymph Node Dissection in Surgery for Lung Cancer: Comparison of Open vs. Video-Assisted vs. Robotic-Assisted Approaches. *Ann. Thorac. Cardiovasc. Surg.* **2016**, *22*, 284–290. [CrossRef]
60. Yang, H.-X.; Woo, K.M.; Sima, C.S.; Bains, M.S.; Adusumilli, P.S.; Huang, J.; Finley, D.J.; Rizk, N.P.; Rusch, V.W.; Jones, D.R.; et al. Long-Term Survival Based on the Surgical Approach to Lobectomy for Clinical Stage I Nonsmall Cell Lung Cancer: Comparison of Robotic, Video-Assisted Thoracic Surgery, and Thoracotomy Lobectomy. *Ann. Surg.* **2017**, *265*, 431–437. [CrossRef]
61. Cerfolio, R.J.; Ghanim, A.F.; Dylewski, M.; Veronesi, G.; Spaggiari, L.; Park, B.J. The Long-Term Survival of Robotic Lobectomy for Non–Small Cell Lung Cancer: A Multi-Institutional Study. *J. Thorac. Cardiovasc. Surg.* **2018**, *155*, 778–786. [CrossRef] [PubMed]
62. Sesti, J.; Langan, R.C.; Bell, J.; Nguyen, A.; Turner, A.L.; Hilden, P.; Leshchuk, K.; Dabrowski, M.; Paul, S. A Comparative Analysis of Long-Term Survival of Robotic versus Thoracoscopic Lobectomy. *Ann. Thorac. Surg.* **2020**, *110*, 1139–1146. [CrossRef] [PubMed]
63. Montagne, F.; Chaari, Z.; Bottet, B.; Sarsam, M.; Mbadinga, F.; Selim, J.; Guisier, F.; Gillibert, A.; Baste, J.-M. Long-Term Survival Following Minimally Invasive Lung Cancer Surgery: Comparing Robotic-Assisted and Video-Assisted Surgery. *Cancers* **2022**, *14*, 2611. [CrossRef]
64. Park, B.J.; Melfi, F.; Mussi, A.; Maisonneuve, P.; Spaggiari, L.; Da Silva, R.K.C.; Veronesi, G. Robotic Lobectomy for Non–Small Cell Lung Cancer (NSCLC): Long-Term Oncologic Results. *J. Thorac. Cardiovasc. Surg.* **2012**, *143*, 383–389. [CrossRef]
65. Kneuertz, P.J.; D'Souza, D.M.; Richardson, M.; Abdel-Rasoul, M.; Moffatt-Bruce, S.D.; Merritt, R.E. Long-Term Oncologic Outcomes after Robotic Lobectomy for Early-Stage Non–Small-Cell Lung Cancer versus Video-Assisted Thoracoscopic and Open Thoracotomy Approach. *Clin. Lung Cancer* **2020**, *21*, 214–224.e2. [CrossRef]
66. Wu, H.; Jin, R.; Yang, S.; Park, B.J.; Li, H. Long-Term and Short-Term Outcomes of Robot- versus Video-Assisted Anatomic Lung Resection in Lung Cancer: A Systematic Review and Meta-Analysis. *Eur. J. Cardiothorac. Surg.* **2021**, *59*, 732–740. [CrossRef] [PubMed]
67. Demmy, T.L.; Nwogu, C. Is Video-Assisted Thoracic Surgery Lobectomy Better? Quality of Life Considerations. *Ann. Thorac. Surg.* **2008**, *85*, S719–S728. [CrossRef]
68. Yamashita, Y.; Mukaida, H.; Harada, H.; Tsubokawa, N. Post-Thoracotomy Pain and Long-Term Survival Associated with Video-Assisted Thoracic Surgery Lobectomy Methods for Clinical T1N0 Lung Cancer: A Patient-Oriented, Prospective Cohort Study. *Eur. J. Cardiothorac. Surg.* **2013**, *44*, e71–e76. [CrossRef]
69. Cerfolio, R.J.; Bryant, A.S.; Skylizard, L.; Minnich, D.J. Initial Consecutive Experience of Completely Portal Robotic Pulmonary Resection with 4 Arms. *J. Thorac. Cardiovasc. Surg.* **2011**, *142*, 740–746. [CrossRef]
70. Asemota, N.; Maraschi, A.; Lampridis, S.; Pilling, J.; King, J.; Le Reun, C.; Bille, A. Comparison of Quality of Life after Robotic, Video-Assisted, and Open Surgery for Lung Cancer. *J. Clin. Med.* **2023**, *12*, 6230. [CrossRef]
71. Lacroix, V.; Kahn, D.; Matte, P.; Pieters, T.; Noirhomme, P.; Poncelet, A.; Steyaert, A. Robotic-Assisted Lobectomy Favors Early Lung Recovery versus Limited Thoracotomy. *Thorac. Cardiovasc. Surg.* **2021**, *69*, 557–563. [CrossRef]

72. Zhou, N.; Niu, J.; Nelson, D.; Feldman, H.A.; Antonoff, M.B.; Hofstetter, W.L.; Mehran, R.J.; Rice, D.C.; Sepesi, B.; Swisher, S.G.; et al. Surgical Approach and Persistent Opioid Use in Medicare Patients Undergoing Lung Cancer Resection. *Ann. Thorac. Surg.* **2023**, *116*, 1020–1027. [CrossRef]
73. Kwon, S.T.; Zhao, L.; Reddy, R.M.; Chang, A.C.; Orringer, M.B.; Brummett, C.M.; Lin, J. Evaluation of Acute and Chronic Pain Outcomes after Robotic, Video-Assisted Thoracoscopic Surgery, or Open Anatomic Pulmonary Resection. *J. Thorac. Cardiovasc. Surg.* **2017**, *154*, 652–659.e1. [CrossRef] [PubMed]
74. Park, B.J.; Flores, R.M.; Rusch, V.W. Robotic Assistance for Video-Assisted Thoracic Surgical Lobectomy: Technique and Initial Results. *J. Thorac. Cardiovasc. Surg.* **2006**, *131*, 54–59. [CrossRef] [PubMed]
75. Subramanian, M.P.; Liu, J.; Chapman, W.C.; Olsen, M.A.; Yan, Y.; Liu, Y.; Semenkovich, T.R.; Meyers, B.F.; Puri, V.; Kozower, B.D. Utilization Trends, Outcomes, and Cost in Minimally Invasive Lobectomy. *Ann. Thorac. Surg.* **2019**, *108*, 1648–1655. [CrossRef] [PubMed]
76. Tupper, H.I.; Lawson, B.L.; Kipnis, P.; Patel, A.R.; Ashiku, S.K.; Roubinian, N.H.; Myers, L.C.; Liu, V.X.; Velotta, J.B. Video-Assisted vs Robotic-Assisted Lung Lobectomies for Operating Room Resource Utilization and Patient Outcomes. *JAMA Netw. Open* **2024**, *7*, e248881. [CrossRef] [PubMed]
77. Deen, S.A.; Wilson, J.L.; Wilshire, C.L.; Vallières, E.; Farivar, A.S.; Aye, R.W.; Ely, R.E.; Louie, B.E. Defining the Cost of Care for Lobectomy and Segmentectomy: A Comparison of Open, Video-Assisted Thoracoscopic, and Robotic Approaches. *Ann. Thorac. Surg.* **2014**, *97*, 1000–1007. [CrossRef]
78. Swanson, S.J.; Miller, D.L.; McKenna, R.J.; Howington, J.; Marshall, M.B.; Yoo, A.C.; Moore, M.; Gunnarsson, C.L.; Meyers, B.F. Comparing Robot-Assisted Thoracic Surgical Lobectomy with Conventional Video-Assisted Thoracic Surgical Lobectomy and Wedge Resection: Results from a Multihospital Database (Premier). *J. Thorac. Cardiovasc. Surg.* **2014**, *147*, 929–937. [CrossRef]
79. Kneuertz, P.J.; Singer, E.; D'Souza, D.M.; Abdel-Rasoul, M.; Moffatt-Bruce, S.D.; Merritt, R.E. Hospital Cost and Clinical Effectiveness of Robotic-Assisted versus Video-Assisted Thoracoscopic and Open Lobectomy: A Propensity Score–Weighted Comparison. *J. Thorac. Cardiovasc. Surg.* **2019**, *157*, 2018–2026.e2. [CrossRef]
80. Verma, A.; Hadaya, J.; Richardson, S.; Vadlakonda, A.; Ramezani, R.; Revels, S.; Benharash, P. The Presence of a Cost–Volume Relationship in Robotic-Assisted Thoracoscopic Lung Resections. *Ann. Surg.* **2023**, *278*, e377–e381. [CrossRef]
81. Patel, Y.S.; Baste, J.-M.; Shargall, Y.; Waddell, T.K.; Yasufuku, K.; Machuca, T.N.; Xie, F.; Thabane, L.; Hanna, W.C. Robotic Lobectomy Is Cost-Effective and Provides Comparable Health Utility Scores to Video-Assisted Lobectomy: Early Results of the RAVAL Trial. *Ann. Surg.* **2023**, *278*, 841–849. [CrossRef] [PubMed]
82. Saji, H.; Okada, M.; Tsuboi, M.; Nakajima, R.; Suzuki, K.; Aokage, K.; Aoki, T.; Okami, J.; Yoshino, I.; Ito, H.; et al. Segmentectomy versus Lobectomy in Small-Sized Peripheral Non-Small-Cell Lung Cancer (JCOG0802/WJOG4607L): A Multicentre, Open-Label, Phase 3, Randomised, Controlled, Non-Inferiority Trial. *Lancet* **2022**, *399*, 1607–1617. [CrossRef] [PubMed]
83. Altorki, N.; Wang, X.; Kozono, D.; Watt, C.; Landrenau, R.; Wigle, D.; Port, J.; Jones, D.R.; Conti, M.; Ashrafi, A.S.; et al. Lobar or Sublobar Resection for Peripheral Stage IA Non–Small-Cell Lung Cancer. *N. Engl. J. Med.* **2023**, *388*, 489–498. [CrossRef] [PubMed]
84. Kneuertz, P.J.; Abdel-Rasoul, M.; D'Souza, D.M.; Zhao, J.; Merritt, R.E. Segmentectomy for Clinical Stage I Non–Small Cell Lung Cancer: National Benchmarks for Nodal Staging and Outcomes by Operative Approach. *Cancer* **2022**, *128*, 1483–1492. [CrossRef] [PubMed]
85. Shapiro, M.; Weiser, T.S.; Wisnivesky, J.P.; Chin, C.; Arustamyan, M.; Swanson, S.J. Thoracoscopic Segmentectomy Compares Favorably with Thoracoscopic Lobectomy for Patients with Small Stage I Lung Cancer. *J. Thorac. Cardiovasc. Surg.* **2009**, *137*, 1388–1393. [CrossRef] [PubMed]
86. Lex, J.R.; Naidu, B. In Patients with Resectable Non-Small-Cell Lung Cancer, Is Video-Assisted Thoracoscopic Segmentectomy an Appropriate Alternative to Video-Assisted Thoracoscopic Lobectomy? *Interact. Cardiovasc. Thorac. Surg.* **2016**, *23*, 826–831. [CrossRef]
87. Zhang, Y.; Chen, C.; Hu, J.; Han, Y.; Huang, M.; Xiang, J.; Li, H. Early Outcomes of Robotic versus Thoracoscopic Segmentectomy for Early-Stage Lung Cancer: A Multi-Institutional Propensity Score-Matched Analysis. *J. Thorac. Cardiovasc. Surg.* **2020**, *160*, 1363–1372. [CrossRef]
88. Caso, R.; Watson, T.J.; Tefera, E.; Cerfolio, R.; Abbas, A.E.; Lazar, J.F.; Margolis, M.; Hwalek, A.E.; Khaitan, P.G. Comparing Robotic, Thoracoscopic, and Open Segmentectomy: A National Cancer Database Analysis. *J. Surg. Res.* **2024**, *296*, 674–680. [CrossRef]
89. Ghaly, G.; Kamel, M.; Nasar, A.; Paul, S.; Lee, P.C.; Port, J.L.; Stiles, B.M.; Altorki, N.K. Video-Assisted Thoracoscopic Surgery Is a Safe and Effective Alternative to Thoracotomy for Anatomical Segmentectomy in Patients with Clinical Stage I Non-Small Cell Lung Cancer. *Ann. Thorac. Surg.* **2016**, *101*, 465–472. [CrossRef]
90. Pardolesi, A.; Park, B.; Petrella, F.; Borri, A.; Gasparri, R.; Veronesi, G. Robotic Anatomic Segmentectomy of the Lung: Technical Aspects and Initial Results. *Ann. Thorac. Surg.* **2012**, *94*, 929–934. [CrossRef]
91. Demir, A.; Ayalp, K.; Ozkan, B.; Kaba, E.; Toker, A. Robotic and Video-Assisted Thoracic Surgery Lung Segmentectomy for Malignant and Benign Lesions†. *Interact. Cardiovasc. Thorac. Surg.* **2015**, *20*, 304–309. [CrossRef]
92. Cerfolio, R.J.; Watson, C.; Minnich, D.J.; Calloway, S.; Wei, B. One Hundred Planned Robotic Segmentectomies: Early Results, Technical Details, and Preferred Port Placement. *Ann. Thorac. Surg.* **2016**, *101*, 1089–1096. [CrossRef] [PubMed]

93. Nguyen, D.; Gharagozloo, F.; Tempesta, B.; Meyer, M.; Gruessner, A. Long-Term Results of Robotic Anatomical Segmentectomy for Early-Stage Non-Small-Cell Lung Cancer. *Eur. J. Cardiothorac. Surg.* **2019**, *55*, 427–433. [CrossRef]
94. Kumar, A.; Deng, J.Z.; Raman, V.; Okusanya, O.T.; Baiu, I.; Berry, M.F.; D'Amico, T.A.; Yang, C.-F.J. A National Analysis of Minimally Invasive vs Open Segmentectomy for Stage IA Non–Small-Cell Lung Cancer. *Semin. Thorac. Cardiovasc. Surg.* **2021**, *33*, 535–544. [CrossRef] [PubMed]
95. Watkins, A.A.; Rizvi, T.Z.; Lopez, E.; Shehata, D.; Ssemaganda, H.; Lin, Z.; Stock, C.T.; Moffatt-Bruce, S.D.; Servais, E.L. Trends and Comparative Outcomes between Operative Approaches for Segmentectomy in Lung Cancer. *J. Thorac. Cardiovasc. Surg.* **2024**, S0022522324006056. [CrossRef]
96. Spaggiari, L.; Galetta, D. Pneumonectomy for Lung Cancer: A Further Step in Minimally Invasive Surgery. *Ann. Thorac. Surg.* **2011**, *91*, e45–e47. [CrossRef] [PubMed]
97. Pan, X.; Gu, C.; Wang, R.; Zhao, H.; Shi, J.; Chen, H. Initial Experience of Robotic Sleeve Resection for Lung Cancer Patients. *Ann. Thorac. Surg.* **2016**, *102*, 1892–1897. [CrossRef] [PubMed]
98. Pan, X.; Chen, Y.; Shi, J.; Zhao, H.; Chen, H. Robotic Assisted Extended Sleeve Lobectomy after Neoadjuvant Chemotherapy. *Ann. Thorac. Surg.* **2015**, *100*, e129–e131. [CrossRef]
99. Watkins, A.A.; Quadri, S.M.; Servais, E.L. Robotic-Assisted Complex Pulmonary Resection: Sleeve Lobectomy for Cancer. *Innov. Technol. Tech. Cardiothorac. Vasc. Surg.* **2021**, *16*, 132–135. [CrossRef]
100. Cerfolio, R.J. Robotic Sleeve Lobectomy: Technical Details and Early Results. *J. Thorac. Dis.* **2016**, *8* (Suppl. S2), S223.
101. Hennon, M.W.; Kumar, A.; Devisetty, H.; D'Amico, T.; Demmy, T.L.; Groman, A.; Yendamuri, S. Minimally Invasive Approaches Do Not Compromise Outcomes for Pneumonectomy: A Comparison Using the National Cancer Database. *J. Thorac. Oncol.* **2019**, *14*, 107–114. [CrossRef]
102. Qiu, T.; Zhao, Y.; Xuan, Y.; Qin, Y.; Niu, Z.; Shen, Y.; Jiao, W. Robotic Sleeve Lobectomy for Centrally Located Non–Small Cell Lung Cancer: A Propensity Score–Weighted Comparison with Thoracoscopic and Open Surgery. *J. Thorac. Cardiovasc. Surg.* **2020**, *160*, 838–846.e2. [CrossRef] [PubMed]
103. Bertolaccini, L.; Batirel, H.; Brunelli, A.; Gonzalez-Rivas, D.; Ismail, M.; Ucar, A.M.; Ng, C.S.H.; Scarci, M.; Sihoe, A.D.L.; Ugalde, P.A.; et al. Uniportal Video-Assisted Thoracic Surgery Lobectomy: A Consensus Report from the Uniportal VATS Interest Group (UVIG) of the European Society of Thoracic Surgeons (ESTS). *Eur. J. Cardiothorac. Surg.* **2019**, *56*, 224–229. [CrossRef]
104. Bulgarelli Maqueda, L.; García-Pérez, A.; Minasyan, A.; Gonzalez-Rivas, D. Uniportal VATS for Non-Small Cell Lung Cancer. *Gen. Thorac. Cardiovasc. Surg.* **2020**, *68*, 707–715. [CrossRef] [PubMed]
105. Bourdages-Pageau, E.; Vieira, A.; Lacasse, Y.; Figueroa, P.U. Outcomes of Uniportal vs Multiportal Video-Assisted Thoracoscopic Lobectomy. *Semin. Thorac. Cardiovasc. Surg.* **2020**, *32*, 145–151. [CrossRef] [PubMed]
106. Harris, C.G.; James, R.S.; Tian, D.H.; Yan, T.D.; Doyle, M.P.; Gonzalez-Rivas, D.; Cao, C. Systematic Review and Meta-Analysis of Uniportal versus Multiportal Video-Assisted Thoracoscopic Lobectomy for Lung Cancer. *Ann. Cardiothorac. Surg.* **2016**, *5*, 76–84. [CrossRef] [PubMed]
107. Paradela, M.; Garcia-Perez, A.; Fernandez-Prado, R.; Torre, M.D.L.; Delgado, M.; Bosinceanu, M.L.; Motas, N.; Manolache, V.; Gallego-Poveda, J.; Gonzalez-Rivas, D. Uniportal Robotic versus Thoracoscopic Assisted Surgery: A Propensity Score-Matched Analysis of the Initial 100 Cases. *Ann. Cardiothorac. Surg.* **2023**, *12*, 23–33. [CrossRef] [PubMed]
108. Manolache, V.; Motas, N.; Bosinceanu, M.L.; De La Torre, M.; Gallego-Poveda, J.; Dunning, J.; Ismail, M.; Turna, A.; Paradela, M.; Decker, G.; et al. Comparison of Uniportal Robotic-Assisted Thoracic Surgery Pulmonary Anatomic Resections with Multiport Robotic-Assisted Thoracic Surgery: A Multicenter Study of the European Experience. *Ann. Cardiothorac. Surg.* **2023**, *12*, 102–109. [CrossRef]
109. Lee, J.H.; Park, T.H.; Kim, H.K. Robotic Thoracic Surgery Using the Single-Port Robotic System: Initial Experience with More than 100 Cases. *J. Thorac. Cardiovasc. Surg.* **2024**, S002252232400206X. [CrossRef]
110. Bagan, P.; De Dominicis, F.; Hernigou, J.; Dakhil, B.; Zaimi, R.; Pricopi, C.; Le Pimpec Barthes, F.; Berna, P. Complete Thoracoscopic Lobectomy for Cancer: Comparative Study of Three-Dimensional High-Definition with Two-Dimensional High-Definition Video Systems. *Interact. Cardiovasc. Thorac. Surg.* **2015**, *20*, 820–824. [CrossRef]
111. Ng, C.S.-H.; Ong, B.-H.; Chao, Y.K.; Wright, G.M.; Sekine, Y.; Wong, I.; Hao, Z.; Zhang, G.; Chaturvedi, H.; Thammineedi, S.R.; et al. Use of Indocyanine Green Fluorescence Imaging in Thoracic and Esophageal Surgery. *Ann. Thorac. Surg.* **2023**, *115*, 1068–1076. [CrossRef] [PubMed]
112. Pardolesi, A.; Veronesi, G.; Solli, P.; Spaggiari, L. Use of Indocyanine Green to Facilitate Intersegmental Plane Identification during Robotic Anatomic Segmentectomy. *J. Thorac. Cardiovasc. Surg.* **2014**, *148*, 737–738. [CrossRef]
113. Geraci, T.C.; Ferrari-Light, D.; Kent, A.; Michaud, G.; Zervos, M.; Pass, H.I.; Cerfolio, R.J. Technique, Outcomes with Navigational Bronchoscopy Using Indocyanine Green for Robotic Segmentectomy. *Ann. Thorac. Surg.* **2019**, *108*, 363–369. [CrossRef] [PubMed]
114. Gangadharan, S.; Sarkaria, I.N.; Rice, D.; Murthy, S.; Braun, J.; Kucharczuk, J.; Predina, J.; Singhal, S. Multiinstitutional Phase 2 Clinical Trial of Intraoperative Molecular Imaging of Lung Cancer. *Ann. Thorac. Surg.* **2021**, *112*, 1150–1159. [CrossRef]
115. Kennedy, G.T.; Azari, F.S.; Bernstein, E.; Marfatia, I.; Din, A.; Deshpande, C.; Galvis, N.; Sorger, J.; Kucharczuk, J.C.; Singhal, S. First-in-Human Results of Targeted Intraoperative Molecular Imaging for Visualization of Ground Glass Opacities during Robotic Pulmonary Resection. *Transl. Lung Cancer Res.* **2022**, *11*, 1567–1577. [CrossRef] [PubMed]
116. Divisi, D.; Barone, M.; Crisci, R. Three-Dimensional Video-Assisted Thoracic Surgery for Pulmonary Resections: An Update. *J. Vis. Surg.* **2017**, *3*, 79. [CrossRef] [PubMed]

117. Hamanaka, K.; Miura, K.; Eguchi, T.; Shimizu, K. Harnessing 3D-CT Simulation and Planning for Enhanced Precision Surgery: A Review of Applications and Advancements in Lung Cancer Treatment. *Cancers* **2023**, *15*, 5400. [CrossRef]
118. Dickhoff, C.; Li, W.W.; Symersky, P.; Hartemink, K.J. Feasibility of 3-Dimensional Video-Assisted Thoracic Surgery (3D-VATS) for Pulmonary Resection. *Ann. Surg. Innov. Res.* **2015**, *9*, 8. [CrossRef]
119. Ujiie, H.; Chiba, R.; Yamaguchi, A.; Nomura, S.; Shiiya, H.; Fujiwara-Kuroda, A.; Kaga, K.; Eitel, C.; Clapp, T.R.; Kato, T. Developing a Virtual Reality Simulation System for Preoperative Planning of Robotic-Assisted Thoracic Surgery. *J. Clin. Med.* **2024**, *13*, 611. [CrossRef]

MDPI AG
Grosspeteranlage 5
4052 Basel
Switzerland
Tel.: +41 61 683 77 34

Cancers Editorial Office
E-mail: cancers@mdpi.com
www.mdpi.com/journal/cancers

www.ingramcontent.com/pod-product-compliance
Lightning Source LLC
Chambersburg PA
CBHW062032220926
51850CB00010B/2522

* 9 7 8 3 7 2 5 8 7 2 9 8 5 *